Public Health Action in Emergencies Caused by Epidemics

A practical guide

Prepared by
P. Brès

Formerly Chief, Virus Diseases,
World Health Organization,
Geneva, Switzerland

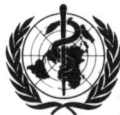

Geneva
World Health Organization
1986

ISBN 92 4 154207 1

TYPESET IN INDIA
PRINTED IN ENGLAND

85/6453—Macmillan/Spottiswoode—7000

CORRIGENDA

Page 278, Section A6.3, Use of rodenticides

Replace lines 1-4 and Table A6.11 by the following:

Several products are available. The first-choice rodenticides against commensal rodents, in most control operations, are the anticoagulant poisons since these are slow-acting compounds. The following anticoagulants are in current use: brodifacoum, bromadiolone, chlorophacinone, coumatetralyl, difenacoum, diphacinone, fumarin, pindone, and warfarin. The manufacturer's instructions should be closely followed in the preparation of baits containing these compounds. The antidote to all the anti-coagulant compounds is vitamin K.

Page 279

Replace Table A6.12 by the following:

Table A6.11. Acute and subacute rodenticides for rapid reduction of rodent populations [a]

Rodenticide	Lethal dose (mg/kg of body weight)[b]	Concentration used in baits (%)	Effective against[c]			Acceptance in baits	Solvent	Antidote
			Rn	Rr	Mm			
Calciferol	40	0.1	+	+	+	Good	Oil	Calcium disodium edetate (orally)
Fluoroacetamide	13-16	2.0	+	+	+	Good	Water	—
Scilliroside	0.42	0.015	+			Fair	Water/oil	—
Sodium fluoroacetate	5-10	0.25	+	+	+	Good	Water	—
Zinc phosphide	40	1.0	+	+	+	Fair	Oil	—

[a] All these compounds are hazardous to man and domestic animals. They should be applied only under controlled conditions by trained operators.

[b] LD_{50} for *R. norvegicus*.

[c] Rn = *R. norvegicus*; Rr = *R. rattus*; Mm = *M. musculus*.

Page 280, lines 7 and 8

Delete   Acute and subacute rodenticides available are shown in Table A6.12.

Insert   Acute and subacute rodenticides available are shown in Table A6.11.

Public Health Action
in Emergencies Caused
by Epidemics

CONTENTS

LIST OF TABLES

Annexes

Acknowledgements

This guide reflects the contributions made by the participants in an Informal Consultation on Strategies for the Control of Emergencies caused by Epidemics of Communicable Diseases, held in Geneva on 9–13 November 1981. The participants are listed in Annex 8.

Special thanks are due to Professor Gelfand and Professor Mattson for their work in preparing Annex 2, and to Miss J. Hargreaves, Division of Communicable Diseases, World Health Organization, for assistance in collating the material from the various sources.

Control of communicable diseases in man, edited by A. S. Benenson and published by the American Public Health Association, has proved to be a most reliable source of information on many diseases and particularly on diagnosis, epidemiological features, and control measures.

*

*   *

The text was reviewed by the individuals listed below and their assistance in this task is gratefully acknowledged.

Dr F. Assaad, Director, Division of Communicable Diseases, World Health Organization, Geneva, Switzerland.

Dr A. S. Benenson, Graduate School of Public Health, San Diego State University, San Diego, CA, USA.

Dr L. J. Charles, formerly Assistant Director for Health Services, World Health Organization, Regional Office for Africa, Brazzaville, Congo.

Dr R. T. D. Emond, Consultant in Infectious Diseases, The Royal Free Hospital, Coppetts Wood, London, England.

Professor F. Fenner, The John Curtis School of Medical Research, The Australian National University, Canberra, Australia.

Professor H. M. Gelfand, Epidemiology-Biometry Program, University of Illinois at Chicago, School of Public Health, Chicago, IL, USA.

Professor D. Mattson, Epidemiology-Biometry Program, University of Illinois, Chicago IL, USA.

Dr D. I. H. Simpson, Special Pathogens Reference Laboratory, Public Health Laboratory Service, Centre for Applied Microbiology and Research, Porton Down, Salisbury, Wiltshire, England.

Dr J. E. M. Whitehead, Director, Public Health Laboratory Service, London, England.

Dr A. Zahra, formerly Director, Division of Communicable Diseases, World Health Organization, Geneva, Switzerland.

1. Introduction

The number of outbreaks of communicable disease has been increasing in recent years. There may be several reasons for this: the increased rapidity of national and international travel and the greater distances travelled; extensive deforestation and irrigation works; neglect of insect and rodent vector control programmes; explosive urbanization and overcrowding associated with poor sanitary conditions; more frequent opportunities for collective gatherings resulting, for example, from improvements in public transport; frequent movements of populations and refugees; social or recreational events; tourism; and large-scale industrial food processing. Some of the increase, however, may be apparent rather than real, since better medical and epidemiological coverage in developing countries has improved the surveillance of these diseases, and outbreaks are now reported that would formerly have gone unnoticed. These reasons may also explain why a disease formerly considered as only occurring sporadically is now endemic or epidemic, although the possibility of changes in pathogenicity or virulence must not be overlooked.

At its foundation in 1948, the World Health Organization was given a mandate by its Member States to help countries facing outbreaks of communicable diseases when they cause problems too great to be dealt with by national resources alone or represent a risk to international health. WHO staff have intervened in epidemics on many occasions and have thereby acquired a great deal of experience based on field operations. An informal consultation on strategies for the control of emergencies caused by epidemics of communicable diseases was convened in Geneva in November 1981. Public health experts from a number of countries exchanged experiences and made recommendations for future WHO activities in this field. They also suggested that WHO should prepare a technical guide to serve as a quick reference on practical measures for public health officers facing an outbreak of a communicable disease, for use primarily under field conditions, in developing countries.

A number of difficulties were encountered in attempting to prepare such a guide, the first being that of defining when an epidemic disease could be considered as constituting an emergency for the public health service, i.e., an "epidemic emergency situation". A definition has been worked out that takes the epidemiological context into account and covers cases when the incubation period of the disease is too long for it to cause panic among the population.

1

The selection of diseases that can cause epidemics also gave rise to difficulty. Some diseases, such as influenza, are well known to cause epidemics in all countries. Other diseases are usually sporadic or endemic but may be able to cause an epidemic in unusual situations, say, in a refugee camp or among a group of tourists, e.g., schistosomiasis or Legionnaires' disease. The increasing frequency of travel and population movements has meant that certain tropical diseases have occurred in temperate regions as imported cases of "exotic" diseases. It is also obvious that an epidemic disease highly prevalent in one part of the world may be rare or absent elsewhere. A decision—perhaps a somewhat arbitrary one—was therefore taken to try and make the coverage as complete as was reasonably possible in order to facilitate differential diagnosis under unusual circumstances, so that certain diseases have been included although they are unlikely to cause emergencies. In contrast, although they may cause epidemics, sexually transmitted diseases have not been included as they do not give rise to emergencies as defined in this guide.

A competent epidemiologist should have an adequate knowledge of other relevant specialities: pathology, microbiology, entomology, veterinary health, and sanitary engineering. It was therefore thought necessary to include some of this diverse background information, but it has been kept within reasonable bounds and limited to what is needed by a reader who is not necessarily a specialist in these disciplines.

References to the many valuable specialized books that might be consulted have been limited, since a sudden outbreak of a communicable disease is not likely to leave much time free for visiting libraries. Where it was felt that further reading could be recommended, preference (purely arbitrary) has been given to widely available WHO documents.

As this guide is intended for practical use, an attempt has been made to arrange the text in the order of the steps that should be taken in an emergency: organizing the emergency health service, following proven procedures for field investigations, analysing methodically the results of investigations, implementing the appropriate control measures and evaluating them. For the reader's convenience in an emergency situation, additional practical information is given in the annexes. Reference should also be made to DUNSMORE, D. J., *Safety measures for use in outbreaks of communicable disease*, published by the World Health Organization.

Many diseases are known under several different names. The guide follows the *International nomenclature of diseases*, published jointly by the Council for International Organizations of Medical Science (CIOMS) and the World Health Organization, for those diseases covered so far, namely diseases of the lower respiratory tract, mycoses, bacterial diseases, and viral diseases. Other common synonyms have been included as appropriate.

2. Explanation of terms and general lines of action

2.1 Explanation of the terms "epidemic" and "emergency"[1]

An *epidemic* of an infectious or parasitic disease is the occurrence of a number of cases of a disease, known or suspected to be of infectious or parasitic origin, that is unusually large or unexpected for the given place and time. An epidemic often evolves rapidly, so that a quick response is required.

A *threatened (or potential) epidemic* is said to exist when the circumstances are such that the epidemic occurrence of a specific disease may reasonably be anticipated; this requires (*a*) a susceptible human population; (*b*) the presence or impending introduction of a disease agent; and (*c*) the presence of a mechanism such that large-scale transmission is possible (e.g., a contaminated water supply, or a vector population).

An *emergency* can be defined only within the context of the social, political and epidemiological circumstances in which it occurs, since such circumstances significantly affect the urgency of the problem, the action that has to be taken and the need for external cooperation.

The characteristic features of an emergency caused by an epidemic or threatened epidemic therefore include the following, although not all need be present and judgement must be exercised in assessing their importance:

(*a*) there is a risk of introduction and spread of the disease in the population;
(*b*) a "large" number of cases may reasonably be expected to occur;
(*c*) the disease involved is of such severity as to lead to serious disability or death;
(*d*) there is a risk of social and/or economic disruption resulting from the presence of the disease;
(*e*) the national authorities are unable to cope adequately with the situation because of a lack or insufficiency of:

—technical or professional personnel;
—organizational experience;

---

[1] For explanation of other terms used in this guide, see Annex 1.

3

—necessary supplies or equipment (drugs, vaccines, laboratory diagnostic materials, vector control materials, etc.);

(*f*) there is a danger of international transmission.

The types of situation that may come within the category of "emergencies" will differ from country to country, depending on two local factors: (*a*) the pre-existing state of endemicity; and (*b*) the presence or absence of a means of transmitting the agent. The examples given in Table 1, for non-endemic and endemic areas, serve to illustrate what may be described as epidemic emergencies for the particular diseases listed.

Epidemic emergencies usually result in human and economic losses, and political difficulties. It is the responsibility of the health services to control or preferably to prevent such situations by the organization of an emergency health service. The general lines of action aimed at achieving this objective are described below and are further discussed in subsequent chapters of the guide.

Table 1. Examples of emergencies related to epidemics or potential epidemics

Disease	In non-endemic areas	In endemic areas
Cholera	One confirmed indigenous case	"Significant" increase in incidence over and above what is normal for the season, particularly if multifocal and accompanied by deaths in children less than 10 years old
Giardiasis	A cluster of cases in a group of tourists returning from an endemic area	A discrete increase in incidence linked to a specific place
Malaria	A cluster of cases, with an increase in incidence in a "defined geographical area"	Rarely an emergency; increased incidence requires programme strengthening
Meningococcal meningitis	An incidence rate of 1 per 1000 in one week in a "defined geographical area" is ominous; the same rate for two consecutive weeks is an emergency	
Plague	One confirmed case	(*a*) A cluster of cases apparently linked by domestic rodent or respiratory transmission; or (*b*) a rodent epizootic
Rabies	One confirmed case of animal rabies in a previously rabies-free country	"Significant" increase in animal and human cases
Salmonellosis	A large cluster of cases in a limited area, with a single or predominant serotype, or a "significant" number of cases occurring in multiple foci apparently related by a common source (not forgetting that several countries may be involved)	

Table 1 (*continued*)

Disease	In non-endemic areas	In endemic areas
Smallpox[a]	Any strongly suspected case	Not applicable
Typhus fever due to *Rickettsia prowazekii*	One confirmed case in a louse-infested, non-immune population	"Significant" increase in the number of cases in a "limited" period of time
Viral encephalitis, mosquito-borne	Cluster of time- and space-related cases in a non-immune population (a single case should be regarded as a warning)	"Significant" increase in the number of cases with a single identified etiological agent, in a "limited" period of time
Viral haemor-rhagic fever	One confirmed indigenous or imported case with an etio-logical agent with which person-to-person transmis-sion may occur	"Significant" increase in the number of cases with a single identified etiological agent, in a "limited" period of time
Yellow fever	One confirmed case in a community with a non-immune human population and an "adequate" vector population	"Significant" increase in the number of cases in a "limited" period of time

[a] The WHO smallpox eradication campaign succeeded in eliminating the disease in 1980; vigilant surveillance of pox-like diseases (e.g., varicella, monkeypox) is maintained during the post-eradication era.

2.2 General lines of action

When an epidemic occurs, the resulting panic among the population and pressures of various kinds leave no time for reflecting on the soundness of the actions necessary to control the situation. Success in dealing with an epidemic therefore depends largely on the state of preparedness achieved in advance of any action. The basic initial step is to institutionalize an emergency health service headed by a coordinator responsible for preparing contingency plans in which all available and necessary resources in different situations are identified. Such plans should be approved by the other public services. Another important step is the establishment of an early warning system to detect any unusual incidence of a communicable disease that could cause an emergency situation. These initial tasks and actions are indicated in Table 2.

An analytical procedure should be followed in investigating epidemics, just as in diagnosing a disease (see also Annex 2). Various sources of information may originate the initial alert, apart from the early warning system, but are not always reliable. The first step is therefore to confirm that an epidemic, or the threat of an epidemic, as defined above, does actually exist. It would be an error to consider as

Table 2. General lines of action

Stage	Action to be taken
Preparedness	1. Constitution of an emergency health service 2. Elaboration of contingency planning 3. Establishment of an early warning system
Intervention	1. Rapid assessment of reality of epidemic 2. Formulation of provisional hypotheses as to its origin 3. Organization of field investigations 4. Analysis of data and determination of causes 5. Implementation of control measures 6. Final evaluation

an epidemic a hitherto unrecognized endemic situation or a mere seasonal increase in the incidence of a disease. It would also be an error to neglect the significance of a single case of a "new" disease in a country, which might well be the prelude to a further dramatic spread. The first data confirming the reality of the epidemic will lead to provisional hypotheses as to the nature of the disease[1] and its epidemiological pattern, which in turn will help to guide thorough field investigations. The objectives are defined, and the most appropriate technique is selected to find cases corresponding to the disease definition (or "case definition") that has been drawn up, at least provisionally to begin with. Observed cases are then located and listed as suspect, presumptive or confirmed, depending on the results of rapid laboratory tests. The analysis of the data collected by the field investigation teams makes it possible to determine the extent of the outbreak in time and place. The incidence of cases in different groups of the population is expressed in terms of the rates defined in Annex 1. The geographical spread of the disease is mapped out. Information on contacts enables the transmission characteristics to be determined and high risk groups identified; they should be placed under close surveillance and protected from the disease.

Although the approach to the understanding of an outbreak should be a systematic one and general advice is given later in this guide, experience shows that each epidemic is different from all the others; this is what, at the same time, causes it to spread among the population and makes it both difficult and interesting for the epidemiologist. This is where the "epidemiological sixth sense", which can be acquired only by personal experience, is so valuable. Above all, an open mind free from any preconceived ideas and a refusal to jump to hasty conclusions are the best safeguards in reaching the correct conclusion.

---

[1] Brief descriptions of diseases that can cause epidemics are given in Annex 3.

3. Organization of an emergency health service

Adequate structures must be established in advance so that a quick response can be made to an epidemic or the threat of an epidemic. The organization of an emergency health service (EHS) should therefore be considered by the health authorities as an integral part of communicable disease prevention and control. Two key steps to be taken to ensure that the EHS will be able to cope rapidly with an outbreak are contingency planning for interventions and the setting up of an early warning system for the detection of epidemics or threatened epidemics. Training and periodic refresher courses are also an integral part in ensuring the necessary preparedness of responsible personnel.

3.1 Structure of an emergency health service

The ultimate responsibility for planning and coordinating emergency operations must rest with a single individual in the health service, identified by title, e.g., the emergency health service coordinator. The EHS coordinator should have the support of an EHS advisory committee, which is indispensable as a permanent source of expertise and a channel for action.

3.1.1 Role of the emergency health service coordinator

The coordinator appointed should be a person of recognized competence and his authority and responsibilities should be clearly defined. He should be either a senior medical officer responsible for the epidemiology service in the ministry of health, or an epidemiologist trained in the newly emerging speciality of disaster preparedness, and should delegate responsibility to appropriate subordinates within the national administrative structure. His field of competence should cover as much as possible of the following:

(*a*) epidemiology, including statistical methods;
(*b*) community medicine;
(*c*) tropical pathology and epidemiology;
(*d*) relevant aspects of microbiology and clinical laboratory diagnosis;
(*e*) the entomology and mammalogy of current reservoirs and vectors;

7

(*f*) sanitary engineering;
(*g*) public health administration.

It is important to ensure that the EHS coordinator's authority to take decisions and institute the necessary action is clearly defined in writing and that the necessary budgetary allocation is made for that purpose. The EHS coordinator should preferably be a member of the national disaster preparedness committee. To ensure the best possible coordination, his position in the health services should be as shown in Fig. 1. The channels linking him to the ultimate authority at ministry of health level for matters relating to epidermics must be short (preferably direct), readily accessible, and capable of producing prompt decisions.

The EHS coordinator should be responsible for:

(*a*) coordinating the emergency services through the EHS advisory committee;
(*b*) establishing an early warning system for epidemics;
(*c*) preparing plans of action for the most probable epidemics;

Fig. 1. Coordination of emergency health services

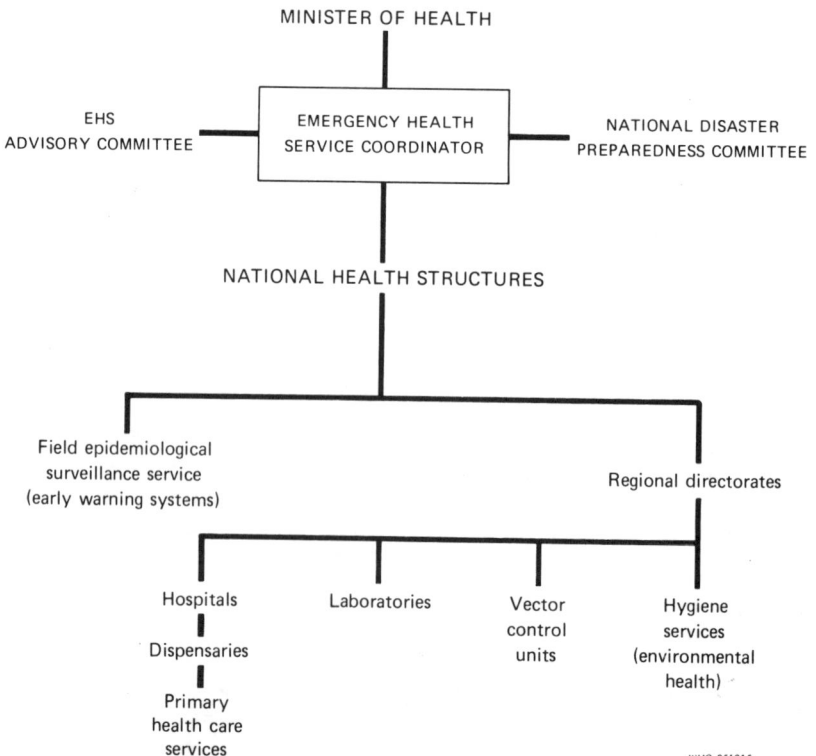

WHO 851015

(*d*) keeping an updated inventory of the national and international resources that may be needed;

(*e*) providing training for emergency operations in epidemics.

3.1.2 The advisory committee

The EHS coordinator should have the support of an EHS advisory committee, whose suggested composition is given in Table 3.

The committee has a very important role during emergencies, and great attention should be paid to its composition with a view to ensuring efficiency. It should consist of about 10–20 persons, representing all the specialities that might have to play an active role during an epidemic, and members should occupy executive positions in their departments of origin. The EHS coordinator should have the power to co-opt representatives from other groups as and when necessary. The committee should meet at regular intervals during the year so as to be ready at all times to take decisions at short notice if an epidemic arises.

Table 3. Suggested composition of an emergency health service advisory committee

---

Health service staff: specialists in different disciplines, e.g., tropical diseases, paediatrics, veterinary health, microbiology, entomology, mammalogy, sanitary engineering, toxicology

Representative of national disaster committee

Senior officials of the public services: finance, transport, communications, public works, police, armed forces, fire service

Representatives of international organizations (UNDP, UNICEF, WHO, Red Cross, etc.)

Representatives of voluntary private organizations

Responsible members of the communities affected

Representatives of the media

3.2 Preparedness measures

A contingency plan must be prepared by the EHS coordinator and approved by the EHS advisory committee and the responsible authority at the ministry of health. It should fit into the normal national administrative structure as an extension of the government's day-to-day dealings with health services, if its provisions are to be acceptable. Furthermore, contingency planning for epidemic-related emergencies should be integrated into any existing national disaster preparedness plan. Pre-planning operations consist of two parts, the first concerning logistics and consisting of an inventory of resources, both existing and required, and the second being technical and consisting of the preparation of investigation and control schemes for the most probable epidemics in the region.

3.2.1 Inventory of existing and required resources

The three essentials are money, manpower and equipment; the relative weight assigned to each will be determined by the local circumstances. The contingency plan should include a directory of addresses and telephone numbers of key persons and alternates, while the status of material in stock for emergencies should be periodically updated. Table 4 shows the most important resources that may be needed.

Budgetary provisions. The rapid implementation of investigation and control operations may involve expenditure of funds over and above those provided in the regular budget, and realistic supplementary estimates will need to be worked out. Since such estimates may be used as the basis for requests for external assistance, it is imperative that they should reflect the actual needs of the impending emergency.

Personnel. Key persons in different specialities, or in executive posts in national services, and their alternates, should be identified and given clear assignments in advance. The nature of the control measures may necessitate the employment of, and crash training courses for, additional staff for field operations, and it is essential that a simple and straightforward method of selecting such personnel should be established.

If it is also necessary to call in external expertise, there are obvious advantages if the international consultants are conversant with the clinical and geopolitical conditions in the region affected, if not

Table 4. Resources needed in emergencies
caused by epidemics

Budgetary provision
Personnel
Medical care
Laboratory support
Field teams
Immunization
Vector control
Environmental sanitation
Supplies
Transport
Communications
Community participation
International aid

specifically with the country itself. Provision should be made for the rapid issue of visas and for arranging travel and insurance for such consultants.

Consideration should be given to immunizing in advance or at short notice the personnel who will be engaged in field operations. Administration of immunoglobulin against hepatitis A, as well as tetanus and poliomyelitis immunizations, should be the first to be considered. The need for immunization against other diseases, such as yellow fever, Rift Valley fever; and Japanese encephalitis, will depend on the local situation. It should be remembered that a week or so is required following immunization for antibodies to appear and thus provide protection. Reimmunization may be needed periodically. Since smallpox has been eradicated, there is no justification for vaccination of team members against that disease unless smallpox-like particles have been seen in specimens by electron microscopy and an experienced clinician strongly suspects a clinical case.

Medical care. Information should be collected in advance on hospitals and other health care centres, as indicated in Table 5.

Irrespective of the nature of the epidemic, some panic may occur and a gradual or sometimes explosive increase in demand for medical care may be expected, even with the best possible public information programme. Although the pressure may first be experienced at peripheral health facilities and by private medical practitioners, the main general hospital(s) will soon be forced to bear the brunt of that demand--whether they normally operate outpatient departments or not. It is advisable, therefore, that every hospital, within the framework of the national disaster preparedness plans, should develop its own emergency plan. As with natural disasters, the plan should include arrangements for expanding the reception and treatment facilities and if necessary for evacuating the surplus inpatients.

While, in epidemics, there may not be the same need for establishing the system of triage essential in disasters associated with

Table 5. Inventory of resources available for medical care

Location of hospitals and other health centres, by category
Catchment areas of hospitals
Usual number of in- and outpatients
Number of beds in infectious disease wards
Type of isolation available for patients
Possibilities for extension of isolation facilities
Facilities for intensive care
Number of ambulances
Requirements for additional personnel
Location of referral hospital
Executive staff to contact in case of emergency
Possible additional facilities available, such as schools, hotels, etc.

large numbers of injuries, a screening mechanism may nevertheless be required to direct patients, as required, to ambulatory or institutional care.

As soon as practicable, however, and again taking into consideration the nature of the epidemic, strenuous efforts must be made to route patients through the normal channels of health care, starting at the peripheral primary health care (PHC) centre, so as to avoid overloading hospitals with mild cases. Both the hospitals under siege and PHC centres where the numbers attending are abnormally high can benefit from the services of voluntary collaborators in maintaining discipline and in keeping simple patient records.

It may be necessary, both for logistical reasons and for ensuring that the limited number of professional personnel are used more efficiently, to establish temporary treatment centres in the epidemic area. Such "field hospitals" may be located in existing facilities (e.g., schools) or may be housed in tents or other temporary structures. Maintenance of the quality of medical care during epidemics may be more difficult but should usually be entirely possible, and such centres may be a great convenience and comfort to the patients and their families.

Highly infectious diseases, such as suspected smallpox-like exanthems and haemorrhagic fevers (Lassa fever, Ebola and Marburg virus diseases), give rise to special safety problems in handling patients. If there is no hospital with a high-security ward, temporary arrangements should be made in advance to admit suspect, highly contagious patients. Although specially designed devices, such as the Trexler plastic film isolator (see Annex 4), ensure the highest level of safety in the management of highly contagious patients by eliminating direct contact with them and reducing the risk of airborne transmission, simpler equipment and good barrier nursing practices may also provide satisfactory protection. The conditions to be satisfied by a high-security ward are summarized in Table 6 and further details are given in Annex 4.

Table 6. Conditions to be satisfied by a high-security ward in a hospital

Direct access for patients to avoid possible contamination of other areas of the hospital

Access to ward restricted to specialized personnel

Anteroom adjacent to each patient-room

Self-contained toilet facilities

Air flow from non-contaminated to contaminated areas and filtration of exhaust to outside

Special waste decontamination and terminal disinfection facilities

Biological barrier equipment (sets of gowns, gloves and masks, disposable or reusable after sterilization) for personnel protection, or bed isolator (if available)

Personnel trained in barrier nursing and kept under medical surveillance

Laboratory support. A directory of laboratories that can be mobilized during epidemics should be kept up to date and should include the information listed in Table 7.

Rapid laboratory support is needed during epidemics to enable the causative agent to be isolated from patients, vectors, and reservoirs, and characterized, and for serological surveys. It must be assumed that laboratories will have to work to the limits of their capabilities in terms of personnel, equipment and reagents. A scheme should be drawn up to use local, regional, central, and WHO reference laboratories, as may be most convenient, depending on the number of specimens and the complexity of the laboratory procedures required.

Extra supplies of current items may have to be provided rapidly to peripheral laboratories to enable them to cope with an unusually large number of specimens and tests, including:

—disposable pipettes, tubes, microplates, syringes, etc.;
—specific reagents;
—ether, acetone, etc.;
—disinfectants;
—refrigerating equipment, liquid nitrogen, dry ice.

When an outbreak is caused by a highly disabling or lethal agent, specimens should be processed in laboratories where the safety equipment and personnel training are appropriate to the risks that the agent represents. Such laboratories should be identified, and special instructions should be circulated in conformity with safety regulations, particularly if specimens have to be sent to foreign laboratories (see Annex 5).

Outbreaks occurring in remote areas may none the less require field laboratory examinations, which may include fluorescent microscopy.

Table 7. Information needed on laboratory support

Network of regional laboratories and referral facilities

For each laboratory:
  —range of infectious agents that can be diagnosed
  —containment level for dangerous pathogens
  —number of specimens that can be processed
  —arrangements for shipment of specimens from periphery
  —executive staff to contact in case of emergency

National and WHO reference laboratories:
  —arrangements and regulations (national, international) for shipment of infectious material
  —contacts to be established in advance of shipment

Reference laboratories for special (highly dangerous) pathogens:
  —special arrangements (contacts through WHO)

Field laboratories:
  —portable equipment for field investigations

Table 8. Resources needed for field teams

Trained personnel

Travel facilities:
—transport, e.g., four-wheel drive vehicles,
—lorries, helicopters, small aircraft
—accommodation, food, etc.
—travel documents

Communications:
—telephone, radio

Equipment for:
—clinical investigations
—collection of laboratory specimens
—emergency control measures, e.g., jet injectors,
  syringes, insecticide sprayers

If the electricity supply is uncertain, a portable generator will be needed. Small portable biosafety cabinets with plastic walls and fixed gloves have been designed for field operations.

Field teams. Mobile teams are necessary to conduct epidemiological investigations and carry out control measures in the field; their composition will vary according to the nature of the outbreak and the local conditions. The resources required by such teams are listed in Table 8.

If the pathogen is suspected of being arthropod-borne, mosquito nets and repellents, or special clothing providing protection against ticks and mites, may also be required by field teams.

If a dangerous pathogen with person-to-person transmission is suspected, the additional resources listed in Table 9 are necessary.

Immunization campaigns. Protection against some of the diseases included in the contingency plan can be provided by immunization. In this case, the resources listed in Table 10 will be necessary.

Table 9. Resources needed for investigation of epidemics caused by dangerous pathogens with person-to-person transmission

---

Adequate number of sets of protective clothing (disposable or reusable after sterilization) (see Annex 4)

Special instructions for dealing with patients, collecting and shipping specimens, and giving supportive care

Protection of team members against local major endemic infections (such as malaria, typhoid, enteric infections, yellow fever) to avoid an intercurrent disease that could arouse suspicion of contamination

Arrangements for responsibility for, and management of, medical evacuation and hospitalization of field team personnel suspected of being infected

Life insurance for team members

Table 10. Resources needed for emergency immunization campaign

---

Directory of suppliers of vaccines

Stocks of vaccine to meet anticipated requirements

Delivery systems:
—syringes (disposable or reusable after sterilization) and sterilization
   equipment, if necessary;
—jet injectors (reserve, maintenance, spare parts, training)

Immunizing teams, transport, cold chain

Voluntary auxiliary personnel, cooperation of mass media

With certain diseases only one injection of vaccine is required (live vaccines), whereas with others (killed vaccines) at least two injections are necessary. The plan should identify sources for the rapid supply of vaccines and injection equipment. In emergency conditions, jet injectors are time-saving (permitting 1000–1500 vaccinations per hour) in comparison with syringes, but require well trained personnel, particular care in maintenance, and good crowd control. Because of possible delays in delivery, a few should be kept as emergency stock. Immunizing teams can benefit greatly from the assistance of voluntary collaborators.

Vector control. Certain preliminary actions must be taken, as indicated in Table 11, before vector control operations can be carried out.

Every health service should possess trained personnel for pest and vector control, whether in a specially designated unit or engaged in environmental sanitation activities. The vector-control unit or environmental health department itself, having been previously alerted to the possibility of an epidemic, and having updated its vector monitoring capabilities as far as practicable, may decide that an impending or actual epidemic either can or cannot be handled

Table 11. Resources needed for vector control operations

Location of vector control units

Mechanisms for rapidly alerting personnel and ensuring their availability

Determination of insecticide resistance

Storage of emergency reserve of recommended insecticides, with turnover
   of stock to keep material fresh

Reserve of air and ground spraying equipment

Contacts with aircraft companies, information on flying regulations

Estimate of additional personnel and ground transport required

Preparation of emergency plans against local potential vectors

---

adequately with the national resources available. In the former case, the necessary field operations should be initiated immediately; in the latter, a request for external collaboration should be sent off without delay.

An inventory of vector control equipment available locally and in operational condition should be updated at the end of each year, items beyond repair being discarded. In addition, data compiled by the WHO regional offices on sources, types and costs of use of other equipment held either by neighbouring countries or the private sector, should be properly filed and easily retrievable for consultation when the need arises.

Insecticides and spraying equipment may be stockpiled, or, preferably, a turnover stock should be kept in order to avoid deterioration on prolonged storage. Insecticides should be selected after determination of possible vector resistance. Different types of equipment (see also Annex 6) may have to be used, as follows:

—hand-operated rotary dusters for powdered insecticides;
—hand-operated back-pack sprayers for liquid insecticides for domestic application;
—power-spray units for large-scale insecticide application.

Environmental sanitation. Among the equipment that may be needed if drinking-water is contaminated, the following should be available in adequate numbers:

—portable water treatment units;
—mobile water tankers;
—mobile chlorinators;
—disinfectants.

Supplies. It may not always be practicable to stockpile the large amounts of equipment and drugs that may be required to combat a major outbreak of a filth-, air-, or vector-borne disease. However, a routine system for monitoring the inventory of the items essential under local conditions would be good practice, and would indicate when normal stocks needed to be replaced or increased.

For each possible epidemic, standardized lists of essential supplies should be prepared in advance, not merely for the country as a whole, but also for the various administrative subdivisions, so as to facilitate the execution of an emergency plan of action, should this become necessary.

To avoid unnecessary delays in delivery, steps should be taken at an early stage to secure either the waiving or at least the simplification of import formalities for emergency equipment and supplies. Standing instructions should also be laid down for the acknowledgement, processing, storage and distribution of such material; the waiving of landing formalities for foreign aircraft hired for disease control purposes may also need to be considered.

Transport. No health service will have sufficient vehicles to meet the needs of an emergency, i.e., additional ambulances, transportation of investigative and operational health personnel, and carriage of equipment and supplies. Assistance may be required from the public works department, utilities, the police, the armed forces and the private sector. Constantly updated information on what may be available, and from whom, is therefore essential. Since such an exercise may already form part of the national disaster committee's preparedness plans, it may be necessary only to ensure that the resources identified for use in disasters can also be called upon to meet the needs of a health emergency, but detailed plans for the use to which each vehicle will be put must be recorded.

In view of possible shortages of petrol, some attention may need to be given to a centrally established system of priorities designed to ensure supplies for transport intended for use in an emergency situation.

Communications. Communication channels normally available to the health services will be inadequate in an emergency. Additional facilities will therefore be required to augment the usual limited two-way radio link between ambulances and the principal hospital. For this purpose, collaboration will be essential—both with the departments responsible for the various facilities that are already available (works, utilities, private) and with those services that are traditionally better served, such as the police and armed forces.

At the headquarters of the EHS coordinator, early installation of additional telephone lines should be envisaged as the emergency situation develops, both for local and overseas calls. All such new numbers should be made widely known to potential users, and one line should perhaps be set aside especially for public inquiries.

For operational purposes, police radio broadcasting services or other networks may have to be used. The usefulness of a suitable receiving and transmitting set at the EHS coordinator's office will be self-evident.

The availability of these supplementary communication channels cannot, however, be left to chance. Their use must be planned well in advance and coordinated if they are to provide a satisfactory service. Finally, the collaboration of any radio communication specialists available in the area should be sought from the outset, so that any emergency network set up will have the benefit of their professional expertise. Although the public services are invariably cooperative in assigning priority in true emergencies, recourse may also be made, by prior arrangement, to private lines at embassies, United Nations offices, or business houses.

Portable transistor radios are to be found in the smallest communities and the fullest use must be made of broadcasting for reaching the population, preferably at the time of popular local transmissions, such as "community news".

To avoid any confusion, all releases must be cleared by the EHS coordinator, and should be factual, accurate, in simple language and, as appropriate, repeated in the commoner local languages. It is obviously better for the public to receive information, advice, and guidance from the responsible health authority rather than be left exposed to false rumours and inaccurate data.

The national newspapers will inevitably report on the various phases of an epidemic, from its initial threat or inception to its subsidence. While the nature of their reporting cannot be controlled, it would be wise to issue, to all of them, formal and accurately documented releases on all aspects of the situation as it evolves, and at intervals and a time of day convenient to them. Interviews of technical staff should preferably be avoided, but if granted by the decision-makers—with adequate briefing and possible participation by the technicians—should be taped so that any significant errors that may inadvertently appear in print can be promptly corrected by mutual agreement.

It must not be forgotten, however, that all releases will normally require clearance at central ministry level. In order to avoid delays, clear policy guidelines must be established in advance on what will be acceptable to the central authorities. Releases may need to be processed by government public information services. If so, agreement must be reached with the responsible officer that material supplied directly by the EHS coordinator will be released promptly, after the necessary clearance.

Failure to supply up-to-date information on the emergency to the media will result in the publication of rumours, inaccuracies, speculation and criticism, all of which will help to undermine public confidence in the health service and reduce enthusiasm and motivation for collaboration with it. On the other hand, the establishment and maintenance of an amicable working relationship with the media can readily provide an opportunity to influence the content and style of reporting on material that may be independently compiled, and thereby minimize or avoid distortion and rank sensationalism on the part of the press.

Community participation. The main obstacles to community participation in a national health programme are the levels of the public's health awareness, the administrator's imagination and the way that he reacts to lay suggestions. All public information activities should therefore be geared not merely to providing enlightenment on the subject, but also to stimulating ideas on ways in which individuals and groups can contribute to the task in hand. This applies both to normal and abnormal situations—such as an emergency caused by an epidemic. Suggestions for local action and the recruitment of voluntary collaborators should be channelled through community health committees, where they exist.

The lessons learned in the global smallpox eradication programme can be applied to case detection during an epidemic, particularly in respect of mild attacks of the disease concerned, the common signs and symptoms of which can be recognized, or arouse suspicion, when observed, for example, by a schoolchild at home. A teacher or district nurse would be a natural point of contact.

At primary health care centres or hospital outpatient departments, selected volunteers can assist in crowd control, simple registration, and as tally clerks and skin swabbers when immunizations are carried out.

Source reduction of domestic mosquito vectors, combined with an environmental clean-up campaign, serves the double purpose of direct vector control and as a practical exercise in health education. In spraying operations, volunteers can help in carrying insecticide, water and equipment in their immediate neighbourhood.

Packaging of supplies at central level for dispatch to the field frequently requires additional manpower, which can be provided by volunteers. It is a common experience that, in times of adversity, there is an upsurge of fellow feeling among the affected population that needs only to be tapped and directed into the right channels.

3.2.2 International aid

International aid may be required when an outbreak develops that cannot be contained with the national resources available. Contingency planning should establish in advance what United Nations agencies might be asked to provide in terms of expertise, equipment, and supplies, and where it can be obtained.

Additional resources may be provided by other countries on a bilateral basis or by regional or intercountry organizations. Other international organizations, such as the International Committee of the Red Cross, may also be able to provide assistance.

United Nations agencies. The United Nations agencies have developed a scheme for cooperation with countries when epidemics occur. Requests may be addressed to the United Nations Disaster Relief Organization (UNDRO) or to the World Health Organization (WHO). Action is taken in collaboration with other organizations, such as the United Nations Children's Fund (UNICEF) and the United Nations Development Programme (UNDP).

WHO emergency technical cooperation. Contingency planning should take into account the additional resources that may be obtained from WHO. In fulfilment of its commitment under Article 2(d) of the Constitution to provide assistance to Member States in dealing with epidemics, WHO has made arrangements for emergency relief, including the establishment of Emergency Relief Operations at headquarters, as shown in Fig. 2. Responsible officers are permanently

Fig. 2. Organization chart of WHO response to requests for cooperation in epidemic emergencies

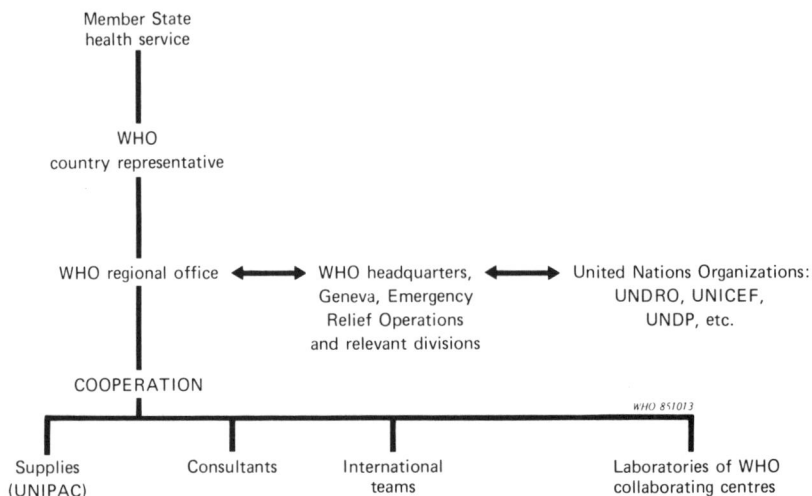

on call at the regional offices and at headquarters in Geneva. The assistance available from WHO includes the provision of WHO experts as short-term consultants, the services of the various WHO collaborating centres, the provision of the WHO emergency health kit, and the procurement of medicines and other health supplies.

General criteria for WHO involvement in emergency relief have been defined and are summarized in Table 12.

Table 12. Criteria for WHO involvement in emergency relief operations

Conditions	Criteria
A request has been received	WHO cooperation is made available if: —the situation is a genuine emergency or threatens to become one if appropriate measures are not taken; —national resources for dealing with the situation are insufficient; —the additional resources likely to be provided by other countries or agencies are also not sufficient to meet the total needs.
No request has been received	WHO may offer technical cooperation to the government when: —it is clear that WHO assistance would materially improve either the physical or the organizational resources locally available for dealing with the situation; —the situation is such that it threatens the public health of the country and of adjoining countries.

Special expertise can be provided by WHO short-term consultants during epidemics, in epidemiological investigations, and in carrying out control measures. Specialists in the following disciplines may be needed: epidemiology, bacteriology, parasitology, malariology, virology, entomology, mammalogy, sanitary engineering, and toxicology; clinical and veterinary expertise for specific diseases may also be required. Under their terms of employment, consultants report only to the ministry of health of the affected countries and to WHO, and not to their country of origin. Up-to-date lists of experts can be obtained from WHO regional offices and headquarters. It may be worthwhile to arrange recruitment formalities in advance, if the experts required are known.

Laboratories designated as WHO collaborating centres for reference and research can help in identifying the disease agent, especially for dangerous pathogens, when high-security laboratories are necessary, in carrying out extensive serological studies with multiple antigens, and in assessing immunity pre- and postimmunization. Such centres can provide experts and also investigative and control teams with the necessary equipment.

Supplies that can be procured at short notice through WHO regional offices and headquarters include:

—drugs and vaccines;
—syringes and injectors;
—standard laboratory equipment;
—insecticides;
—spraying equipment;
—protective clothing;
—sanitation equipment.

Most of this equipment is also kept in stock by UNICEF in the UNIPAC programme for procurement at short notice in emergencies.

3.2.3 Contingency planning

Contingency planning should include the identification of potential epidemic diseases and the preparation of the corresponding plans for action.

Identification of potential epidemic diseases. The diseases for which special plans of action should be prepared may be selected on the basis of the following criteria:

—epidemic diseases capable of causing an emergency as defined in Chapter 2;
—epidemic diseases known to have caused emergencies locally in the past;
—locally endemic diseases that may become epidemic;
—diseases that may be imported.

For each potential epidemic disease selected, a study should be carried out to establish, for the locality concerned, the nature of:

—the source(s) (reservoirs) of the infectious agent;
—the vehicle(s) of transmission;
—the receptive host(s).

A potential epidemic agent may exist locally in an endemic or sporadic condition, as shown by a past history of epidemics. It may also be uncovered by means of a systematic multipurpose serological survey. In both cases, the serological survey will also indicate the existence and proportion of susceptible persons in different population groups. The reservoir of the agent may be human, animal, or in the environment, the last being the most difficult to identify. The cooperation of veterinarians and entomologists is necessary in studies of diseases that can be transmitted directly or indirectly by animals, or by insects.

Not all epidemic diseases can be imported into a given country. A careful assessment of the conditions necessary for the importation of a particular disease may avoid useless and expensive preventive measures. Such conditions include:

—a way in which the disease can be introduced;
—the existence of a susceptible population;
—an environment favourable to the rapid establishment of the disease;
—factors favourable to the long-term maintenance of the disease locally.

The probability of importation will depend on the existence of good communications with countries where the disease is present either permanently or occasionally. The transit time between the two countries should be shorter than the incubation period of the disease, and this is usually the case nowadays with air travel. Travellers who have taken connecting flights in non-infected transit countries are less likely to be identified as originating from an endemic zone and the risk of importation of disease may then be overlooked. The international exchange of sanitary information increases the awareness of the risk of importation of exotic disease. WHO provides such information through the *Weekly epidemiological record* and the automatic telex reply service.

Preparation of plans of action. Plans of action against potential epidemic diseases should be prepared. It is essential that the arrangements should be reviewed regularly, so that they can be implemented promptly in any affected area at any time.

Up-to-date general information on communicable diseases and on methods of controlling them is necessary if such plans are to be satisfactory. References to relevant WHO and other publications are given in the bibliography to this chapter. The information needed in

Table 13. Information needed in drawing up plans
of action against epidemic diseases

Baseline data on occurrence

Definition of epidemic threshold

Indications expected from the early warning system

Population groups at risk

Possible socioeconomic effects

Emergency clinical, laboratory, epidemiological
    investigations to be performed

Safety measures necessary

Possible emergency control measures

National resources required

International cooperation required

Follow-up measures

drawing up such plans of action is summarized in Table 13. Most of the items concerned will be discussed in greater detail in the different sections of this guide.

Criteria for determining the threshold between endemicity and epidemicity vary for each disease and also depend on the usual seasonal variations in incidence in the locality concerned. Relevant data for defining such seasonal variations may be obtained from routine surveillance and should be recorded annually. An illustration of the seasonal threshold problem is given for influenza in Fig. 3, which shows clearly when the seasonal threshold has been passed and the excess mortality may be attributed to the disease.

3.3 Early warning system for epidemics

An early warning system to detect outbreaks is of fundamental importance in preparedness for epidemics and its functioning is the responsibility of the EHS coordinator. Outbreaks may be detected by routine epidemiological surveillance and, when justified, by special additional active surveillance of those diseases representing the greatest potential danger.

3.3.1 Routine epidemiological surveillance

In routine epidemiological surveillance, statistics on morbidity and mortality are usually collected at all levels of the health services for certain specified diseases, not all of which may cause epidemics. It would be desirable for outbreaks to be detected directly by the

Fig. 3. Use of seasonal mortality curves for respiratory disease in identifying epidemics due to influenza

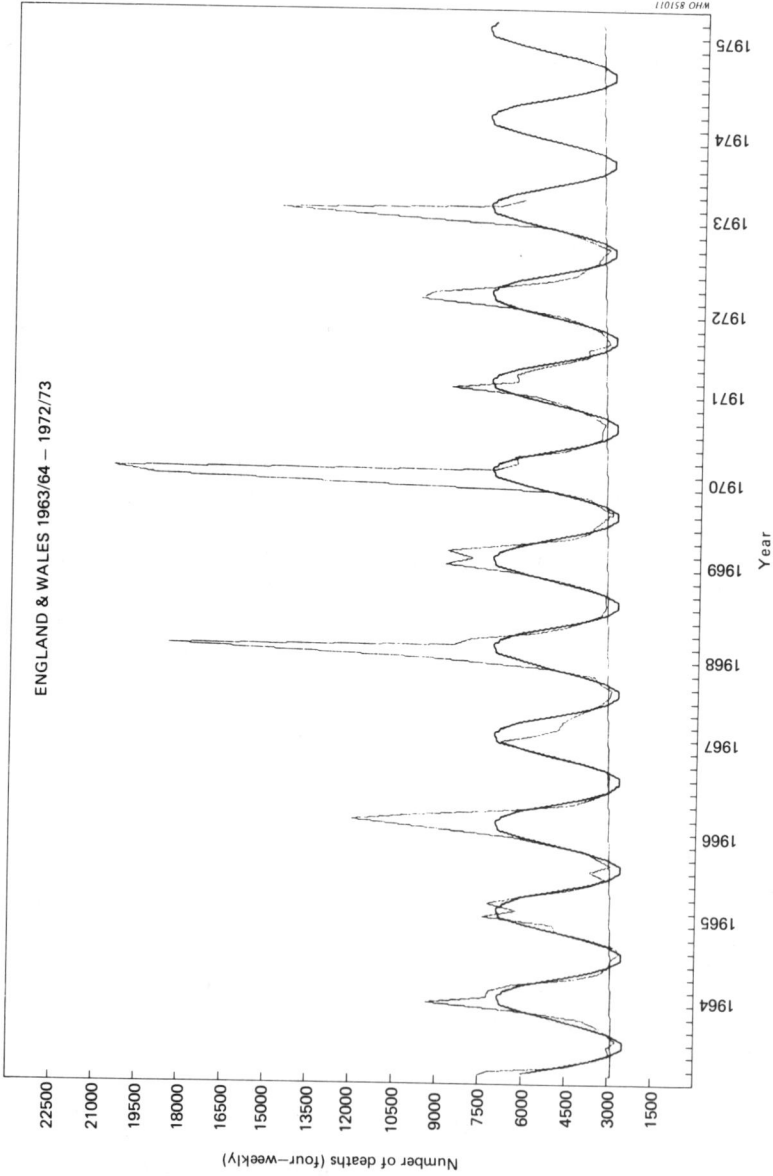

ENGLAND & WALES 1963/64 – 1972/73

The two curves, plotted by computer for four-week periods, represent (*a*) the expected seasonal curve constructed from deaths in the years of low mortality when no sizeable outbreaks of influenza occurred; and (*b*) the curve of actual numbers of deaths. It is clear that influenza epidemics occurred in 1966, 1968, 1970 and 1973. (Source: ASSAAD, F. ET AL. Use of excess mortality from respiratory diseases in the study of influenza. *Bulletin of the World Health Organization*, **49**: 219–233 (1973))

peripheral health units, and ideally at the primary health care level. However, this is often difficult because each peripheral unit sees relatively few patients and covers only a limited area. One or two patients with a particular set of symptoms and signs may not be enough to make the local nurse aware that an epidemic has begun. This may be especially true for outbreaks of enteric diseases, or for diseases presenting as "flu-like" or "malaria-like", or as "fever" or "jaundice". A small cluster of patients may not at first arouse any suspicion. If each health worker has been taught the definition of an epidemic and the locally applicable criteria for their initial detection, however, suspicion can be aroused promptly at the peripheral level.

However, in most instances, "epidemics" are first recognized at the intermediate health unit level (district, province, region). This is the level where reports are received from a number of dispensaries or small hospitals, summarized and forwarded to a higher level. The number of cases in each area should be plotted for each disease together with baseline data derived from routine surveillance during previous years and showing expected seasonal variations. The criteria for the epidemic threshold should be established and peripheral health centres informed of them so that they know precisely when they should notify higher levels of the excess occurrence of any disease.

Weekly rather than monthly reporting is needed in detecting outbreaks. Weekly reports must be completed promptly, and the appropriate authority should be alerted if and when there is evidence of an increase in incidence over and above normal trends. Routine surveillance must be intensified when epidemiological information from neighbouring countries warrants such action. Feedback of information to peripheral staff through periodic health service bulletins on infectious diseases has a stimulating effect by showing the staff concerned the value and utility of their contribution.

Even if reporting is prompt, a serious deficiency of routine surveillance is that patients who do not attend medical facilities are not covered and that diseases that are difficult to diagnose may be assigned to the wrong category, particularly if an unusual disease occurs.

3.3.2 Active epidemiological surveillance

Active epidemiological surveillance consists of frequent in-depth searches for cases of a few selected diseases likely to cause severe epidemics in a region so that rapid action can be taken or, preferably, any spread from the initial cases prevented. Permanent arrangements are necessary such that suspect cases can be further investigated immediately in order to uncover rapidly the source of infection, as well as other possible secondary cases. In addition, the occurrence of the selected disease must be assessed at convenient intervals by means of serological multipurpose surveys, as well as surveys of vectors and reservoirs, if any.

Active surveillance is based on existing health institutions and/or special mobile field teams. It is more reliable than routine surveillance but is more expensive and the vigilance of the volunteers ("spotters") used must be continuously monitored. It should therefore be limited to a restricted list of diseases of particular importance or to limited periods when a special temporary watch is justified.

Selection of diseases to be monitored. Criteria for the selection of diseases for which active surveillance is justified give greater weight to those of major public health importance and to others that may appear when there are unusually favourable circumstances. These criteria are summarized in Table 14.

Health-institution-based active surveillance. Active surveillance is based on "sentinel" hospitals and on spotters in small communities or villages.

A number of sentinel hospitals should be selected, located preferably in the endemic zone or at points of entry to the country. In such hospitals, a physician should be made responsible for:

(1) inspection of the data on daily admissions and attendances at outpatient clinics, and reporting to the EHS weekly, or immediately if there is any suspicion of an outbreak, on the presence (or absence) of any disease on the priority list or any other disease of interest;

(2) inquiring about the place and source of infection;

(3) collecting appropriate specimens in consultation with the laboratory.

The physician in charge should be provided with the relevant documentation concerning the diseases under active surveillance and use a form for reporting that can be based on the suggested model shown later in Table 25 (p. 45).

Spotters at the community level should detect outbreaks earlier than hospitals and also record cases that are not hospitalized. Motivated spotters can be recruited among private practitioners, primary health care workers in villages, or trained members of staff in schools, industry, public services, etc. A strategy should be developed to locate these spotters in the most suitable places. They should

Table 14. Criteria for active surveillance of certain diseases

Great public health importance

Local endemicity or close links with an external active focus in another country

Appearance or risk of a "new" disease (e.g., Ebola haemorrhagic fever) with unknown local transmission potential

Absence or low level of immunity in certain human (or animal) population groups

Large local population of potential insect and animal vectors and reservoirs

Unusual ecological (irrigation, deforestation), climatic (droughts, floods) or population (immigration) conditions favourable to transmission

Table 15. Surveillance of animal reservoirs and vectors

Identification of species, subspecies or biotypes, if any
Population density
Seasonal/annual density variations
Breeding habits
Feeding habits
Period of infectivity
Factors determining contacts with man
Laboratory detection of infection
Control measures (e.g., sensitivity to insecticides or rodenticides and method of choice for application)

normally report weekly and should contact a designated responsible person immediately if they suspect an outbreak. The report form should again be the same as that shown later in Table 25. Spotters should be provided with training material concerning the diseases under active surveillance and should receive feedback information on the activities of the system.

Weekly reports should be prepared by sentinel hospitals and spotters, even in the absence of outbreaks, so as to ensure that vigilance is maintained at all times.

Active surveillance by mobile field team(s). A mobile emergency health service team should visit sentinel hospitals and community spotters as often as possible. Active surveillance can also benefit greatly from serosurveys and special ecological surveys.

The initial serosurvey is aimed at determining the prevalence of priority diseases in an area or community. Subsequent periodic surveys can indicate the number of seroconversions if the same persons are bled or if the two samples of the population can be compared statistically. Serosurveys should be carried out in close collaboration with a laboratory and a statistician.

The active surveillance of certain epidemic diseases may require the ecological surveillance of their reservoirs and vectors, such as rodents and arthropods. The general ecological surveillance procedures carried out by specialists (entomologists, mammalogists) in field visits are shown in Table 15.

3.3.3 International notifications

WHO provides information on epidemics through:

—an automatic telex reply service (No. 28150 Geneva);
—the *Weekly epidemiological record*, mailed each Friday to all ministries of health and official health institutions;

—inquiries to the Secretariat in Geneva (telephone 91 21 11, telex 27821, cables UNISANTE GENEVA) and to the Regional Offices for: Africa (P.O. Box No. 6, Brazzaville, Congo, telephone 81 38 60, telex 5217, cables UNISANTE BRAZZAVILLE); the Americas (Pan American Sanitary Bureau, 525 Twenty-third Street N. W., Washington, DC, USA, telephone 861–3200, telex 248338, cables OFSANPAN WASHINGTON); the Eastern Mediterranean (P.O. Box 1517, Alexandria-21511, Egypt, telephone 49–300 90, telex 54028, cables UNISANTE ALEXANDRIA); Europe (8 Scherfigsvej, DK-2100 Copenhagen Ø, Denmark, telephone 29 01 11, telex 15348, cables UNISANTE COPENHAGEN); South-East Asia (World Health House, Indraprastha Estate, Mahatma Gandhi Road, New Delhi-110002, India, telephone 331 7804, telex 65031, cables WHO NEW DELHI); and the Western Pacific (P.O. Box 2932, Manila 2801, Philippines, telephone 59 20 41, telex 27652, cables UNISANTE MANILA).

The *Weekly epidemiological record* publishes detailed accounts of epidemics as soon as they are available from Member States, whereas the automatic telex reply service provides information on brief urgent notifications.

Conversely, when an epidemic occurs, Member States should inform WHO without delay. WHO Member States have an obligation to notify the following diseases:

(*a*) Diseases subject to the International Health Regulations, namely cholera, plague and yellow fever. Each health administration must notify the Organization by telegram or telex within 24 hours of its being informed that the first case of a disease subject to the Regulations, that is neither an imported nor transferred case, has occurred in its territory. The purpose is to ensure maximum security against the international spread of disease with the minimum interference with world traffic.

(*b*) Diseases under international surveillance, namely typhus fever due to *Rickettsia prowazekii*, relapsing fever due to *Borrelia recurrentis*, paralytic poliomyelitis and viral influenza. Health administrations must inform the Organization promptly by telegram or telex of the occurrence of any outbreak. This does not imply any quarantine measures.

Although not included in these lists, other diseases such as meningococcal meningitis, dengue, viral haemorrhagic fevers, Legionnaires' disease, and food-borne epidemics, are also important, and information on outbreaks is useful and should be shared among countries on a cooperative basis through rapid notification in the *Weekly epidemiological record*.

Rather than a tiresome obligation, notifications should be regarded as good epidemiological practice. In order to avoid creating panic, information is released by WHO only when the existence and nature of an outbreak have been confirmed, initial containment measures taken, and the government concerned has agreed to its release. In the meantime, the government can benefit from rapid assistance from WHO and other international organizations.

3.4 Training

Training of national staff at different levels in conducting emergency operations during epidemics is an important responsibility of the EHS coordinator. A suggested curriculum for the training of district medical officers is given in Table 16.

In addition to the training of newly recruited personnel, periodic workshops and simulation exercises are useful. Training may have to be repeated because of changes in personnel and in the epidemiological situation, and advances in technology. Periodic meetings of personnel and/or site visits by the EHS coordinator are recommended. The relevant documentation should be updated periodically.

Table 16. Suggested curriculum for training of district medical officers in conducting emergency operations during epidemics

A. Theory

Clinical, epidemiological and control aspects of locally prevalent epidemic diseases, or those likely to occur; preparation of plans of action

Methodology of epidemiological surveillance and early warning systems

General methodology of epidemiological investigations during epidemics

Laboratory support for surveillance and investigations

Analysis of epidemiological data: statistical significance, transmission patterns

General and specific methodology for control of epidemics

Administrative organization of emergency health service

B. Practical work

Participation in surveillance activities, responsibility for a given problem

Simulation exercises for different kinds of outbreaks, including:

   —hospital survey
   —population survey and interviews
   —collection and shipment of specimens
   —safety precautions
   —improvisation of patient isolation
   —immunization, cold chain
   —medical evacuation
   —vector control and sanitation
   —disinfection
   —reporting
   —dealing with the media

Planning and evaluating operations

Maintenance of vehicles, refrigerators, etc.

An epidemic may often involve a number of countries. Joint training programmes might be conducted by neighbouring countries in order to solve immediate problems in the border areas as well as to ensure the exchange of epidemiological information and thus contain epidemics more effectively and economically. Such training programmes can be coordinated by WHO.

BIBLIOGRAPHY

BARKER, D. J. P. & BENNETT, F. J. *Practical epidemiology.* Edinburgh, Churchill Livingstone, 1982.

CENTERS FOR DISEASE CONTROL. Viral hemorrhagic fever: initial management of suspected and confirmed cases. *Morbidity and mortality weekly report,* **32**: 27S–39S (1983).

Communicable diseases in disasters. *Weekly epidemiological record,* **54**: 355–357 (1979).

CRUICKSHANK, R. ET AL. *Epidemiology and community health in warm climate countries.* Edinburgh, Churchill Livingstone, 1976.

DEPARTMENT OF HEALTH AND SOCIAL SECURITY. *Memorandum on the control of outbreaks of smallpox.* London, HMSO, 1975.

DEPARTMENT OF HEALTH AND SOCIAL SECURITY AND THE WELSH OFFICE. *Memorandum on Lassa fever.* London, HMSO, 1976.

Disaster prevention and mitigation. Vol. 8. Sanitation aspects. New York, United Nations, 1982.

DUNSMORE, D. J. *Safety measures for use in outbreaks of communicable disease.* Geneva, World Health Organization, 1986.

Emergency health management after natural disasters. Washington, DC, Pan American Health Organization, 1981 (Scientific Publication No. 407).

FAO Expert Consultation on Emergency Disease Control. Rome, Food and Agriculture Organization, 1981 (Report AGA 801).

Dengue haemorrhagic fever: diagnosis, treatment and control. Geneva, World Health Organization, 1986.

International Health Regulations (1969), 3rd ed. Geneva, World Health Organization, 1983.

Management of suspected cases of smallpox in the post-eradication period. Unpublished WHO document, WHO/SE/80.157/Rev.1.

MONATH, T. P. Lassa fever and Marburg virus disease. *WHO Chronicle,* **28**: 212–219 (1974).

MONATH, T. P. & CASALS, J. Diagnosis of Lassa fever and the isolation and management of patients. *Bulletin of the World Health Organization,* **52**: 707–715 (1975).

Planning and organization of emergency medical services. Copenhagen, WHO Regional Office for Europe, 1981 (EURO Reports and Studies No. 35).

Procedures for the surveillance and management of monkeypox and viral haemorrhagic fevers (yellow fever, Lassa fever, Ebola and Marburg virus diseases). Unpublished WHO document, CDS/80.2.

Report of the informal consultation on the Marburg virus-like disease outbreaks in the Sudan and Zaire in 1976. Unpublished WHO document, VIR/77.1.

Report of the Working Group on Haemorrhagic Fever with Renal Syndrome. WHO Regional Office for the Western Pacific, unpublished document, WPR/RPD/WG/(HFRS)/82.16.

Rift Valley fever: an emerging human and animal problem. Geneva, World Health Organization, 1982 (Offset Publication No. 63).

SIMPSON, D. I. H. *Marburg and Ebola virus infections: a guide for their diagnosis, management and control.* Geneva, World Health Organization, 1977 (Offset Publication No. 36).

Strategies for the control of emergencies caused by epidemics of communicable diseases. Unpublished WHO document, CDS/MTG/82.1.

Technical guide for a system of cholera surveillance. *Weekly epidemiological record,* **46**: 393–396 (1971).

Technical guide for a system of influenza surveillance. *Weekly epidemiological record,* **46**: 65–68 (1971).

Technical guide for a system of louse-borne typhus surveillance. *Weekly epidemiological record,* **46**: 273–275 (1971).

Technical guide for a system of malaria surveillance. *Weekly epidemiological record,* **46**: 329–333 (1971).

Technical guide for a system of plague surveillance. *Weekly epidemiological record,* **48**: 149–160.

Technical guide for a system of poliomyelitis surveillance. *Weekly epidemiological record,* **50**: 205–209 (1975).

Technical guide for a system of yellow fever surveillance. *Weekly epidemiological record,* **46**: 493–500 (1971).

The long-term future of the International Health Regulations. *WHO Chronicle,* **32**: 439–447 (1978).

The management of emergencies caused by "unusual" diseases. Unpublished WHO document, WHO/SMM/80.16.

TYRELL, D. A. J. ET AL. *Microbial diseases: the use of the laboratory in diagnosis, therapy and control.* London, Edward Arnold, 1979.

Vaccination certificate requirements for international travel and health advice to travellers. Geneva, World Health Organization (issued annually).

WHO emergency health kit. Geneva, World Health Organization, 1984.

WHO regional and inter-regional seminar on methods of epidemiological surveillance of zoonoses, foodborne infections and the communicable diseases. *Weekly epidemiological record,* **49**: 25–29 (1974).

WHO technical guidelines on Japanese encephalitis. WHO Regional Office for South-East Asia, unpublished document, SEA/CD/79.

4. Procedures for epidemiological investigations

When an epidemic occurs, it is first necessary to carry out a thorough epidemiological investigation; this is the responsibility of the emergency health service. The success of the investigation will depend on the methodical organization of operations both at central level and in the field.

4.1 Operations at central level

As soon as the initial information on an outbreak reaches the central level, the EHS coordinator must determine whether the information is correct. If the existence of an epidemic is confirmed— or even pending confirmation—the coordinator must analyse the situation and initiate the decision-making processes at the central level. Thanks to the advance planning, there should be very little delay in setting up the epidemiological team(s) for on-the-spot investigations and in giving them clear instructions.

4.1.1 Checking of initial information on an epidemic

The information on an outbreak may come initially from routine or emergency reports from medical facilities, epidemiological surveillance and the early warning system described in section 3.3, or from other sources, such as veterinary services, laboratories, or, as frequently happens, from rumours disseminated rapidly by the media. An epidemic may also first be detected by a village official or local administrator who senses that a problem exists. The role of the EHS coordinator is to check carefully the validity of the information on the outbreak. The procedure is shown diagrammatically in Fig. 4.

Comparison of the information obtained from a number of different sources will indicate whether the initial reports are reliable. The situation may also require a rapid site visit by a competent person who should have both clinical and epidemiological experience of the suspected disease. It is important: (1) that he or she is aware of the other possible diseases that may be involved; and (2) that laboratory specimens are collected to confirm the tentative clinical diagnosis. The

32

Fig. 4. Checking the validity of information about an epidemic and immediate action to be taken

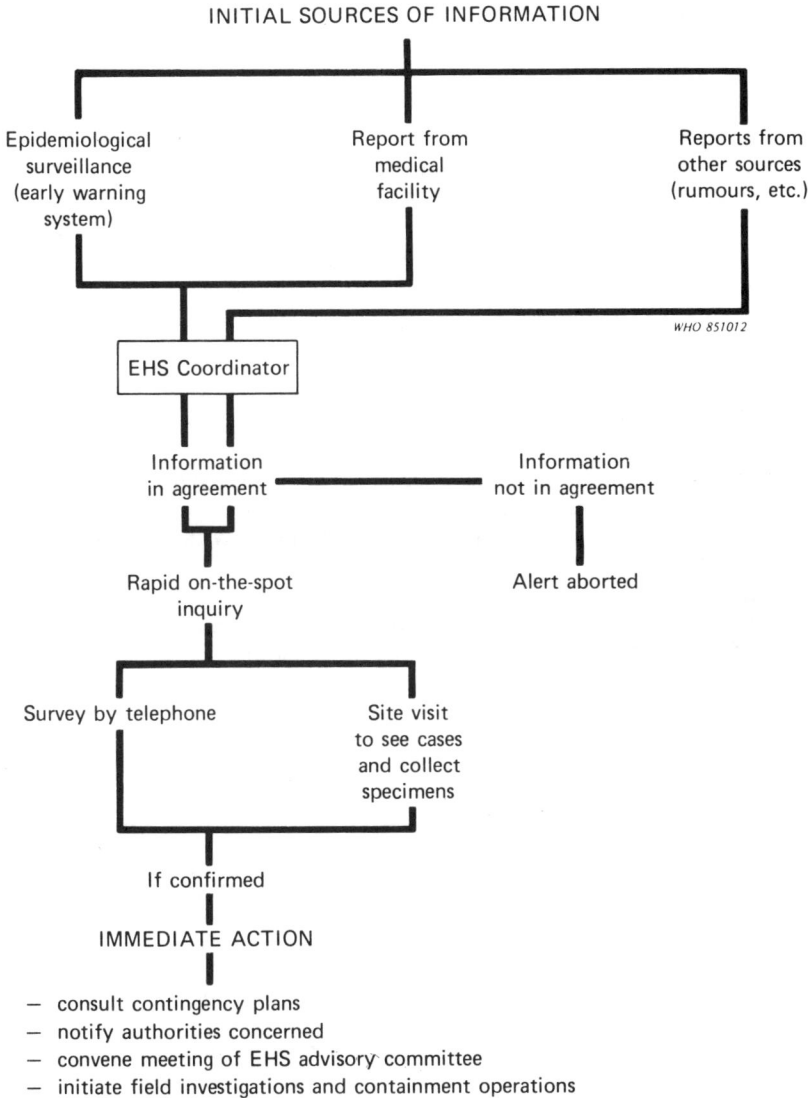

INITIAL SOURCES OF INFORMATION

| Epidemiological surveillance (early warning system) | Report from medical facility | Reports from other sources (rumours, etc.) |

WHO 851012

EHS Coordinator

| Information in agreement | Information not in agreement |

Rapid on-the-spot inquiry | Alert aborted

Survey by telephone | Site visit to see cases and collect specimens

If confirmed

IMMEDIATE ACTION

— consult contingency plans
— notify authorities concerned
— convene meeting of EHS advisory committee
— initiate field investigations and containment operations

analysis of the initial data may appear to provide strong evidence implicating a particular disease, but special attention should be paid to the differential diagnosis and a sufficient number of cases should be examined before any definite conclusion is reached.

4.1.2 Preliminary analysis of the situation

As a first step, it is necessary:

—to establish a clear definition of the disease (case definition);
—to formulate initial hypotheses as to the nature of the agent and the cause of the outbreak;
—to formulate the objectives and strategy of the epidemiological investigations.

Case definition. The wording of the case definition is very important as it will serve as a guide to the field investigation teams in case finding. It should satisfy two conditions: it must be precise but at the same time not too exclusive. The provisional case definition will be based on the examination of the earliest cases seen and' will have to be amended as soon as more precise clinical and epidemiological data become available. A final case definition should contain the following:

—the name of the disease (it may be described as " . . . -like" until more precise data are available);
—the most frequent and the occasional signs and symptoms in both mild and severe cases;
—the epidemiological circumstances associated with the occurrence of cases;
—a confirmatory laboratory test, if any;
—the criteria for "confirmed", "presumptive", and "suspect" levels of certainty, and "primary" or "secondary" positions in the transmission chain.

Table 17. Grading of cases

Type of case	Criteria
Confirmed	Definite laboratory evidence (serological, biochemical, bacteriological, virological, parasitological) of current or recent infection, *whether or not* clinical signs or symptoms are or have been present
Presumptive	Signs and symptoms compatible with the illness, and suggestive but not conclusive laboratory evidence indicative of recent infection (e.g., a single serological test)
Suspect	Signs and symptoms compatible with the illness, but no laboratory evidence of infection (negative, absent, or pending)

Since not all cases will be investigated with the same degree of thoroughness, a grading system is necessary to indicate the certainty with which the diagnosis is made. The criteria for confirmed, presumptive and suspect cases are shown in Table 17.

The following is an example of a case definition in an outbreak of a suspected food-borne disease to which the name dysentery-like syndrome was given:

Initial definition: a person having diarrhoea and one or more of the following signs and symptoms: fever, nausea, vomiting, abdominal cramps, tenesmus, blood in the stools.

Final definition:

—by severity:
A severe case is one with fever above 38 °C and bloody diarrhoea, with or without other signs and symptoms as indicated above.
A mild case is one fitting the initial definition, but without high fever and bloody diarrhoea.

—by level of certainty:
A confirmed case is one from which a strain of *Shigella* has been isolated and identified, with or without clinical signs or symptoms.
A presumptive case is one where no agent has been isolated but where the faecal exudate is rich in polymorphonuclear leukocytes or macrophages.
A suspect case is one with a compatible clinical picture, but without positive laboratory findings.

—by epidemiological associations:
A primary case is someone who ate at a certain restaurant on a given date and became ill (or from whom the agent was isolated) within seven days.
A secondary case is someone who had contact with a primary case and became ill (or from whom the agent was isolated) within seven days of that contact (tertiary or higher-level contact cases may also exist).
A non-associated case is someone who did not eat at the suspect restaurant and did not have direct or indirect contact with a primary case.

Initial hypotheses. It is important that initial hypotheses should be formulated as to (1) the nature of the disease; and (2) the origin of the outbreak and the mode of transmission. Such hypotheses are necessarily based on incomplete information but are essential as a guide to further investigations. They are subject to modification, refinement, or total change as the study proceeds.

The approach by syndrome to the etiological diagnosis of epidemic diseases, recommended in Chapter 5, facilitates a comprehensive

Table 18. Field investigations: information sought and procedures

Information sought	Procedures
Nature of the disease	Case finding Clinical examinations Laboratory examinations (agent isolation, serology) Listing of cases
Extent of the outbreak and population group(s) affected	Establishment of epidemic curves Case mapping Determination of population sub- group incidence rates Retrospective survey Serological survey Prospective surveillance
Source of infection and mode of transmission	Contact tracing Laboratory examination of source material
Areas and persons at continued risk	Information on previous occurrence of epidemics Immunization status Immunity survey (serological)

review of the different agents that should be considered in the differential diagnosis, and which are listed later in Tables 31 and 32 (see pp. 61 and 64).

Objectives and strategy of field investigations. The exact nature of the disease, the extent of the outbreak, the population group(s) affected, the source of infection and the mode of transmission must be established by further field investigations in order to define the appropriate control measures. The objectives of such investigations and the procedures necessary are listed in Table 18 and are further described in the section on field investigations (section 4.2).

A number of different strategies are possible in the conduct of epidemiological investigations and case-finding; they are enumerated in Table 19. One such strategy may be considered sufficient or several may be tried together. The choice will depend on the nature of the outbreak and the local resources.

4.1.3 Emergency health service advisory committee meeting

The objectives of the first meeting of the committee, convened by the EHS coordinator, are:

—discussion of situation analysis (presented by the EHS coordinator);

Table 19. Strategies for use in case finding and epidemiological investigations

Strategy	Advantages	Disadvantages
Rapid and complete reporting from all medical facilities	Rapidity	Biased sample of cases
Visits to hospitals and other medical facilities	Ease of access to patients and contacts	Only severe cases are seen
Telephone survey	Rapidity	Biased population sample
Distribution of questionnaries	Rapidity, no bias in access to population	Misunderstandings, incomplete answers
Absenteeism in schools, factories, etc.	Ease of access to patients and contacts	Biased sample (special risk of infection or special condition)
Community surveys (household visits)	Exact picture of incidence, severity and epidemiology	Requires special organization (field teams), slow
Contact tracing	Specific leads are provided by known cases	Time-consuming and limited to known cases
Survey for etiological agent, by isolation or serology	Precise information on infection; only way to identify subclinical infections	Expensive and time-consuming; requires laboratory support

—adoption of general strategy;
—preparation and approval of a plan of operations;
—allocation of responsibilities according to specialities;
—time schedule for completion of tasks.

When the nature of the outbreak and its extent require the cooperation of teams of experts from outside the country, those responsible for such teams should be included, together with the WHO representative, in the EHS advisory committee. The terms of reference for the experts brought in should be such as to ensure that their activities are in conformity with the practices of the host country.

The outcome of the EHS advisory committee meeting should be a plan of action, based on the analysis of the situation and taking technical, economic and political factors into account; much of this will have already been considered in the course of the contingency planning (section 3.2). Table 20 shows what such a plan of action should generally include.

During the first few days of operations, daily reports from field investigative teams will progressively produce more precise clinical and epidemiological data. Further meetings of the EHS advisory committee or its subgroups will enable the coordinator to adjust the

Table 20. Items to be included in a plan of action

Initial case definition

Hypotheses as to the nature and extent of the outbreak

Objectives of the investigations

Investigation and control strategy

Assignment of personal responsibilities and time schedule for completion
   of tasks

Strengthening of EHS headquarters' operational facilities

Chains of command and reporting, channels of communication for coordination,
   delegation of responsibilities, persons on permanent duty

Mobilization of internal resources

Organization of investigative and control teams

Arrangements for hospital and laboratory support

Financial provisions

Notification to WHO

Mobilization of external resources

Statements to information media (designation of spokesman)

Periodicity of EHS advisory committee meetings

---

case definition, the plan of action, and the control measures
accordingly.

4.1.4 Organization of field operations

The arrangements for the organization of field operations should be
annexed to the plan of action. Field teams may be easy to organize in
countries where access to the epidemic focus is easy, but the
organization is obviously more complicated and requires more
detailed attention when such access is difficult, as will be envisaged
here. Field teams have to carry out two functions simultaneously:
investigation and control. (For further details on control operations,
see Chapter 6.) In organizing field teams, attention must be paid to
the following:

—definition and allocation of sectors;
—selection of personnel;
—instructions to team leaders;
—equipment and logistic support;
—safety precautions;
—medical evacuation.

Definition and allocation of sectors. Each team is allocated a
sector, the size of which will depend on:

(a) ease of access and ease of movement within the sector;
(b) the transport available and its speed;
(c) the population density;
(d) the time required to find and examine a patient;
(e) the time required to collect laboratory specimens;
(f) the time required for completing emergency control measures;
(g) ease of telecommunications.

Each sector must be carefully defined, and the number of sectors must be such that teams will be able to cover the area affected by the suspected epidemic in the shortest possible time.

Selection of personnel. The specialists and other personnel to be included in the field team will depend on the initial hypotheses considered most credible by the EHS advisory committee; a typical example of team composition is shown in Table 21.

Table 21. Composition of typical field team

Category	Profession
Specialists	Epidemiologist
	Clinician (pathologist)
	Veterinarian
	Microbiologist
	Entomologist
	Mammalogist
	Sanitary engineer
	Toxicologist
Auxiliaries	Nurses
	Specialist assistants
	Secretary/interpreter
	Driver

Instructions to team leaders. It may be difficult to foresee all the conditions under which field teams may have to operate and the difficulties they may have to face. The task may be complicated by rains, floods, panic, the establishment of a *"cordon sanitaire"*, quarantine requirements, population movements, shortage of certain supplies, and difficulties in transport and communications. Team leaders will need initiative in addition to technical competence and should have the necessary mental resilience and physical strength. Although they should have the power to take instant decisions, they should also be given written instructions by the EHS coordinator (see Table 22), together with other documentation, much of which should already have been prepared as part of the contingency planning.

Table 22. Instructions and other documentation to be given to field team leaders

Objectives
Copy of plan of action
Features of area to be investigated
Official travel documents
Tentative time schedule and itinerary
Time schedules and itineraries of other teams in adjacent areas
Schedule for regular communications with EHS headquarters
Arrangements for communication with other teams
Strategy to be adopted in investigations
Investigative procedures to be used
Instructions on use of report forms (see section 4.2.2)
Instructions for collection and shipment of laboratory specimens
Instructions for emergency control measures
Safety precautions and instructions on medical evacuation of team members
Inventory of equipment

Equipment and logistic support. Rapidity and efficacy are essential to successful emergency investigation and control operations. Here too, contingency planning should help in making available in the shortest possible time all the equipment and logistic support needed by field teams. The types of equipment that may be required will depend on local conditions. The EHS coordinator must ensure that the equipment is not so heavy that it slows down movement, but that all essential items are included, particularly in regions where communications are difficult. The check list in Table 23 may be useful in selecting the necessary equipment; certain items of information needed by teams are also included.

Safety precautions. The initial data on the case-fatality rate will give some indication of the risk to which field teams are exposed. The mode of transmission of the disease is the key to the precautions that the EHS coordinator should recommend. However, this may at first be unknown and precautions may initially have to be taken against a number of different possible modes of transmission. Recommended precautions for different suspected modes of transmission are shown in Table 24.

Maximum protection, including respiratory precautions, may be necessary in examining highly contagious patients, and in high-risk operations, such as post-mortems or the processing of dangerous laboratory specimens. Protective equipment and procedures are

Table 23. Equipment and information needed by field teams

Travel documents, maps

Money (cash)

For travel by land: petrol, oil, vehicle spare parts

For travel by air: flight authorizations, length and accessibility of landing strips, types of aircraft, permitted dimensions of crates, possibilities of refuelling, cost of operations, insurance, utilization for medical evacuation

Radio sets, authorization to transmit (and, if possible, spare parts)

Electric generator(s) and/or batteries, lamps, gas lamps

Cold chain: refrigerators, dry ice or liquid nitrogen and appropriate insulated containers

Bedding, mosquito-nets, insect repellents

Canned food, drinks, water filters and tablets for water purification

Prophylactic drugs for team members (against malaria, enteric infections)

Rehydration fluid (oral, intravenous)

Medicines for population

Special protective equipment, e.g., protective clothing (see Annex 4)

Special equipment for collecting laboratory specimens, e.g., syringes, Vacutainers, tubes (see Annex 5)

Special equipment for control measures, e.g., insecticides, sprayers, chlorinators, injectors, syringes (see Annex 6)

---

described in Annex 4. Protective clothing may be disposable or reusable; if it is not available, plastic bags can be used.

Disposable clothing is expensive but may be necessary whenever teams have to move around rapidly and see many patients in different places. (WHO keeps a stock for use in emergencies.) Clothing made of waterproof polyethylene fibre may be uncomfortable if worn for long periods in hot climates. In principle, every person carrying out examinations must have a separate suit for each person to be examined, so that quite a large number may be required.

Ordinary reusable gowns, gloves and surgical masks can be effective in preventing disease transmission. Latex gloves can be used if carefully checked for cuts and cracks.

Effective protection can also be provided by using improvised water-resistant clothing made from large plastic bags or plastic sheets. Smaller plastic bags can be used instead of boots, hoods and even gloves.

Medical evacuation. Medical evacuation of team members falling ill during field operations should be arranged in advance so as to ensure compliance both with national procedures and with those of the team members' countries of origin. The first difficulty encountered may be that of deciding, when a team member suddenly falls ill, whether his

Table 24. Safety precautions for field teams according to mode of transmission of disease

Mode of transmission of disease	Precautions
Water-borne	Use boiled or disinfected water for drinking and preparing meals, disinfected water for washing; filters require special attention
Food-borne	Use canned food; no vegetables, no fruit, no pre-cooked food
Insect-borne	Repeated applications of repellents on exposed skin, long sleeves, mosquito nets, antimalarials if indicated
Direct contact (faecal–oral)	Wash hands after contact with suspected cases (and carriers); surgical masks may be necessary if the agent is also transmissible by air (e.g., some enteroviruses)
Droplet and aerosol	Use surgical cotton half-face mask (not effective when moist); highly lethal agents (e.g., Ebola virus) require maximum safety precautions with protective clothing and full-face biological masks (see Annex 4)

Note. When collecting and handling laboratory specimens and at post mortem examinations: precautions against contact with skin erosions and cuts, or with mucous membranes (contact of fingers with eyes, nose), pricks, aerosols, splashes, inhalation; avoid pipetting by mouth and use protective clothing and biological mask for necropsies if a highly lethal agent is suspected

illness is caused by the agent responsible for the outbreak or has an intercurrent cause. For this reason, it is recommended that team members should be immunized against locally endemic diseases, whenever vaccines exist, and that prophylactic drugs (e.g., anti-malarials, standard immune globulin) should be administered before field operations are begun.

The decision to evacuate is most often taken on the third day after the onset of the disease when the systemic symptoms are replaced by the specific symptoms of the disease concerned. Those responsible for evacuation should be alerted and preliminary arrangements made during this observation period. If the outbreak is caused by a highly contagious agent, protective clothing must be provided for those accompanying the patient or a special stretcher with plastic isolation tent used in the ambulance or aircraft. Replacement of fluids by infusion may be necessary during long journeys, as may safe disposal of excreta. The driver or pilot may have to be given the same protective clothing as the nurses if the agent is highly contagious. Accompanying persons may have to be quarantined on arrival.

4.1.5 Arrangements for laboratory support

The contingency plan should identify laboratories in the country, and their special fields of expertise, as well as those that can be contacted through the network of WHO collaborating centres for reference and research. In deciding to which laboratory, or laboratories, specimens should be sent, the following should be taken into consideration:

—the nature of the suspected agent, bacterium, parasite, virus, or toxic substance;
—the level of expertise required and available;
—the types of protective equipment available;
—the facilities for the shipment of specimens;
—the delays expected in receiving results.

Identification of the agent may require sophisticated techniques if it is to be fully characterized. For example, it is necessary to differentiate between the Marburg and Ebola viruses, which appear very similar when viewed by electron microscopy; there is, however, an antigenic difference that influences the choice of immune plasma to be administered to patients. The identification of an agent may require an extensive battery of specific antisera, or serological tests may require an extensive battery of antigens. Such batteries of reagents are available in only a few laboratories, designated as WHO collaborating centres for this reason. It is good practice to divide the specimens collected into two aliquots, one for local examination, and the other to be sent for reference purposes to a WHO collaborating centre.

Whenever patient mortality is high, maximum precautions should be taken in collecting, packaging and shipping the specimens (see Annex 5). They should be sent to one of the appropriate WHO collaborating centres for reference and research after preliminary agreement has been reached with the centre, through WHO, to that effect.

4.2 Field investigations

Investigative teams should be given precise instructions covering their activities, including safety precautions, methods of case finding, contact tracing, special investigations, and collection and shipment of laboratory specimens

4.2.1 Safety precautions

The principles guiding safety precautions in the field and criteria for deciding whether medical evacuation of sick field team members is necessary have already been discussed (see pp. 40–42). Unnecessary protective measures slow down the progress of investigations and make them substantially more expensive. Ignorance or contempt of danger, however, may lead to a disaster for team members. Sound judgement is needed in deciding on adequate protective measures in dealing with contagious patients, their excreta and other sources of infection, but until the mode of transmission of the agent causing the outbreak has been definitely determined, the decision is not easy.

4.2.2 Case finding

The procedures used to identify as many as possible of the affected persons are listed in Table 19 (p. 37). Records of cases should be based on precise definitions and the findings systematically validated. The use of a carefully designed survey form is necessary to ensure accurate and rapid investigation.

Case description and recording (Form A). A standard case investigation form is needed to ensure that complete information is obtained for each case. The type of information needed is the same for all diseases and epidemics, but specific details must be adapted to the individual disease and to the unique circumstances of each epidemic situation and each location. It is impossible, therefore, to devise a form that can be used in all epidemics. The best that can be done here is to provide a *model* form that can be adapted rapidly for use in any situation. This will be referred to as Form A, and is shown in Table 25.

Despite the pressure of time, great attention must be given to patient identity, the serial numbers allocated to cases, forms and specimens, and the labelling of specimens. Important data are too often rendered meaningless or misleading because of errors.

Medical centre surveys. An institution-based survey should not be restricted to hospitals but should cover other health centres, including dispensaries. The survey should include:

—a search for suspected cases during the visit to the centre;
—a retrospective survey;
—the establishment of prospective surveillance.

The search for suspected cases corresponding completely or in part to the case definition should not be limited to patients in the infectious diseases ward of the medical centre but should be extended to other wards, such as the paediatric or surgical ward, to which patients might have been admitted because of apparent complications: "bleeding ulcer" may be confused with the haematemesis of an infectious disease; shock may be confused with coma. The survey should also be extended to cover recent sickness among hospital personnel, including cleaners. Examination of laboratory records may uncover suspect cases admitted with vague or incorrect diagnoses,

Table 25. Model form for case description and recording (Form A)

Identifying information

Case number
Source of report (e.g., community, clinic, or hospital)
Person who prepared report (name, title, address)
Place report prepared
Date report prepared

Personal (case) data

Name, age, sex
Name of head of household
Residence
Place where patient became ill, if different from residence
Immunizations (only if relevant to disease being investigated)

Clinical information

Check-list of signs and symptoms (relevant to the disease, always including space for
  "others")
Degree of severity (severe or mild)
Date of onset (and time of day, if relevant)
Date of end of illness, if now recovered
Date of death, if deceased

Laboratory examination

List of laboratory specimens, including for each:
  type of specimen(s) and serial number(s)
  type of test
  date collected
  storage temperature
  date shipped
  route of shipment
  laboratory
  date results reported
  results

Treatment

Antibiotics and other drugs used

Exposure history (see section 4.2.3)

Relevant dates (i.e., of time interval between maximum and minimum incubation
  periods)
Relevant activities (depending on disease):
  Travel
  Contacts with known cases
  Source of food and water
  Exposure to animals and animal products
  Exposure to disease vectors or reservoirs, etc.
Laboratory examination of possible sources (details as for laboratory examination of
  case)

e.g., jaundice, albuminuria, or viral hepatitis, instead of yellow fever.
Suspect patients should be examined according to the procedure
described in the previous section and Form A completed for each
case. The overall results of a visit to a hospital or health centre

should be entered in a different form, a model of which is shown in Table 26 (Form B).

A retrospective survey should be conducted using records of inpatients, outpatients and laboratory results going back over the previous three months or so. Special attention should be given to cases that might have been misdiagnosed, such as those for which the records show:

—"cause of death unknown";
—patient removed from hospital;
—symptomatic diagnoses: fever, influenza, vomiting, diarrhoea, jaundice, haematemesis, conjunctivitis, headache;
—unconfirmed diagnoses: "malaria", "dengue", "typhoid", "pneumonia", "varicella".

In any case, an increase in the number of consultations or admissions should arouse suspicion. It should be remembered that, in endemic areas, malaria may be associated with another disease, yet often the only diagnosis reported is malaria.

Whenever the hospital or health centre visited is located in the epidemic zone or in an area where spread of the disease may occur, the investigative team must draw up a prospective surveillance scheme based on the procedures indicated in Table 27.

Prospective surveillance should be encouraged by feedback of information, visits at frequent intervals, and supply of drugs (or insecticides, disinfectants, etc.) if they are not locally available.

Table 26. Model of medical centre investigation form (Form B)

INVESTIGATOR: Date of investigation:

MEDICAL CENTRE: Outpatient clinic   ☐

                                 or inpatient ward   ☐

---

1. LINE LISTING OF CASES

Make sure that the addresses of contacts and the serial numbers of laboratory specimens have been recorded on Form A.

Serial No.	Form A No.	Name	Age	Sex	Address	Date of onset	Laboratory specimen(s)	
							Nature	Container No.
1								
2								
3								
4								
etc.								

---

2. GENERAL COMMENTS

Attach relevant Form A

Table 27. Prospective surveillance scheme

Criteria for identifying disease and grading cases

Safety precautions

Procedures for collection and shipment of laboratory specimens

Investigation of contacts (household, school, work-place, travel)

Recording on Forms A and B

Establishment of reporting channels to EHS coordinator

Recommended containment measures

Treatment of patients and contacts

Community survey (Form C). The need for a community survey may be indicated by the addresses of contacts seen at health centres or reports emanating from the population or the authorities, or from the early warning system. The community may be a city, district, village or camp, depending on the circumstances. The aim is not only to discover suspected cases but also to investigate the epidemiological factors that may have contributed to the spread of the causative agent in the community. The characteristics of interest in the community investigated are listed in Table 28.

A case-finding strategy should be developed in the community concerned, using one or more of the following procedures:

—visits to local health facilities;
—interviews with key persons (doctors, pharmacists, nurses, veterinarians, and veterinary health personnel);

Table 28. Community characteristics of epidemiological significance

---

Geographical location

Climatic conditions

Economic resources

Socioeconomic status

Hygiene standards in households

Medical surveillance and prophylaxis

Potable water distribution and surveillance

Sewage collection system

Food supplies

Population movements

Contacts with animals (including insects)

Recent disease outbreaks and endemic diseases

—interviews with a random statistical sample of the population or with the population at points where people gather together;
—visits to known contacts of inpatients and outpatients who reported to hospitals and health centres (Forms A and B);
—systematic house-to-house visits (extensive or to a random statistical sample).

Warnings broadcast by radio and television, the distribution of questionnaires, displays of pictures, conferences, mobilization of schoolchildren, and provision of incentives such as drugs may help in obtaining assistance from the population. Individual cases should be recorded on Form A, and the results of community surveys on the suggested Form C (Table 29).

More useful data will be provided by a community survey if it is organized as a case-control study for statistical analysis (see Annex 2).

A prospective surveillance scheme should be put into effect in the community if suspect cases have been found or if the community is considered to be at risk. One or more resident investigators should be given the task of ensuring that the community participates in the scheme. The instructions to be provided are similar to those recommended for health-centre-based prospective surveillance (see Table 27).

4.2.3 Search for source of infection and contact tracing

The primary purpose of searching for the source of infection, either of an individual case or of the entire group of cases, is to eliminate, terminate, or isolate the source so that similar circumstances do not occur again or are less likely to do so in the future.

General method. The methods used for identifying sources and tracing contacts will differ according to whether an individual case or an outbreak is being investigated, whether the relevant infection is transmitted from person to person or by some other means, and whether transmission is continuous or of common source origin. However, the steps to be taken and the order in which they are taken will remain the same:

—identify the date (or time) of disease onset;
—ascertain the range of incubation periods for the disease in question;
—look for a source of infection in the time interval between the maximum and minimum incubation periods.

Incubation periods vary from as little as a few hours (e.g., salmonellosis), to days (e.g., influenza), weeks (e.g., hepatitis A), and even months (e.g., rabies). It is necessary, therefore, to diagnose the disease under investigation in order to determine the relevant period of time. In addition, since the incubation period varies, it is useful to know not only the most common one, but also the maximum and

Table 29. Model form for community investigation (Form C)

INVESTIGATOR: Date of investigation

PLACE:

1. COMMUNITY PROFILE

Type: ☐ Urban ☐ Rural ☐ Other (specify):

Geography:

Economy:

Social classes:

Endemic diseases:

Epidemics (dates):

Immunizations (dates, groups):

Water sources:

Food:

Waste treatment:

Rodents:

Arthropods:

Rains (seasonal):

Other (floods, drought, immigration, overcrowding, etc.):

2. CENSUS

Date and origin

Sex	Age group (years)							
	<1	1–4	5–9	10–19	20–39	40–59	≥60	Total
Male Female								
Total								

3. LINE LISTING OF CASES

Make sure that the addresses of contacts and the serial numbers of laboratory specimens have been recorded on Form A.

Serial No.	Form A No.	Name	Age	Sex	Address	Date of onset	Laboratory specimen(s)	
							Nature	Container No.
1								
2								
3								
4								
etc.								

4. GENERAL COMMENTS

Attach relevant Form A.

minimum. Incubation periods are shown later in Table 32 (p. 64) for most common epidemic diseases and in Annex 3 for other diseases that need to be considered in the differential diagnosis.

Outbreaks with continuous person-to-person transmission. A case of meningitis due to *Neisseria meningitidis*, where the onset of symptoms was on 20 February, may be taken as an example. The incubation period of this disease varies from 2 to 10 days, so that a search must be made for contact with another case or a carrier during the period 10–18 February. Since the most frequent incubation period for this type of meningitis is 3–4 days the search should be focused on the period 16–17 February.

The example just given is for an infection usually transmitted from person to person, and the process described is referred to as "contact tracing". In order to avoid confusion the case under investigation will henceforward be referred to as the "index case", and the contact being searched for in the period 10–18 February as the retrospective or "source" contact. If this contact is found and the retrospective search is to be continued still further, the first contact found may be referred to as the primary source contact, the one before that as the secondary source contact, and so on.

Contact tracing can also be done prospectively, i.e., a search is made for cases *produced* by the index case. Such contacts may be called prospective or "potential case" contacts. These relationships are shown diagrammatically in Fig. 5.

Contact tracing, i.e., establishing the pathway of person-to-person transmission, is very difficult, and often not very useful, when there are large numbers of cases in a community. It is particularly important, however, when movement from one community to another is involved, and transmission is to be prevented. Travel history is therefore of extreme significance.

Outbreaks with a common source of infection. When the disease under study may be transmitted by some other mechanism, a search should be made at the times indicated by the incubation period for the presence of vectors, reservoir animals, environmental contamination, or whatever is the appropriate source of infection.

If the analysis provides grounds for suspecting that a common source was involved, the search for that source is basically the same as in person-to-person transmission. The period of time during which the common exposure might have taken place is determined by the range of the incubation period and this in turn defines the period to be covered by the search. The common source may have been an individual, and the mechanism of transmission person-to-person, as in a school-wide epidemic caused by a pupil in a contagious state, or a hospital outbreak of tuberculosis or Lassa fever originating from a single patient. If some other mechanism of transmission has been

Fig. 5. Contact tracing in diseases with person-to-person transmission

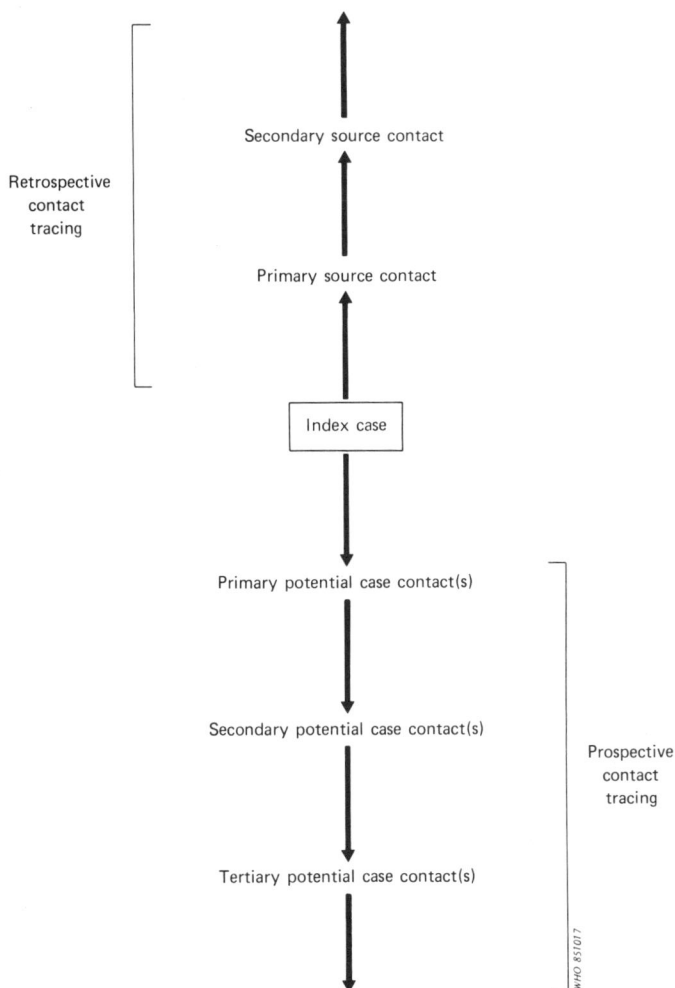

```
                          ↑

                  Secondary source contact
                          ↑
   Retrospective
      contact
      tracing
                  Primary source contact
                          ↑


                      ┌──────────────┐
                      │  Index case  │
                      └──────────────┘
                          ↓

                  Primary potential case contact(s)
                          ↓                              ┐

                                                         Prospective
                  Secondary potential case contact(s)      contact
                          ↓                                tracing

                  Tertiary potential case contact(s)
                          ↓

                          ↓
```

WHO 851017

involved, special investigations must be undertaken, as suggested in section 4.2.5.

Information on exposure history is obtained from the index case (or another informant) at the time that individual cases are investigated, and is recorded on Form A (Table 25). As previously mentioned, this section of the case investigation form must be specially designed for a particular disease outbreak; the dates relevant to the retrospective search (based on the incubation period) must be filled in for each separate case.

4.2.4 Search for continued transmission

Prospective or potential case contact tracing was mentioned in the previous section. This is the converse of retrospective tracing, and its purpose is the identification of new cases that may already have occurred or may still result from contact with the source of infection. Whether the mechanism of spread is person-to-person, via insect vectors, or contamination of food or the environment, the investigation should be based on the infective period, i.e., the time during which a case is shedding the infectious agent (or is carrying it in a site accessible to a vector, or disseminating it in the environment).

The infective period may be brief (e.g., three days from the onset of influenza), a few weeks (e.g., from about midway in the incubation period to a few days after the onset of hepatitis A), a year or more (e.g., malaria), or lifelong (in chronic carriers of hepatitis B). In all instances, however, the maximum duration of the infective period defines the time during which a search for new cases, through contacts, the infection of new vectors, or the contamination of new environments, should be conducted. It is important to recognize that not only does the duration of the period of communicability vary, but also that this period may or may not begin before the appearance of signs and symptoms, and may or may not continue for a variable time after they have appeared. Infectious periods are given later in Table 32 (p. 64) for the most common epidemic diseases that must be considered in differential diagnosis. The ways in which the incubation and infective periods can vary are illustrated in Fig. 6.

Forward (prospective) tracing of contacts has two main purposes: (1) to identify continuing chains of infection and/or contamination, in order to interrupt them; and (2) to locate new cases, so that they can be treated. It is particularly important if the patient has travelled outside his own community, and may therefore have introduced infection some distance away from his home.

The primary information is recorded on Form A (Table 25), which, as for retrospective tracing, must be specially adapted for the particular disease outbreak under study, and the dates relevant to the prospective search (based on the contagious period) must be filled in for each separate case.

4.2.5 Special investigations for common-source infections

Whenever there is some evidence of a common source of infection, special investigations must be carried out. Such sources may include arthropods, vertebrate animals, food, beverages and the environment.

Arthropod-borne diseases. Numerous blood-sucking insects (the term is also used here to designate arthropods not belonging to the class Insecta, e.g., ticks, which belong to the class Arachnida) are able to transmit diseases from man or from animal reservoirs to a

Fig. 6. Incubation, infective, surveillance and quarantine periods. The infective period may begin one day before the clinical onset of the disease. The length of the isolation period varies according to the disease

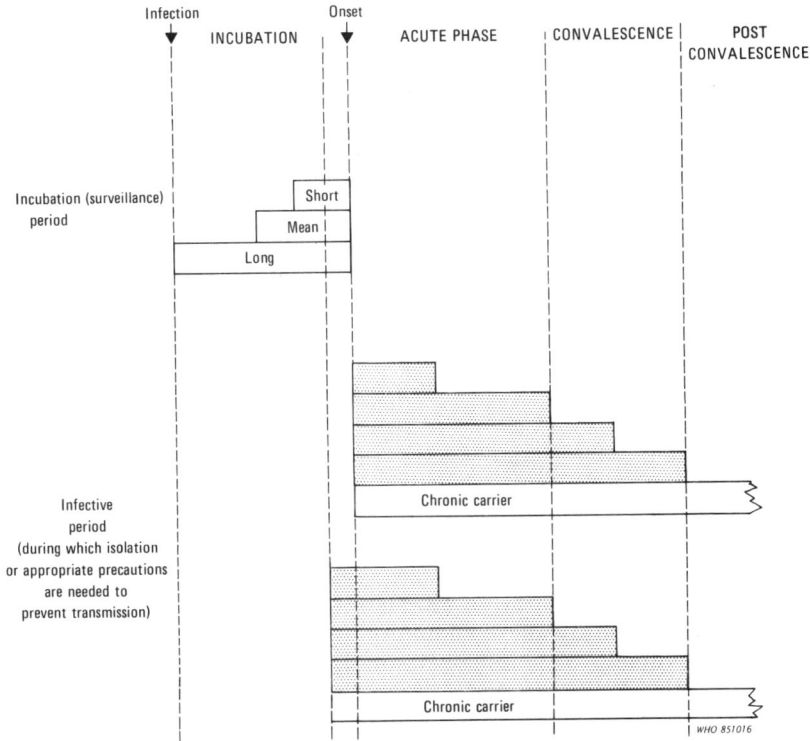

receptive person: *Chrysops* (horse flies), culicoides (biting midges), fleas, glossines (tsetse flies), body lice, mites, mosquitos, phleboto-mines (sand flies), reduviids (kissing bugs), *Simulium* (blackflies), and ticks. They are most often specialized in the diseases that they can transmit and this knowledge, plus their abundance at the time of the outbreak, can lead to a particular insect being incriminated as the mode of transmission (see list given later in Table 34, p. 90).

The possible role of insects is best confirmed by a specialist entomologist–epidemiologist, who will also know how best to collect specimens for laboratory examination. Methods of identifying insects and collection procedures are described in Annex 6.

Zoonoses. Zoonoses may be transmitted from vertebrate animals to man both by arthropod bites and by contamination of food and the environment. Direct contact with sick domestic or wild animals or healthy carriers, such as horses, cattle, sheep, goats, pigs, dogs, cats, poultry, monkeys, rodents, and birds, may cause the epidemic diseases listed later in Table 36 (see p. 95).

Proof that infection in an animal species is related to the human disease may require the assistance of the veterinary services.

Epidemic food-borne diseases. A food-borne disease will obviously be suspected when a number of persons who have eaten a meal together fall ill. Finding the infected dish responsible is more difficult and all those who ate the meal should be classified into subgroups according to the dishes that they consumed. Tracing the source of infection is even more difficult if the incriminated food has been eaten intermittently in different places, or if the contaminated product is mixed with different kinds of food or beverages. Food contamination may originate from infected animals, food handlers, flies and the environment.

Contaminating agents are listed later in Table 37 (see p. 96) and information on sampling suspected food with a view to laboratory examinations is given in Annex 5. Investigations may have to be carried out on:

—the conditions under which the food concerned is grown, produced and consumed;
—the handling and storage of foodstuffs, with particular reference to conditions known to be potentially hazardous;
—the domestic storage of water;
—the sanitary condition of restaurants, tea-stalls, snack-bars, etc., and their use by the community;
—the possibility of cross-contamination from raw food to cooked food, the packages, bags, or containers in which the food has been transported, and the cooking utensils and working surfaces associated with its preparation;
—the health status and hygienic practices of food handlers.

The assistance of the veterinary services may also be needed here.

Diseases orginating in the environment. Common-source-infection may originate in the environment if water, soil or air are contaminated; the source of such contamination may be man or animals. In addition, certain agents of mycotic diseases may be present in soil. Several modes of transmission may be involved:

—water (water-borne diseases): transmission via beverages, contaminated food, or from bathing in recreational waters;
—soil: transmission by direct contact, or contact of dust with mucous membranes (respiratory tract, eyes);
—air: inhalation of droplets or aerosols.

The list of epidemic diseases that can be transmitted in such ways is given later in Table 38 (see p. 99). Proof of causation should be carefully established, and this may be very difficult. It may be necessary to investigate water-treatment systems, sewage systems, possible contamination of water and soil by human faeces and animal dung, use of night soil as fertilizer, water recycling, and air-conditioning systems.

4.2.6 Collection and shipment of laboratory specimens

As has been noted in previous sections, laboratory support is essential in clinical and epidemiological investigations. The value of the results obtained will depend on:

—correct sampling of appropriate specimens;
—correct storage, packaging, and shipment;
—appropriate formulation of requests for laboratory examinations;
—the speed with which the laboratory responds to such requests.

If possible, therefore, the field team should include a microbiologist, or seek the advice of one whenever necessary.

Sampling of specimens. Laboratory specimens from the human population exposed to the outbreak should be collected in such a way that significant statistical comparisons are possible (see Annex 2).

If a common source of infection is suspected, in addition to samples taken from the human population, samples should be taken from the suspected source (arthropods, vertebrate animals, food, environment). The collection of the specimens required for isolation of the agent or for serological diagnosis, depending on the source of infection, is described in Annex 5.

Storage, packaging and shipment. Recommended procedures are described in Annex 5. Special care should be taken with specimens that may contain a highly infectious agent.

Requests for examination. If the team does not include a microbiologist, the team leader should follow the instructions given by the EHS coordinator and, if necessary, divide the specimens aseptically into aliquot parts for tests for bacteria, viruses and parasites. These aliquots should then be sent to the different laboratories indicated in the instructions for field teams. Each laboratory should receive a copy of the information recorded on the special part of Form A (Table 25).

Speed of response. Isolation of the agent by classical methods may be rapid or may require a week or more; such isolation may be necessary to confirm the diagnosis.

Serological tests usually provide an answer in 24 hours and enable a larger segment of the population to be examined, if the antigen is available; however, results may be difficult to interpret (see Chapter 5), particularly with single serum samples.

New rapid laboratory techniques have been developed in many

fields of microbiology that can provide an answer in a few hours. Collecting specimens for tests using these techniques may require special procedures and should be carried out in close consultation with the competent laboratory. Some of these techniques are even applicable in the field, which enormously increases both the speed and accuracy of clinical and epidemiological investigations.

BIBLIOGRAPHY

ASSAAD, F. ET AL. Use of excess mortality from respiratory diseases in the study of influenza. *Bulletin of the World Health Organization*, **49**: 219–233 (1973).

BRAM, R. A. *Surveillance and collection of arthropods of veterinary importance.* Washington, DC, Animal and Plant Health Inspection Service, US Department of Agriculture, 1978 (Agriculture Handbook No. 518).

DUNSMORE, D. J. *Safety measures for use in outbreaks of communicable disease.* Geneva, World Health Organization, 1986.

MADELEY, C. R. *Guide to the collection and transport of virological specimens.* Geneva, World Health Organization, 1977.

Manual of basic techniques for a health laboratory. Geneva, World Health Organization, 1980.

Manual on food virology. Unpublished WHO document, VPH/83.46.

Procedures to investigate arthropod-borne and rodent-borne illness. Ames, IA, International Association of Milk, Food and Environmental Sanitarians Inc., 1982.

SERVICE, M. W. A critical review of procedures for sampling populations of adult mosquitos. *Bulletin of entomological research*, **67**: 343–382 (1977).

SUDIA, W. D. & CHAMBERLAIN, R. W. *Methods for collection and processing of medically important arthropods for virus isolation.* Atlanta, GA, US Department of Health, Education, and Welfare, 1967.

SUDIA, W. D. ET AL. *Collection and processing of vertebrate specimens for arbovirus studies.* Atlanta, GA, US Department of Health, Education, and Welfare, National Communicable Disease Center, 1970.

THATCHER, F. S. ET AL. *Microorganisms in foods. Sampling for microbiological analysis: principles and specific applications.* Toronto, University of Toronto Press, 1974.

US DEPARTMENT OF HEALTH, EDUCATION, and WELFARE. *Guidelines for confirmation of foodborne disease outbreaks*, Washington, DC, US Government Printing Office, 1981 (DHEW Publication No. (CDC) 81-8185).

5. Analysis of investigation data

After the field teams have started their investigations, the EHS coordinator should hold frequent meetings with specialists on the EHS committee, together with the team leaders whenever feasible, to compile and analyse the clinical, epidemiological and laboratory data as soon as they become available.

The data collected by means of forms A, B and C are used to arrive at a probable clinical diagnosis of the disease, define the epidemiological characteristics of the outbreak, confirm the identity of the causative agent, and identify the appropriate control methods. These steps are shown in Fig. 7.

5.1 Clinical data

The clinical data, i.e., the signs and symptoms recorded for each patient on Form A, are tabulated, the more precise picture of the disease thus obtained enabling the provisional case definition to be revised and providing a clinical approach to an etiological diagnosis.

5.1.1 Compilation of data

A disease is generally described either in terms of the relative frequency of the various signs and symptoms that have been observed, or by drawing curves showing the way that these frequencies change during the course of the disease. The two methods are particularly useful if the disease happens to be unusual.

Tabulation of frequency of signs and symptoms. Frequency is defined as the number of times a sign or a symptom has been observed in a group of at least 30 patients, and preferably more if the results are to be reasonably accurate. The examination procedure should not vary too greatly from day to day and from one examiner to another. If the number of persons examined is large enough, the data for suspected, presumptive, and confirmed cases, or for mild and severe forms of the disease, can be tabulated separately. Data for the full range of signs and symptoms characterizing the disease can usually be obtained in 2–4 days of investigations. An example of such a tabulation for Lassa fever is given in Table 30.

Fig. 7. Steps in the analysis of investigation data

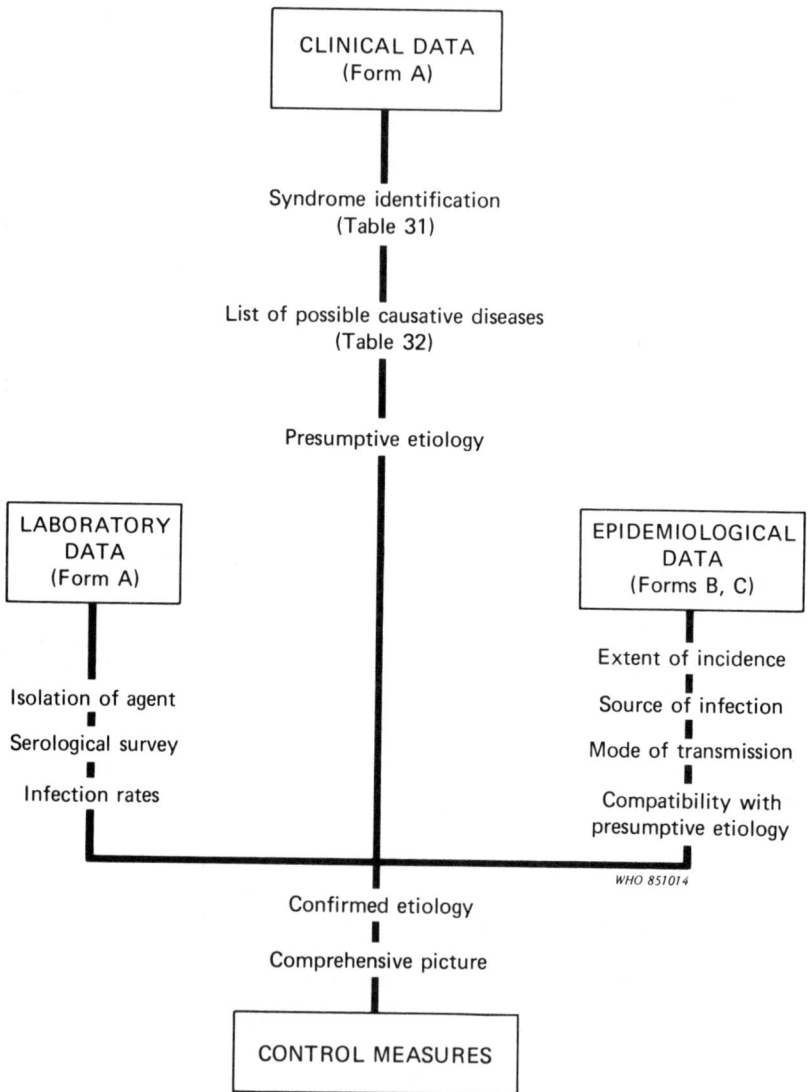

Syndrome identification
(Table 31)

List of possible causative diseases
(Table 32)

Presumptive etiology

LABORATORY DATA (Form A)

EPIDEMIOLOGICAL DATA (Forms B, C)

Isolation of agent

Serological survey

Infection rates

Extent of incidence

Source of infection

Mode of transmission

Compatibility with presumptive etiology

WHO 851014

Confirmed etiology

Comprehensive picture

CONTROL MEASURES

Representation of the course of the disease. It is important to note the date of onset of the disease when a patient is examined. If a sufficient number of patients are examined, the frequency of signs and symptoms can be tabulated at serial intervals of 3 or 5 days after onset for the period up to convalescence, which may be as long as 3 weeks. The frequency of signs and symptoms during the course of the disease may be represented by means of curves, as shown in Fig. 8.

Table 30. Lassa fever: frequency of symptoms and signs[a]

Symptom	Frequency (%)[b]	Sign	Frequency (%)[b]
Nausea/vomiting	80	Fever	100
Sore throat	80	Pharyngitis	79
Cough	68	Reduced blood pressure	
Headache	57	and pulse pressure	66
Abdominal pain	57	Abdominal tenderness	53
Myalgia	46	Albuminuria ($\geqslant 2 +$)	52
Diarrhoea	43	Lymphadenopathy	48
Chest pain	39	Leukopenia (< 4000	
Dizziness	25	leukocytes/mm^3 of blood)	41
Deafness	18	Puffiness of face or neck	36
Tinnitus	16	Coated tongue	36
Constipation	5	Conjunctivitis	34
		Bleeding	32
		Rales	25
		Muscle tenderness	21
		Petechiae	12
		Rash	7
		Convulsions	5

[a] After MONATH, T. P. & CASALS, J. *Bulletin of the World Health Organization*, **52**: 707–715 (1975).
[b] Based on 34–44 patients; the denominator is variable because of incomplete recording of information on specific symptoms or signs.

5.1.2 Clinical diagnosis

The approach follows the steps indicated in Fig. 7: syndrome identification, list of *possible* causative diseases, determination of presumptive etiology.

Syndrome identification. The case definition and the compilation of signs and symptoms will point to one or a number of clinical syndromes and thus to a list of diseases to be considered in the differential diagnosis. The following syndromes are most frequently encountered during epidemics:

—febrile systemic disease without characteristic rash
—febrile rash
—haemorrhagic fever
—febrile lymphadenopathy
—febrile neurological disease
—febrile respiratory tract disease
—febrile gastrointestinal disease
—febrile icterus
—afebrile disease

A definition of each syndrome is given in Table 31.

Fig. 8. Diagram showing chronology of symptoms of Lassa fever (after MONATH, T. P. & CASALS, J. *Bulletin of the World Health Organization,* **52**: 707–715 (1975))

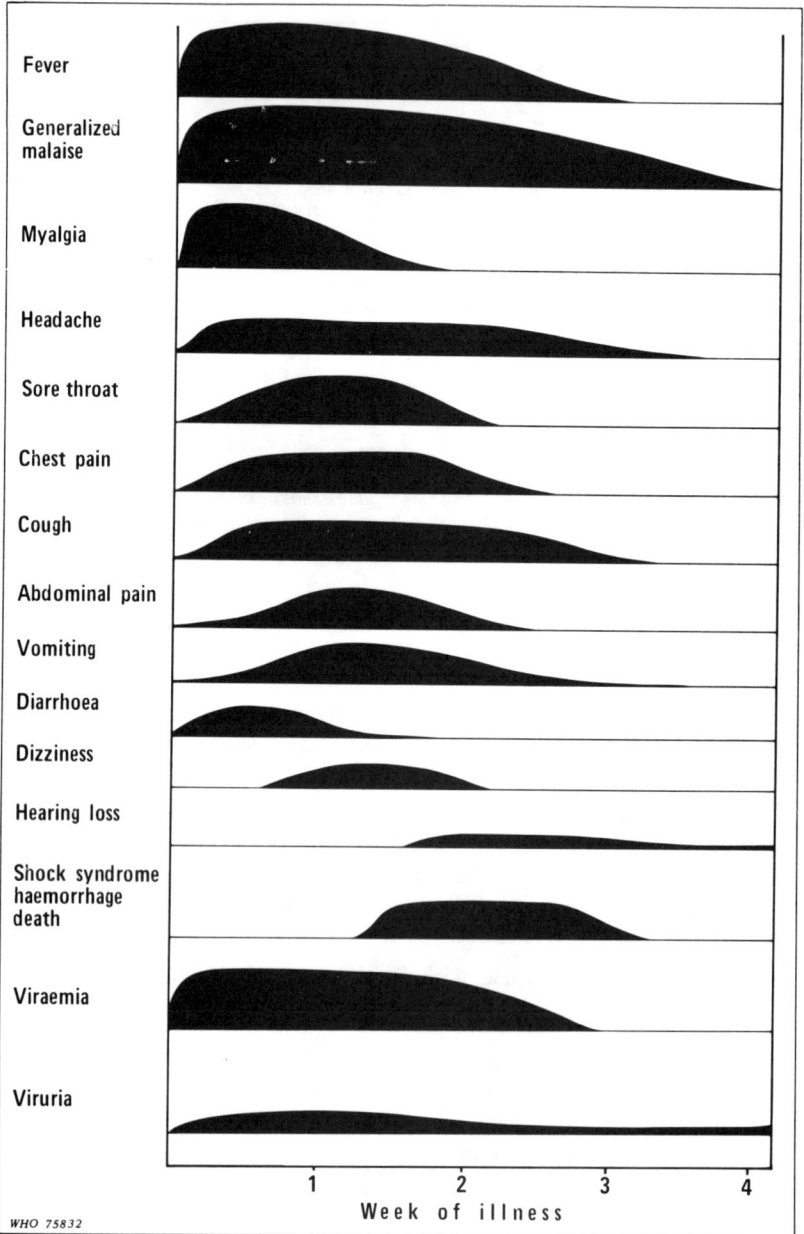

Table 31. Syndrome characteristics

Syndrome	Characteristics
1. Febrile systemic disease without characteristic rash	Sudden or progressive onset with fever, headache, muscle and joint pains; occasionally gastrointestinal symptoms; no detectable specific localization; occasionally polyadenopathy, arthritis; may be biphasic or recurrent
2. Febrile rash	Onset with fever and systemic symptoms; generalized eruption (macular, papular, vesicular, pustular) or eruption localized to parts of skin and/or mucous membranes; if haemorrhagic, see syndrome 3
3. Haemorrhagic fever	Onset with fever and systemic symptoms; second phase after 3–5 days with cutaneous bleeding (petechiae, ecchymoses, puncture oozing), internal bleeding (vaginal, haematemesis, melaena, haematuria), occasionally jaundice, with or without terminal shock syndrome
4. Febrile lymphadenopathy	Onset with fever and systemic symptoms; suppurative or non-suppurative, localized or generalized glandular swelling
5. Febrile neurological disease	Occasionally onset with fever and systemic symptoms; signs of meningitis, encephalitis, paralysis
6. Febrile respiratory tract disease	Fatigue; cough, thoracic pain, dyspnoea; purulent or blood-stained sputum
7. Febrile gastrointestinal disease	Systemic symptoms may be absent or mild; nausea, vomiting, abdominal cramps; diarrhoea with or without mucus, blood; occasionally followed by neurological signs and symptoms (see syndrome 5) or rash (see syndrome 2) (note: food poisoning may be afebrile)
8. Febrile icterus	Initial phase with systemic symptoms (see syndrome 1) but may be without; jaundice; if haemorrhagic, see syndrome 3
9. Afebrile disease	Some of the signs and symptoms of the preceding syndromes but without fever

List of possible causative diseases. A list of diseases that should be considered in the differential diagnosis within each syndrome is given in Table 32. The list includes diseases that are normally endemic or only sporadic, but that may become epidemic under unusual conditions. It is not rare nowadays for "new" epidemic diseases to appear, as happened in the case of Legionnaires' disease, and acquired immunodeficiency syndrome (AIDS), which is now affecting certain population groups. Furthermore, in the natural focus of a disease, epidemics may be "usual", whereas in other regions the disease may considered "exotic" and epidemics are "unusual". This is the case for diseases having a discrete occurrence zone, e.g., many parasitic diseases. Tropical diseases, such as schistosomiasis or malaria, may regularly give rise to a certain number of cases in endemic zones but also to unusual epidemics in newcomer groups, such as tourists or refugees. Finally, certain common diseases, e.g., tuberculosis or sexually transmitted diseases, can cause epidemics and emergencies only rarely, in exceptional situations. Because of all these possibilities, the epidemiologist must keep an open mind in considering critically all possible differential diagnoses, even the highly unlikely ones, to avoid the pitfall of an *a priori* hasty clinical diagnosis.

Also in connection with the list in Table 32, several other points must be borne in mind:

—the list is not exhaustive and is intended only for quick reference;
—the same agent may cause different syndromes;
—at the onset of a disease, the clinical picture may consist only of systemic signs and symptoms, becoming more specific only after a few days;
—some signs and symptoms, such as rash and jaundice, may be transient or difficult to detect;
—the full clinical picture may be evident only in some of the infected persons, the others having mild forms or subclinical infections;
—an outbreak of enteric or respiratory diseases may sometimes be caused *simultaneously* by more than one agent.

Presumptive etiology. Geographical considerations and the initial data on the mode of occurrence of the disease make it possible to eliminate from the list of possible diseases, at least provisionally, certain diseases that are unlikely to have the same epidemiological characteristics as those seen in the outbreak. Table 32 has been prepared to enable the reader to survey rapidly the epidemiological characteristics of the diseases included in the list. Further details are given for each disease in Annex 3. The outcome of this survey should be a short list of a few diseases that are compatible with the given epidemiological situation. Such a short list will also be useful in determining whether the laboratory results, which may be subject to errors of omission or commission, are compatible with the situation and have discriminated between other possible agents.

5.2 Epidemiological data

A good epidemiological description is urgently required for two reasons:

1. so that the size of the outbreak, the population groups most severely affected, and the likelihood of continued spread can be determined; this is necessary for planning the provision of medical care;
2. so that a hypothesis can be formulated as to the causative agent, the mode of transmission, and the probable further progress of the outbreak; this is necessary to guide control efforts.

5.2.1 Compilation of data

In compiling data, the epidemiologist should remember to use the correct definitions of the different parameters, as given in Annex 1.

Unless the number of cases is very small, it is difficult to assemble case data directly from Forms A, B and C. Some method of summarizing the most important facts is therefore needed to highlight the pattern of occurrence of cases.

If a computer is available, data on individual cases can be coded on Form A and later retrieved by the use of an appropriate data-processing programme. Even where computer facilities and personnel are available, the investigator will probably frequently need to update, change, re-examine and compile the data, and a simple method may still prove useful. Furthermore, rapid compilation of data on the spot may be necessary in the field. Procedures for line-listing of cases and preparation of hand-sorted cards are described in Annex 2 in which a dysentery epidemic is taken as an example.

5.2.2 Assembling data to show case distribution

General procedures for assembling epidemiological data and formulating and testing hypotheses of causation are described in Annex 2, but the following considerations should be borne in mind.

Data on the *numbers* of persons affected are relatively meaningless for the purposes of epidemiological analysis if the size of the population or subgroups concerned is not known. *Rates* must therefore be calculated but are only as accurate as the numerators (numbers of cases) and denominators (populations at risk). Case counts must be as complete as possible and census data must be as accurate as possible.

(*Text continues on page 82.*)

Table 32. Epidemic diseases grouped by clinical syndrome, with main epidemiological features

1. Febrile systemic disease without characteristic rash[a]

1.1 All climates

Disease	Agent[b]	Occurrence	Mode of transmission[c]	Incubation period[d]	Infective period[e]
Arthropod-borne viral fever, not otherwise specified	V	Worldwide, discrete foci	A(m,p,t)	2–15 (3–6)	—
Brucellosis	B	Worldwide	Z(d) E(f)	5–30 or longer	—
Epidemic myalgia	V	Worldwide	P(d, i)	3–5	Acute stage
Leptospirosis	B	Worldwide	Z(d, r, w) E(f, w)	4–19 (10)	—
Non-pneumonic Legionnaires' disease	B	USA, probably more widespread	E(a)	5h–3 days (1–2)	—
Paratyphoid fever	B	Worldwide	P(d, i) E(f, w) A(f)	7–21	1–2 weeks or carrier state
Trench fever	R	Europe	Lice	7–30	—
Trichinosis	P	Worldwide	E(f)	1–45 (10–14)	—
Typhoid fever	B	Worldwide	A(f) E(f, w) P(d)	7–21	Chronic carrier state possible

1.2 Warm climates or seasons

Acute schistosomiasis	P	Discrete foci	E(w)	4–6 weeks	—
Dengue fever	V	All continents	A(m)	3–15 (5–6)	—
Heat stroke	nil	Dry zones	Nil	Short	—
Malaria	P	Extensive foci	A(m)	12 days–10 m	—
Relapsing fever	B	Limited foci in all continents	A(lice, ticks)	5–15(8)	—
Rift Valley fever	V	Africa south of Sahara, Egypt	Z(d) A(m)	2–7 (3)	—
Sandfly fever	V	All continents	A(p)	3–4	—

[a] See also: gammaherpesviral mononucleosis (infectious mononucleosis) (4); Lassa fever (3); listeriosis (5); melioidosis (6); Q fever (6); trypanosomiasis (4); tularaemia (4) (number of syndrome in parentheses).

[b] B: bacteria; C: chlamydia; F: fungus; P: parasite; R: rickettsia; V: virus.

[c] A: arthropod-borne: (f) houseflies; (m) mosquitos; (p) phlebotomines (sandflies); (t) ticks; (o) others;
E: environment: (a) air or dust; (f) food; (s) soil; (w) water;
P: person-to-person: (d) direct; (i) indirect;
Z: zoonotic: (d) domestic animal; (r) rodent; (w) wild animal.

[d] In days unless otherwise stated (h: hours; w: weeks; m: months); average incubation period in parentheses.

[e] When direct person-to-person transmission occurs.

Table 32 (continued)

2. Febrile rash or localized eruption[a]

Disease	Agent[b]	Occurrence	Mode of transmission[c]	Incubation period[d]	Infective period[e]
2.1 Generalized rash (macular or petechial)					
Enteroviral exanthematous fever	V	Worldwide, warm season	P(d) A(f) E(f)	3–5	Acute phase and longer
Erythema infectiosum	V(?)	Worldwide	P(d)	5–10	Acute phase
Measles	V	Worldwide	P(d, i) E(a)	8–13 (10)	1 week before, 4 days after onset of rash
Meningococcal bacteraemia	B	Worldwide	P(d, i)	2–10 (3–4)	Until 24 hours after treatment
Rat-bite fever	B	Worldwide	Z(r) E(f)	3–10	—
Roseola infantum	V(?)	Worldwide	P(d)	5–15(10)	—
Rubella	V	Worldwide	P(d, i) E(a)	14–21 (16–18)	1 week before, 4 days after onset of rash
Scarlet fever	B	Worldwide	P(d)	1–3	10–21 days, treated 2 days
Spotted fever group:					
Boutonneuse fever	R	Africa, south-west Asia, Mediterranean, India	A(t)	5–7	—
Rocky Mountain SF	R	Americas	A(t)	3–14	—
Toxic shock syndrome due to Staphylococcus aureus	B	America, Europe	Vaginal tampons	short	—
Typhus fever:					
due to Rickettsia typhi	R	Worldwide	A(fleas) E(a)	7–14 (12)	—
due to Rickettsia prowazekii	R	Worldwide	A(lice)	7–14 (12)	—
due to Rickettsia tsutsugamushi	R	Asia	A(mites)	6–21 (10–12)	—

2.2 Generalized rash (vesicular or pustular)

Monkeypox	V	Africa, equatorial forest	Z(w)	?	—
Rickettsialpox	R	Africa, USA, USSR	A(mite)	7–10	—
Smallpox[f]	V	Eradicated	P(d, i) E(a)	7–17 (10–12)	Few days before rash to 3 weeks after
Varicella	V	Worldwide	P(d, i) E(a)	14–21 (13–17)	2 days before rash onset, 6 days after

2.3 Localized eruption (any aspect)

Anthrax, cutaneous	B	Worldwide	Z(d) E(s, a)	2–5	—
Dracontiasis	P	Africa, south-west Asia, India, discrete foci	E(w)	12m	—
Enteroviral vesicular stomatitis with exanthem	V	Worldwide	P(d)	3–5	Acute stage and longer
Erythema chronicum migrans due to *Borrelia burgdorferi*	B	USA	A(t)	3–21	—
Herpesviral gingivostomatitis	V	Worldwide	P(d)	2–12	Acute stage and longer
Mucocutaneous lymph node syndrome	?	Europe, Japan	?	?	—
Poxviral local cutaneous infections	V	Worldwide, discrete foci	Z(d, w)	7–14	—

[a] See also: bartonellosis (4); coccidioidomycosis (6); gammaherpesviral mononucleosis (4); leishmaniasis, cutaneous (9); meningococcal meningitis (5); pharyngitis (6); paratyphoid fever (1); relapsing fever (1); sporotrichosis (9); swimmers' itch (9); swimming-pool-associated dermatitis (9); tularaemia (4); trypanosomiasis (4); typhoid fever (1); viral haemorrhagic fever (3) (number of syndrome given in parentheses).

[b] B: bacteria; C: chlamydia; F: fungus; P: parasite; R: rickettsia; V: virus.

[c] A: arthropod-borne: (f) houseflies; (m) mosquitos; (p) phlebotomines (sandflies); (t) ticks; (o) others;
E: environment: (a) air or dust; (f) food; (s) soil; (w) water;
P: person-to-person: (d) direct; (i) indirect;
Z: zoonotic: (d) domestic animal; (r) rodent; (w) wild animal.

[d] In days unless otherwise stated (h: hours; w: weeks; m: months); average incubation period in parentheses.

[e] When direct person-to-person transmission occurs.

[f] Now considered to have been eradicated.

Table 32 (continued)

3. Haemorrhagic fever (HF)[a]

Disease	Agent[b]	Occurrence	Mode of transmission[c]	Incubation period[d]	Infective period[e]
3.1 Mosquito-borne					
Chikungunya HF	V	South-East Asia	A(m)	?	—
Dengue HF	V	South-East Asia	A(m)	?	—
Yellow fever	V	Tropical areas of Africa and Americas	A(m)	3-6	—
3.2 Tick-borne					
Crimean-Congo HF	V	Africa, Europe	A(t) P(d)	7-12	Exceptional
Kyasanur Forest disease	V	India	A(t)	3-7	—
Omsk HF	V	USSR	A(t)	3-7	—
3.3 Rodent-borne					
Haemorrhagic fever with renal syndrome	V	Worldwide	Z(r)	7-35 (14-21)	—
Junin and Machupo HF	V	South America	Z(r)	7-16	Occasional for Machupo HF
Lassa fever	V	Tropical Africa	Z(r) P(d)	7-21	Acute stage up to 60 days

3.4 Unknown vector

Ebola and Marburg virus diseases	V	Tropical Africa	Z(?) P(d)	2–21(3–7)	Up to 2 months

[a] See also: leptospirosis (1); measles (2); meningococcaemia (2); plague, bubonic (4); relapsing fever (1); Rift Valley fever (1); smallpox (2) (number of syndrome in parentheses).

[b] B: bacteria; C: chlamydia; F: fungus; P: parasite; R: rickettsia; V: virus.

[c] A: arthropod-borne: (f) houseflies; (m) mosquitos; (p) phlebotomines (sandflies); (t) ticks; (o) others;
E: environment: (a) air or dust; (f) food; (s) soil; (w) water;
P: person-to-person: (d) direct; (i) indirect;
Z: zoonotic: (d) domestic animal; (r) rodent; (w) wild animal.

[d] In days unless otherwise stated (h: hours; w: weeks; m: months): average incubation period in parentheses.

[e] When direct person-to-person transmission occurs.

Table 32 (continued)

4. Febrile lymphadenopathy[a]

Disease	Agent[b]	Occurrence	Mode of transmission[c]	Incubation period[d]	Infective period[e]
4.1 General lymphadenopathy					
Acquired immunodeficiency syndrome	V	Americas, Europe	Sexual, blood	?	?
Bartonellosis	P	South America	A(p)	16–22, up to 4 m	—
Filariasis	P	Warm humid regions	A(m)	3 m and longer	—
Leishmaniasis, visceral	P	Discrete foci in warm climates	A(p)	10 days–2 years (2 m–4 m)	—
Toxoplasmosis	P	Worldwide	E(f, w)	5–23 or longer	—

4.2 Regional lymphadenopathy

Gammaherpesviral mononucleosis	V	Worldwide	P(d)	4–6 w	—
Plague, bubonic	B	Discrete foci in all continents	A(fleas)	2–6	See plague, pneumonic (syndrome 6)
Tularaemia	B	America, Asia, Europe	Z(w) A(o) E(f, w)	2–10 (3)	—
Trypanosomiasis, African	P	Tropical Africa	A(o)	14–21 or months	—
Trypanosomiasis, American	P	Americas	A(o)	5–14	—

[a] See also: arthropod-borne viral fever (1); chancroid (9); mucocutaneous lymph node syndrome (2); rubella (2); sandfly fever (1); syphilis (9) (number of syndrome in parentheses).

[b] B: bacteria; C: chlamydia; F: fungus; P: parasite; R: rickettsia; V: virus.

[c] A: arthropod-borne: (f) houseflies; (m) mosquitos; (p) phlebotomines (sandflies); (t) ticks; (o) others;
E: environment: (a) air or dust; (f) food; (s) soil; (w) water;
P: person-to-person: (d) direct; (i) indirect;
Z: zoonotic: (d) domestic animal; (r) rodent; (w) wild animal.

[d] In days unless otherwise stated (h: hours; w: weeks; m: months); average incubation period in parentheses.

[e] When direct person-to-person transmission occurs.

Table 32 (continued)

5. Febrile neurological disease[a]

Disease	Agent[b]	Occurrence	Mode of transmission[c]	Incubation period[d]	Infective period[e]
5.1 Paralysis					
Enteroviral encephalo-myelitis	V	Worldwide	P(d)	?	?
Poliomyelitis	V	Worldwide	P(d) E(f)	3–35(7–14)	1 week for throat, 6 weeks or longer for faeces
5.2 Meningitis					
Angiostrongyliasis	P	Egypt, South Pacific	E(f)	7–21 or longer	—
Lymphocytic choriomeningitis	V	Worldwide, discrete foci	Z(r) E(a)	15–21	—
Meningitis due to *Haemophilus influenzae*	B	Worldwide	P(d)	2–4	May be prolonged
Meningitis, viral	V	Worldwide	Depends on agent	Depends on agent	Depends on agent
Meningococcal meningitis	B	Worldwide	P(d)	2–10(3–4)	Until 24 hours after treatment, carriers possible
Mumps	V	Worldwide	P(d)	14–21(18)	6 days before onset of parotitis to 9 days after

5.3 Encephalitis

Arthropod-borne viral encephalitides	V	Worldwide, discrete foci	A(m, t)	5–15	—
Cryptococcosis	F	Worldwide	E(a)	?	—
Encephalitis, viral	V	Worldwide	Depends on agent	Depends on agent	Depends on agent
Listeriosis	B	Worldwide	P(d) E(a, f) (?)	4–21 (?)	?
Meningoencephalitis due to miscellaneous infectious agents	B, V, P	Worldwide	Depends on agent	Depends on agent	Depends on agent
Rabies	V	Worldwide	Z(d, w)	10 days–12 m or longer (30–50)	—

[a] See also: botulism (9); enteroviral exanthematous fever (2); leptospirosis (1); erythema chronicum migrans due to *Borrelia burgdorferi* (2); malaria (1); mumps (9); Reye's syndrome (9); tetanus (9); trypanosomiasis, African (4); typhoid fever (1); typhus (2) (number of syndrome in parentheses).

[b] B: bacteria; C: chlamydia; F: fungus; P: parasite; R: rickettsia; V: virus.

[c] A: arthropod-borne: (f) houseflies; (m) mosquitos; (p) phlebotomines (sandflies); (t) ticks; (o) others; E: environment: (a) air or dust; (f) food; (s) soil; (w) water; P: person-to-person: (d) direct; (i) indirect; Z: zoonotic: (d) domestic animal; (r) rodent; (w) wild animal.

[d] In days unless otherwise stated (h: hours; w: weeks; m: months): average incubation period in parentheses.

[e] When direct person-to-person transmission occurs.

Table 32 (*continued*)

6. Febrile respiratory tract disease[a]

Disease	Agent[b]	Occurrence	Mode of transmission[c]	Incubation period[d]	Infective period[e]
6.1 Upper respiratory tract (larynx, trachea, bronchi)					
Acute viral pharyngitis	V	Worldwide	Depends on agent	Depends on agent	Depends on agent
Acute viral rhinitis	V	Worldwide	P(d)	1–3	Acute phase
Bronchitis	B, V	Worldwide	P(d, i)	Depends on agent	Depends on agent
Diphtheria	B	Worldwide	P(d)	2–5	2 weeks, or longer (chronic carriers)
Enteroviral lymphonodular pharyngitis	V	Worldwide	P(d, i)	5	Acute phase for the throat, longer for faeces
Enteroviral vesicular pharyngitis	V	Worldwide	P(d, i)	3–5	Acute phase for the throat, longer for faeces
Laryngotracheobronchitis, viral	V	Worldwide	P(d, i)	Depends on agent	Depends on agent
Pertussis	B	Worldwide	P(d)	7–21 (7)	3 weeks
Streptococcal pharyngitis	B	Temperate zones	P(d) E(f)	1–3	Untreated 21 days, treated 2 days

6.2 Lower respiratory tract (bronchioles, alveoli)

Disease	[b]	Geographical distribution	[c]	Incubation period [d]	Communicable period [e]
Anthrax, pulmonary	B	Worldwide, discrete foci	P(d) E(a)	2–7 (2–5)	Acute phase
Bronchiolitis	B	Worldwide	P(d, i)	Few days to a week	Acute phase
Coccidioidomycosis	F	Americas, arid zones	E(a)	7–28	—
Histoplasmosis	F	Worldwide, discrete foci	E(a)	5–18 (10)	—
Influenza	V	Worldwide	P(d) E(a)	1–3	3 days from onset
Legionnaires' disease	B	North America, Europe	E(a)	2–10 (5–6)	—
Melioidosis	B	Africa, South-East Asia, Europe	E(s, w)	2 days to several months	—
Ornithosis	B	Worldwide	E(a) P(d)	4–15 (10)	Acute phase
Plague, pneumonic	B	All continents, discrete foci	P(d, i)	2–3	Acute phase
Pneumonia, bacterial	B	Worldwide	P(d, i)	1–3	Acute phase
Pneumonia due to *Mycoplasma pneumoniae*	B	Worldwide	P(d, i)	14–21	Less than 10 days but occasionally longer
Pneumonia due to *Streptococcus pneumoniae*	B	Worldwide	P(d, i)	1–3	Acute phase
Pneumonia due to other infectious agents	P, F, C	Depends on agent	Depends on agent	Depends on agent	Depends on agent
Pneumonia, viral	V	Worldwide	P(d, i)	1–3	Acute phase
Q fever	R	Worldwide	E(a) Z(d)	14–21	—
Tuberculosis	B	Worldwide	P(d) E(f)	4w–12w	—

[a] See also: capillariasis (9); epidemic myalgia (1); non-pneumonic Legionnaires' disease (1); tularaemia (4) (syndrome number in parentheses).

[b] B: bacteria; C: chlamydia; F: fungus; P: parasite; R: rickettsia; V: virus.

[c] A: arthropod-borne: (f) houseflies; (m) mosquitos; (p) phlebotomines (sandflies); (t) ticks; (o) others;
E: environment: (a) air or dust; (f) food; (s) soil; (w) water;
P: person-to-person: (d) direct; (i) indirect;
Z: zoonotic: (d) domestic animal; (r) rodent; (w) wild animal.

[d] In days unless otherwise stated (h: hours; w: weeks; m: months): average incubation period in parentheses.

[e] When direct person-to-person transmission occurs.

[f] Now considered to have been eradicated.

Table 32 (continued)

7. Febrile gastrointestinal disease[a]

Disease	Agent[b]	Occurrence	Mode of transmission[c]	Incubation period[d]	Infective period[e]
7.1 Diarrhoea					
Acute viral gastro-enteropathy	V	Worldwide	P(d) E(f, w)	1–2	Acute stage, possibly more
Campylobacter enteritis	B	Worldwide	E(f, w) Z(d, w)	1–10(3–5)	7 weeks
Cholera (non–01 Vibrio cholerae gastroenteritis)	B	Americas, Africa, Asia, Europe	E(w, f)	1–5(2–3)	—
Diarrhoea due to parasites	P	Depends on agent	Depends on agent	Depends on agent	Depends on agent
Enteritis due to Escherichia coli	B	Worldwide	E(f, w) P(d)	12h–3	Several weeks
Rotaviral enteritis	V	Worldwide	P(d)	2	Until eighth day of illness
Salmonellosis	B	Worldwide	E(f, w) P(d)	6 h–72 h (12 h–36 h)	Carrier state of variable duration
Traveller's diarrhoea	B	Tropical areas	E(f, w)	12 h–72 h	Several weeks or longer
Yersiniosis	B	Worldwide	E(f, w) P(d)	3–10(3–7)	Chronic carriers possible

7.2 Dysentery

Amoebiasis	P	Worldwide, predominant in tropical areas	E(w, f) P(d) A(f)	14-28 or longer	Not during acute phase but chronic carriers exist
Anthrax, intestinal (rare)	B	Worldwide	E(f)	1-3	—
Shigellosis	B	Worldwide, temperate and tropical areas	P(d, i) E(f, w) A(f)	1-7(1-3)	Up to 4 weeks or carrier state

7.3 Other

Anisakiasis	P	Asia, Europe, South America	E(f)	Few hours–few weeks	—

a See also: clonorchiasis (9); fascioliasis (9); food poisoning (9); paratyphoid fever (1); schistosomiasis, intestinal (9); trichinosis (1); typhoid fever (1); tularaemia (4) (number of syndrome in parentheses).

b B: bacteria; C: chlamydia; F: fungus; P: parasite; R: rickettsia; V: virus.

c A: arthropod-borne: (f) houseflies; (m) mosquitos; (p) phlebotomines (sandflies); (t) ticks; (o) others;
E: environment: (a) air or dust; (f) food; (s) soil; (w) water;
P: person-to-person: (d) direct; (i) indirect;
Z: zoonotic: (d) domestic animal; (r) rodent; (w) wild animal.

d In days unless otherwise stated (h: hours; w: weeks; m: months); average incubation period in parentheses.

e When direct person-to-person transmission occurs.

Table 32 (continued)

8. Febrile icterus[a]

Disease	Agent[b]	Occurrence	Mode of transmission[c] (2)	Incubation period[d]	Infective period[e]
Viral hepatitis A	V	Worldwide	P(d) E(w, f)	15–50(28–30)	Latter half of incubation period and few days after onset
Viral hepatitis B; non-A, non-B; delta virus	V	Worldwide	Blood, blood products, sexual	45–160 (60–90)	Weeks before onset, possible chronic carrier state
Viral hepatitis, non-A, non-B, epidemic	V	Worldwide	P(d) E(w)	14–180	?

[a] See also: capillariasis (9); gammaherpesviral mononucleosis (3); leptospirosis (1); malaria (1); yellow fever (3).
[b] B: bacteria; C: chlamydia; F: fungus; P: parasite; R: rickettsia; V: virus.
[c] A: arthropod-borne: (f) houseflies; (m) mosquitos; (p) phlebotomines (sandflies); (t) ticks; (o) others;
E: environment: (a) air or dust; (f) food; (s) soil; (w) water;
P: person-to-person: (d) direct; (i) indirect;
Z: zoonotic: (d) domestic animal; (r) rodent; (w) wild animal.
[d] In days unless otherwise stated (h: hours; w: weeks; m: months; average incubation period in parentheses).
[e] When direct person-to-person transmission occurs.

9. Afebrile diseases[a]

Disease	Agent[b]	Occurrence	Mode of transmission[c]	Incubation period[d]	Infective period[e]
9.1 Rash					
Leishmaniasis, cutaneous	P	Africa, south-west Asia, Mediterranean basin, Central and South America	A(p)	Few days to several months	—
Sporotrichosis	F	Worldwide	E(s)	7 days to months	—
Swimmers' itch	P	Discrete foci in all climates	E(w)	Short	—
Swimming-pool-associated dermatitis	B	Worldwide	E(w)	Hours	—
Yaws	B	Humid tropical areas, Africa, Americas	P(d)	2 w–3 m	Several years
9.2 Neurological					
Guillain-Barré syndrome	—	—	—	—	—
Reye's syndrome	—	—	—	—	—
Tetanus	B	Worldwide	E(s)	4–21(10)	—
9.3 Respiratory					
Paragonimiasis	P	Asia, Africa, west coast of South America	E(f)	Variable, long	—

Table 32 (continued)

9. Afebrile diseases[a]

Disease	Agent[b]	Occurrence	Mode of transmission[c]	Incubation period[d]	Infective period[e]
9.4 Gastrointestinal					
Balantidiasis	P	Worldwide	E(w, f) P(d) A(f)	?	May be prolonged
Capillariasis	P	All continents	E(f)	3 w–4 w	—
Cholera (epidemic *Vibrio cholerae* O-groups)	B	Africa, Asia, eastern Europe	A(f) E(w, f)	1–5 (2–3)	—
Clonorchiasis	P	West Pacific	E(f)	About 1 m	—
Fasciolopsiasis	P	Asia	E(f)	About 1 m	—
Giardiasis	P	Worldwide	E(w, f) P(d)	7–28 (14)	May be prolonged
Schistosomiasis, intestinal	P	Africa, South America, west Pacific	E(w)	4–6 w	—
9.5 Food poisoning caused by:					
Bacillus cereus	B	Mainly in Europe	E(f)	1 h–16 h	—
Clostridium botulinum	B	Worldwide	E(f)	12–36 or several days	—
Clostridium perfringens	B	Worldwide	E(f)	6–24 (10–12 h)	—
Staphylococcus aureus	B	Worldwide	E(f)	1–6 (2–4 h)	—
Toxic substances	Toxins, chemicals	Worldwide	A(f)	Depends on agent	—
Vibrio parahaemolyticus	B	Worldwide	E(f)	4 h–96 h (12 h–24 h)	—

9.6 Jaundice

Fascioliasis	P	All continents	E(f)	Variable	—

9.7 Conjunctivitis

Acute bacterial conjunctivitis	B	Worldwide, frequent in warm climates	P(d, i)	1–3	Acute phase
Adenoviral conjunctivitis	V	Worldwide	P(d, i)	5–12	14 days
Chlamydial conjunctivitis	C	Worldwide	P(d) E(w)	5–12	Carrier state possible
Enteroviral haemorrhagic conjunctivitis	V	Worldwide	P(d, i)	1–2	1–2 weeks

9.8 Urinary tract disease

Schistosomiasis, urinary	P	Africa, south-west Asia	E(w)	4w–6w	—

a For food poisoning, see also: clonorchiasis (9.4); for conjunctivitis, see also arthropod-borne fevers (1); measles (2) (number of syndrome in parentheses).

b B: bacteria; C: chlamydia; F: fungus; P: parasite; R: rickettsia; V: virus.

c A: arthropod-borne: (f) houseflies; (m) mosquitos; (p) phlebotomines (sandflies); (t) ticks; (o) others;
E: environment: (a) air or dust; (f) food: (s) soil; (w) water;
P: person-to-person: (d) direct; (i) indirect;
Z: zoonotic: (d) domestic animal; (r) rodent; (w) wild animal.

d In days unless otherwise stated (h: hours; w: weeks; m: months): average incubation period in parentheses.

e When direct person-to-person transmission occurs.

As far as the numerator is concerned, it should be remembered that:

—case counts based on reporting will almost inevitably be incomplete and their accuracy will depend on the effort put into reporting;

—case counts based on hospital reports will include only the most severely affected persons and will produce artificially high case-fatality rates;

—case counts for clinically overt illness will be complete only if based on a total or random sample population survey for illness;

—case counts including overt illness and subclinical infections can be complete only if they are based on a total or random sample population survey for illness *and* on laboratory evidence of infection.

Before it is realized that an epidemic exists, cases will be reported at whatever level of completeness is characteristic of the reporting system in the area. After an epidemic is known to exist, case reporting often becomes more complete, and much more so if active case finding is introduced as part of an investigation. The plotted epidemic curve thus exaggerates the change from the endemic to the epidemic level. This is true even if retrospective case finding is undertaken, since this is rarely, if ever, as complete as concurrent case finding.

The value of the case-fatality rate (CFR) found will depend on whether retrospective or concurrent case finding is used. Severe and fatal cases are more readily detected retrospectively than mild ones, so that retrospective case finding will give a higher CFR than concurrent case finding, which enables a higher proportion of mild cases to be detected. The apparent decline in the CFR in going from retrospective to concurrent case finding may give the false impression that a treatment programme has been successful.

Incidence (attack) rates by personal characteristics. The purpose of calculating attack rates separately for different population subgroups is to identify those at greatest risk, and thereby to guide control efforts.

As will be seen from Annex 2, the attack rates by personal characteristics most frequently used are for age and sex, and occupation. Other subgroups may be found to be of interest during an investigation (e.g., ethnic groups). Investigation of a food-borne outbreak may require the division of those affected into a number of subgroups based on the composition of the meals consumed.

Incidence (attack) rates by locality. The location of cases can be conveniently displayed on "spot maps" as shown in Annex 2. A difficulty with such maps is that they only show the location of cases (numerators) and not the intensity of infection by locality, which is indicated only by incidence rates. Maps should therefore be used to supplement tables, not to replace them.

Spot maps may be considered to be "working" maps; they are started early in the course of an investigation and are kept up to date by inserting new cases as they are added to the list. After an investigation has been completed, the final report may include maps to illustrate other important features of the outbreak, such as attack rates, other quantitative indices, communication lines, vector densities (Fig. 9), house-to-house communications (Fig. 10), sewage systems, or progress of the epidemic with time (Fig. 11).

Distribution of cases in time. The third and equally important epidemiological indicator is time. The distribution of cases in time is best shown by a graph (histogram), as described in Annex 2. This may also show possible relationships between incidence and factors such as age, sex, occupation, the effect of control measures (Fig. 12) or the outcome of cases (fatal cases).

Fig. 9. Vector densities and geographical distribution of cases of yellow fever during an outbreak in Senegal in 1965 (after *Bulletin of the World Health Organization*, **36**: 113–150 (1967))

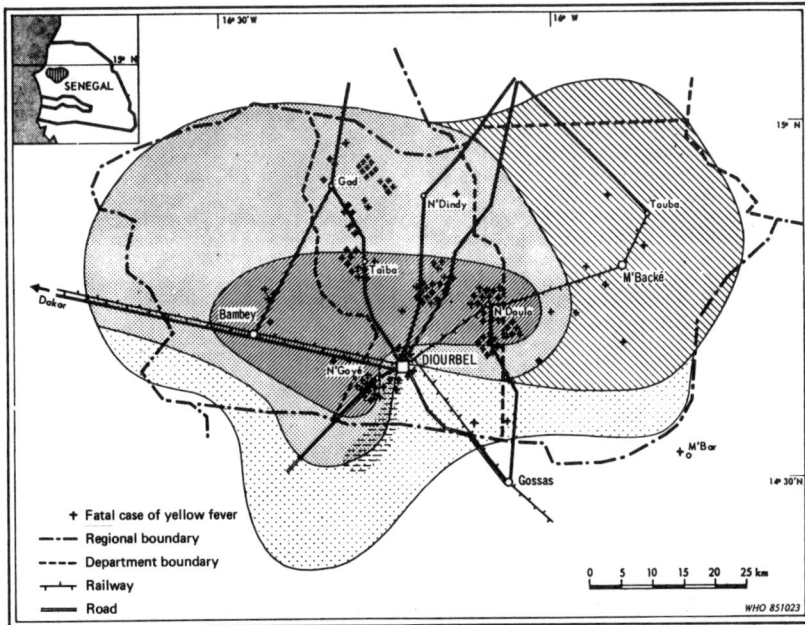

Percentage of earthen jars containing Aedes aegypti larvae:

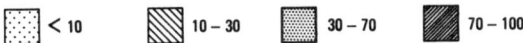

< 10 $10 - 30$ $30 - 70$ $70 - 100$

Fig. 10. Ebola haemorrhagic fever cases by household in Zaire in 1976 (after BREMAN, J. G. ET AL. The epidemiology of Ebola haemorrhagic fever in Zaire, 1976. In: Pattyn, S. R., ed., *Ebola virus haemorrhagic fever*, Amsterdam and New York, Elsevier/North Holland Biomedical Press, 1978, p. 116)

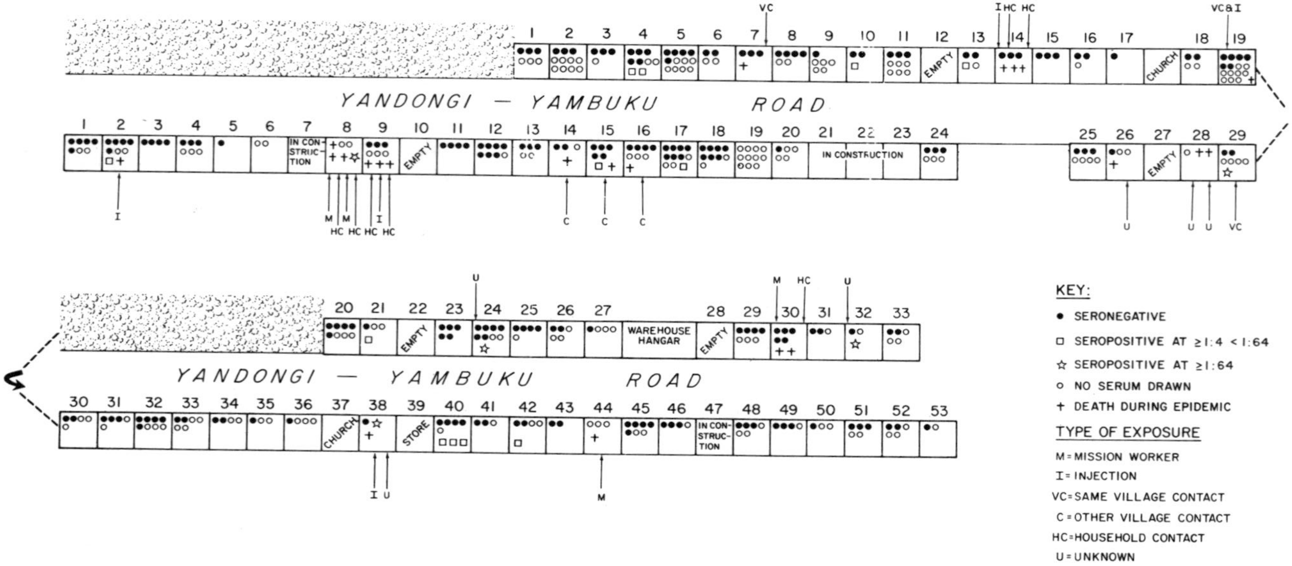

Fig. 11. Progress of outbreak of yellow fever in the Gambia, 1978–1979 (after MONATH, T. P. ET AL. *American journal of tropical medicine and hygiene*, **29**(5): 912–928 (1980))

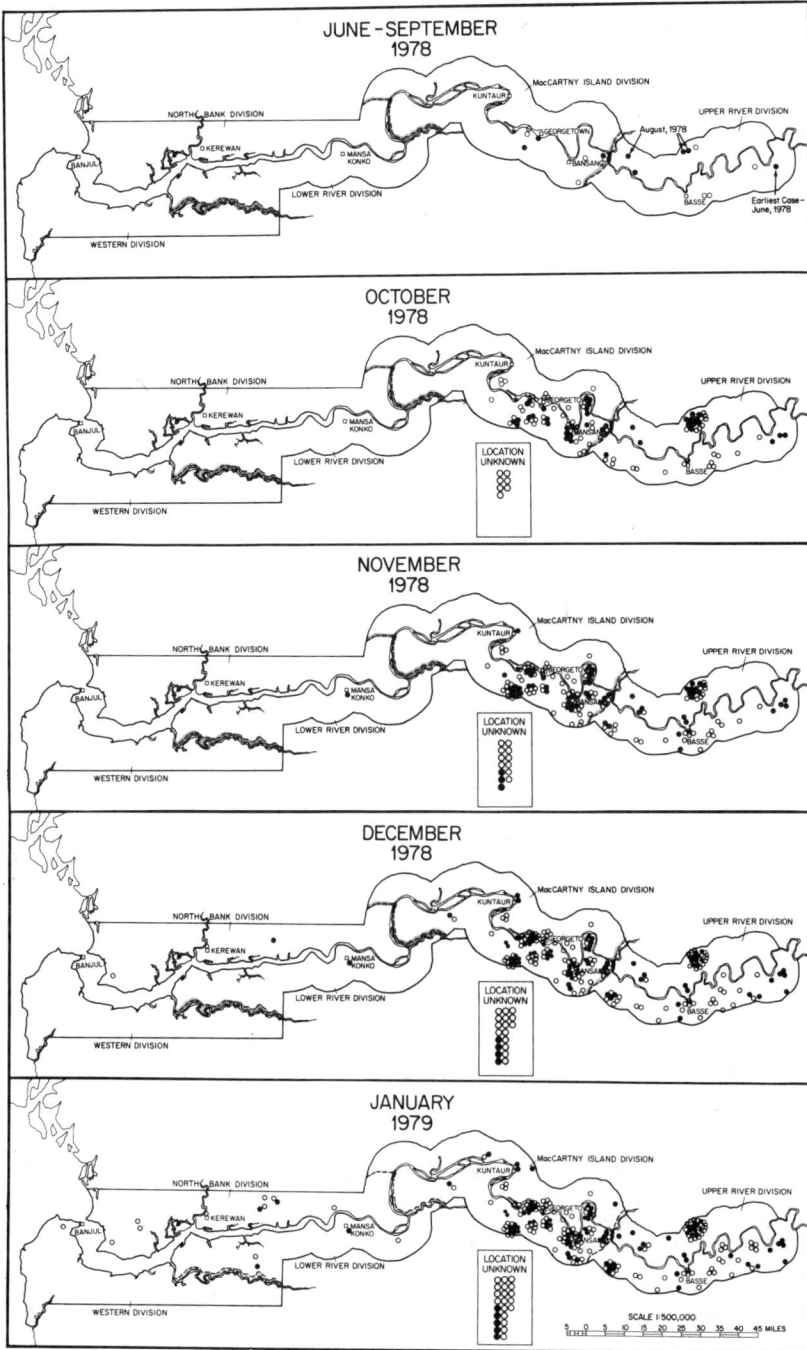

Fig. 12. Number of cases of Ebola virus disease in Zaire in 1976 by day of onset and by probable type of transmission (after *Bulletin of the World Health Organization*, **56**: 271–293 (1978)). The epidemic was largely the result of the use, for parenteral injections in a hospital, of syringes that were not properly sterilized. The most effective control measure was therefore closure of the hospital on 3 October, after which the outbreak ended.

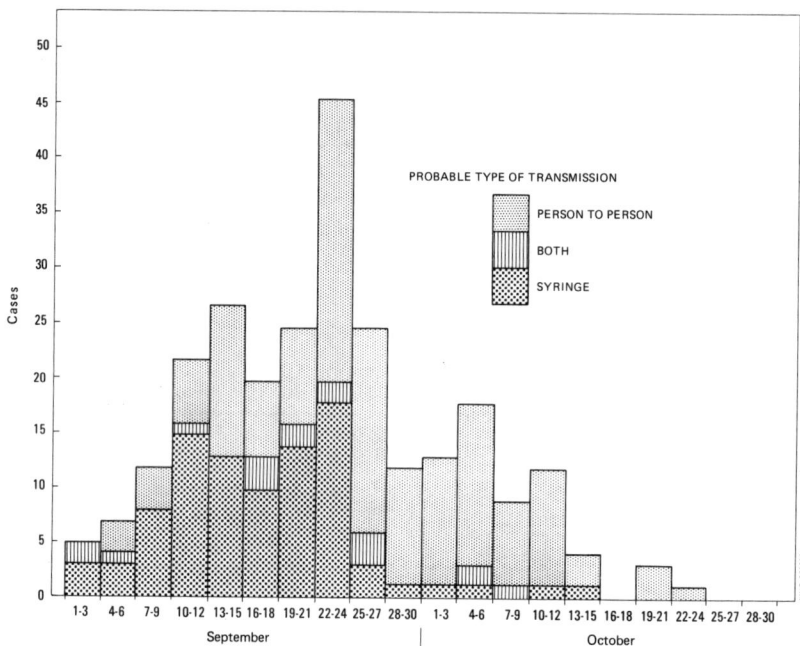

Case-fatality rate. Assuming that the cause of death of each patient can be related to the cause of the outbreak, the case-fatality rate (CFR) will differ, depending on the population subgroup considered, e.g., hospitalized cases, all overt cases, all infected cases (overt cases plus subclinical infections detected by laboratory examination of the entire population at risk, or of a randomized sample of it, due attention being paid to age, sex, occupation and place of residence). In yellow fever outbreaks, the CFR may be as high as 80 % of severe hospitalized cases and as low as 1 % of all infected persons.

5.2.3 Formulating and testing hypotheses of causation

Contact tracing (see section 4.2.3) usually points to one of the following transmission patterns:

(*a*) transmission from person to person, originating from a single index case (which may not be recognized);

(*b*) transmission from a common source (point source), which may be infected arthropods, animals, food or the environment, with no further person-to-person transmission;

(*c*) common-source transmission, followed by person-to-person transmission, e.g., water-borne typhoid fever.

One or several hypotheses of causation will be deduced from the critical analysis of the observed transmission pattern and will have to be confirmed by statistical analysis. Detailed information procedures for assembling epidemiological data and formulating and testing hypotheses of causation are given in Annex 2.

Person-to-person transmission pattern. The transmission pattern may be characterized by the following three indicators.

(*a*) *The route of transmission*

Direct and/or indirect transmission may occur by different routes (see Table 33). Knowledge of the route is of great importance in deciding on the control measures to be taken.

(*b*) *The period of contagiousness*

Careful case interviews will determine the dates of infective contact with confirmed cases. The investigator can then establish the incubation and infective periods of the disease (see section 4.2 and

Table 33. Routes of person-to-person transmission

| Excretion route | Infection route | |
	Direct	Indirect
Respiratory (speaking, sneezing, coughing)	"Face-to-face" contact (less than 1 m)	Aerosols, toilet articles
Saliva	Mouth-to-mouth contact	Glass vessels, toothbrushes, towels, forks and spoons
Faecal	Dirty hands	Water, food, toilet articles
Urine	Dirty hands	Aerosols, splashes during nursing
Eye secretions	Dirty hands	Ophthalmic instruments, toilet articles
Cutaneous and mucous membrane lesions, genital infections	Skin abrasions or cuts; sexual intercourse	Toilet articles, bed linen, dressings

Fig. 6), which are important in determining the duration of precautionary or isolation measures.

(c) The chain of cases

It is sometimes possible to discover the index case and establish the sequence of secondary and further generations of cases (see Fig. 5, p. 51). This is of little importance in outbreaks of diseases such as influenza but for others, such as Lassa fever, tertiary cases are less severe than secondary ones. The length and multiplicity of chains of cases give some indication of how widely the disease is likely to spread, which is also useful in deciding on the control measures necessary. An example of the reconstitution of the chain of cases in an epidemic of Ebola virus disease in the Sudan is given in Fig. 13.

Common-source transmission pattern. Infectious and parasitic agents may also be transmitted to man from non-human sources and may cause outbreaks when transmission occurs in a cluster of cases over a limited period of time. The formulation of hypotheses as to the causation of the outbreak will depend on the date of common-source exposure, which has first to be determined, and also on the transmission characteristics of the incriminated disease. The possible common sources for such diseases are arthropods (insects), domestic and wild animals, food and drink, and the environment.

(a) Determining the date of common-source exposure

If the dates of onset for many cases are almost identical, there may be a common source (point source) of infection, taking into account the possible variations in the length of the incubation period (see Fig. 6). This pattern may be clear-cut for some food-borne or water-borne diseases. However, cases may be in contact with the source of infection over a period of several days and the scattered dates of case onset may resemble the pattern seen with person-to-person transmission. This is the case with arthropod-borne diseases, when a population may be bitten by infected insects over a number of days.

(b) Transmission by arthropods

The list of arthropods of medical importance and the diseases they transmit is given in Table 34.

The arthropod-borne viral diseases deserve special mention. They are transmitted to man by mosquitos, ticks, phlebotomines and *Culicoides*, after multiplication of the virus in them, and cause a variety of syndromes: arthritis and rash, encephalitis, fever with systemic symptoms, and haemorrhagic fever. Arthropod-borne viral diseases have a characteristic distribution and require specific vector species for their transmission. The most important ones in man are listed in Table 35.

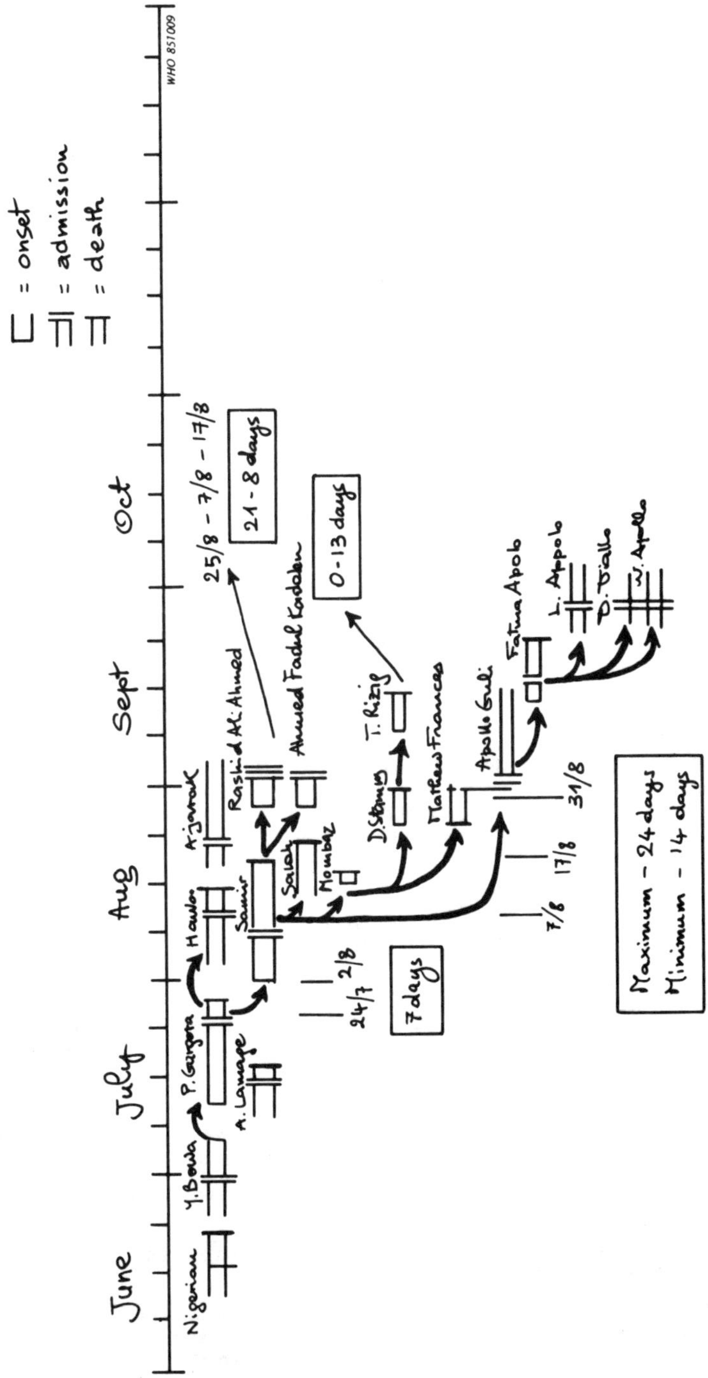

Fig. 13. Example of chart prepared in the field showing chain of cases of Ebola virus disease in the Sudan in 1976

Table 34. Arthropod-borne diseases

Arthropod	Disease		
	Bacterial or rickettsial (R)	Parasitic	Viral
Chrysops (horse flies)	Tularaemia	—	—
Cockroaches[a]	Typhoid fever,[b] shigellosis,[b] salmonellosis[b]	Toxoplasmosis, intestinal parasitic diseases	Lymphocytic choriomeningitis
Crustaceans, crabs, crayfish, cyclops	—	Paragonimiasis, dracontiasis	
Culicoides (biting midges)	—	Filariasis	Arbovirus[c] infections
Fleas	Plague,[b] tularaemia, typhus fever due to *Rickettsia typhi* (R)	—	—
Flies (houseflies)	Typhoid fever,[b] shigellosis,[b] salmonellosis,[b] cholera,[b] yaws[b]	Intestinal parasitic diseases	Poliomyelitis,[b] other enteric viral diseases[b]
Glossina (testse flies)	—	African trypanosomiasis (sleeping sickness)	—
Lice (body)	Epidemic relapsing fever, typhus fever due to *Rickettsia prowazekii* (R), trench fever (R)	—	—
Mites	Typhus fever due to *Rickettsia tsutsugamushi* (R), rickettsialpox (R)	—	—
Mosquitos: *Aedes*	—	Filariasis	Arbovirus infections (especially dengue, yellow fever)
Anopheles	—	Malaria, filariasis	Arbovirus infections
Culex	—	Filariasis	Arbovirus infections
Phlebotomines (sandflies)	—	Leishmaniasis	Sandfly fever
Reduviids (kissing bugs)	—	American trypanosomiasis (Chagas' disease)	—

Table 34 (*continued*)

Arthropod	Disease: Bacterial or rickettsial (R)	Disease: Parasitic	Disease: Viral
Ticks	Endemic relapsing fever, spotted fevers, tularaemia, erythema chronicum migrans due to *Borrelia burgdorferi*, Q fever (R)		Arbovirus infections, Colorado tick fever, tick-borne haemorrhagic fevers

[a] Occasional mechanical vector, no proven role in epidemics.
[b] Possible person-to-person transmission.
[c] Acronym for a group of arthropod-borne viruses belonging to different genera but all transmitted by biting insects.

An arthropod may be incriminated for the following reasons:

—it belongs to a species and biotype (subspecies distinguished by particular characteristics) known to be a vector, and is at the right stage of development (larva, nymph, adult);
—it is sufficiently abundant (although the most abundant species is not necessarily the one responsible for the epidemic);
—its behaviour (breeding and feeding habits) establishes a close relationship between the vertebrate reservoir of pathogens (the arthropod may itself be a reservoir) and receptive individuals (host specificity);
—a sufficient number of individuals of the incriminated species carry the agent, as determined by laboratory examination.

There are two transmission patterns. Some arthropods are simply passive mechanical vectors, e.g., houseflies, but in others the agent multiplies; the latter are thus amplifier hosts in the transmission cycle of the agent. This second category of arthropods becomes infected by biting an infected vertebrate host, which may be man or a domestic or feral animal. Once infected, after an appropriate incubation period (called the extrinsic incubation period), these arthropods excrete the infective agent through saliva, coelomic fluids or faeces, depending on the type of agent and the vector insect. A vector insect may also act as an effective reservoir if it remains infected for a long period, and/or if it transmits the agent to its progeny (transovarial transmission). Transmission cycles involving insects may be represented as follows:

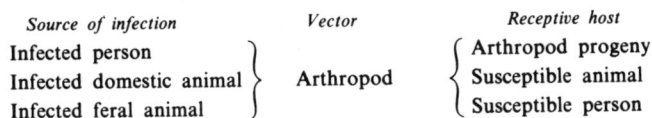

Source of infection	*Vector*	*Receptive host*
Infected person		Arthropod progeny
Infected domestic animal	Arthropod	Susceptible animal
Infected feral animal		Susceptible person

Table 35. Arthropod-borne viral diseases[a]

Syndrome	Vector	Disease	Occurrence
Arthritis and rash[b]	Mosquito	Ross River disease	Australia, Papua New Guinea, Pacific islands
Encephalitis[b]	Mosquito	California encephalitis	Canada, USA
		Eastern equine encephalomyelitis	Americas
		Japanese encephalitis	Asia, Pacific islands
		Murray Valley encephalitis	Australia, Papua New Guinea
		Rocio virus disease	Brazil
		St Louis encephalitis	Americas, Jamaica
		Venezuelan equine encephalitis	South and Central America, Mexico, USA
		Western equine encephalomyelitis	Americas
	Tick	Central European tick-borne encephalitis	Europe
		Far eastern tick-borne encephalitis	Europe, Asia
		Louping ill	United Kingdom
		Powassan virus encephalitis	Canada, USA
Fever[c]	Mosquito	Bunyamwera virus disease	Africa
		Bwamba virus disease	Africa
		Chikungunya virus disease	Africa, south-east Asia, Philippines
		Dengue fever	Africa, Asia, Australia, Caribbean, Indian subcontinent, Pacific islands, Papua New Guinea, South America
		Group-C viral fevers	South America
		Mayaro virus disease	South America
		O'nyong-nyong	Africa
		Oropouche virus disease	South America
		Rift Valley fever	Africa
		West Nile fever	Africa, south-west Asia, Europe, Indian subcontinent

Table 35 (*continued*)

Syndrome	Vector	Disease	Occurrence
	Phleboto-mine	Sandfly fever	Africa, South and Central America, Asia, Europe
	Tick	Colorado tick fever	USA
Haemorrhagic fever[b]	Mosquito	Chikungunya virus disease	South-west Asia
		Dengue haemorrhagic fever	South-east Asia, Caribbean, Pacific islands
		Yellow fever	Africa, South America
	Tick	Crimean-Congo haemorrhagic fever	Africa, central and south-west Asia, Europe
		Kyasanur Forest disease	India
		Omsk haemorrhagic fever	USSR

[a] Further information on some of these diseases will be found in Annex 3 and will generally be applicable to others in the same category.
[b] Characteristic signs and symptoms are often preceded by fever, headache, and muscular and joint pains. The same virus may cause only systemic symptomatology.
[c] Fever only, or associated with different degrees of headache, and muscular and joint pains.

The arthropod-borne agents of the diseases listed in Tables 34 and 35 have both specific vectors and specific hosts. The amplification of transmission cycles depends on the seasonal or occasional increase in numbers of vectors, infected hosts, and receptive hosts; such increases are regulated by climatic and epidemiological factors. Entomological studies of the factors influencing the transmission capacity of arthropods are necessary in order to understand how unusual circumstances have caused an outbreak. Such factors include:

—species and biotype;
—climatic and other conditions;
—effect of temperature on extrinsic incubation period;
—breeding habits (types of breeding site, periodicity);
—duration of developmental stages (larval, nymphal, adult);
—distance that the species is capable of travelling, with or without human assistance;
—resting places;
—feeding habits (preference for certain animals, times, places);
—tropisms (attraction to specific objects);
—biting activity (periods, stimulation);
—longevity;
—resistance to chemical insecticides, sensitivity to biological insecticides.

The distance that an arthropod is capable of travelling influences the pattern of spread of the outbreak. Insects capable of travelling only short distances cause a slowly extending outbreak of the "oil stain" type, e.g., yellow fever transmitted by the domestic *Aedes aegypti* mosquito, which has an average flight range of 300 m. Flying insects capable of travelling long distances may create secondary foci far from the original one. Arthropods may also be carried by vehicles or be transported as parasites on migrating animals, e.g., domestic flocks and herds, rodents, birds. Flying insects may be carried over long distances by high-altitude winds.

(c) Transmission by vertebrate animals (zoonoses)

Some animal pathogens may also be infectious to man and cause what are called zoonoses; these are listed in Table 36.

Zoonoses may be transmitted by direct contact with an infected animal or indirectly through insect vectors, food and contamination of the environment.

Transmission by direct contact occurs among those engaged in certain occupations (farmers, hunters, veterinary public health personnel) or as a result of poor hygiene when animals and people share a dwelling (this may also occur in camp and on safaris). One infected animal can infect a number of people over a short or long period.

Infected animals may be sick or healthy carriers. As in human disease, the incubation and excretion periods must be determined, and this may require the assistance of a veterinarian. A knowledge of the ecology and behaviour of wild animals and their taxonomy may also be necessary, in which case the assistance of a mammalogist may be required.

Outbreaks resulting from direct contact with animals are usually confined to a restricted area, but may spread with migration of these animals, unusual pullulation, or transport of the animals by man. For example, an epidemic was caused by Marburg virus in the Federal Republic of Germany after the introduction of infected African green monkeys.

(d) Transmission by food

Epidemic food-borne diseases are listed in Table 37; two different transmission mechanisms exist, as follows:

—poisoning: a toxic substance is introduced into food or is secreted by a bacterium, which may thereafter disappear as a result of death or sterilization (certain toxins are thermolabile, others are thermoresistant);
—infection: food is contaminated by a bacterium, virus or parasite, which develops the usual infectious pathology when ingested by consumers.

Table 36. Epidemic zoonoses transmitted by direct contact

Animal	Bacterial, chlamydial (C) or rickettsial (R)	Parasitic	Viral
		Disease	

	A. Domestic animals		
Cats	Yersiniosis	*Pneumocystis* pneumonia,[a] toxoplasmosis	—
Cattle, sheep, goats	Anthrax, brucellosis, *Campylobacter* enteritis, leptospirosis, tuberculosis (*Mycobacterium bovis*), Q fever (R)	—	Poxviral local cutaneous infections, rabies, Rift Valley fever
Dogs	Brucellosis (rare), leptospirosis, yersiniosis	*Pneumocystis* pneumonia[a]	Rabies
Hamsters	—	—	Lymphocytic choriomeningitis
Pigs	Anthrax, brucellosis, leptospirosis, tuberculosis	—	—
Poultry	Salmonellosis, *Campylobacter* enteritis, ornithosis (C)[a]	—	—

	B. Wild animals		
Birds	Ornithosis (C)	—	Influenza A
Monkeys	Tuberculosis	—	Herpesviral encephalitis, viral hepatitis A,[a] monkeypox,[a] poxviral local cutaneous infections, Marburg virus disease
Rodents	Leptospirosis, plague, rat-bite fever, tularaemia, yersiniosis, murine typhus (R)	*Pneumocystis* pneumonia[a]	Lymphocytic choriomeningitis, Lassa fever,[a] Junin haemorrhagic fever, Machupo haemorrhagic fever, haemorrhagic fever with renal syndrome
Wild carnivores	—	Trichinosis	Rabies[b] and rabies-like diseases

[a] Person-to-person transmission possible.
[b] Also transmitted by bats in the Americas.

Table 37. Epidemic food-borne diseases

Source	Food poisoning	Food-borne infection		
		Bacterial	Parasitic	Viral or rickettsial (R)
Eggs and egg products	—	Salmonellosis[a] Streptococcal pharyngitis[a]	—	—
Meat and meat products	Bacillus cereus food poisoning Botulism Clostridium perfringens food poisoning Staphylococcal food poisoning	Anthrax, intestinal Campylobacter enteritis Salmonellosis[a] Tularaemia Yersiniosis[a]	Toxoplasmosis Trichinosis	Hepatitis A[a]
Milk and dairy products	Bacillus cereus food poisoning Staphylococcal food poisoning	Brucellosis Campylobacter enteritis Enteritis due to Escherichia coli[a] Diphtheria (rare) Listeriosis Paratyphoid fever[a] Rat-bite fever Salmonellosis[a] Shigellosis[a] Streptococcal pharyngitis[a] Scarlet fever[a] Tuberculosis Typhoid fever[a] Yersiniosis[a]	Giardiasis[a]	Hepatitis A[a] Q fever (R) Tick-borne encephalitis
Salads	Staphylococcal food poisoning	Cholera O-group 1 Cholera-like disease (non-O1) Enteritis due to Escherichia coli[a] Paratyphoid fever[a] Typhoid fever[a]	—	Hepatitis A[a]
Seafood	Botulism Ichthyosarcotoxism Shellfish poisoning Vibrio parahaemolyticus food poisoning	Cholera O-group 1 Cholera-like disease (non-O1) Paratyphoid fever[a] Salmonellosis[a] Shigellosis[a] Typhoid fever[a]	Angiostrongyliasis Anisakiasis	Hepatitis A[a] Poliomyelitis[a] Acute viral gastroenteropathy[a]

Table 37 (*continued*)

| Source | Food poisoning | Food-borne infection | | |
		Bacterial	Parasitic	Viral or rickettsial (R)
Vegetables	*Bacillus cereus* food poisoning Pesticide intoxication	Cholera O-group 1 Cholera-like disease (non-O1) Leptospirosis Listeriosis Paratyphoid fever[a] Salmonellosis[a] Shigellosis[a] Typhoid fever[a]	Amoebiasis[a] Angiostron-gyliasis Giardiasis[a]	
Other sources: Contamination by food handlers	Staphylococcal food poisoning	Paratyphoid fever[a] Shigellosis[a] Typhoid fever[a]	Amoebiasis[a] Giardiasis[a]	Hepatitis A[a]
Contamination by flies	—	Cholera O-group 1 Cholera-like disease (non-O1) Paratyphoid fever[a] Shigellosis[a] Typhoid fever[a]	Amoebiasis[a]	—
Contamination by rodents	—	Leptospirosis	—	Lassa fever[a] Lymphocytic chorio-meningitis
Honey	—	Botulism, infant	—	—
Mushrooms	Intoxication (muscarine or phalloidine)	—	—	—
Unspecified	Chemical intoxication	—	—	Acute viral gastroenter-opathy (Norwalk-type)[a]

[a] Person-to-person transmission is also possible.

Food-borne infections may result from:

—consumption of insufficiently cooked meat (smoked meat), undercooked eggs;
—consumption of raw shellfish, untreated milk, dairy products or raw vegetables;
—inadequate refrigeration during storage;
—cross-contamination of properly processed food by contaminated raw food or utensils;
—infected food handlers in combination with poor personal hygiene;
—adulteration of food;
—use of contaminated wrappings during transport and storage;
—contact with flies, crawling insects, rodents;
—contamination of crops by night soil used as fertilizer, sewage, or contaminated recycled water.

Outbreaks of food-borne disease are increasing in frequency in developed countries because of the increasing extent of industrial food processing, factory farming, mass catering and extensive use of refrigeration. The origin of an outbreak is obvious when a single dish has been contaminated and causes illness in a group of people who have eaten a meal together, but is less so when the contaminated food has been sent to a number of different places remote from one another or when secondary foci are less severe than the primary one and are not immediately recognized, or if victims disperse after consuming the contaminated food.

(e) Transmission of diseases originating in the environment
The epidemic diseases that can result from the environment are listed in Table 38.

Water, soil and air may serve as vehicles for infectious agents and poisons. They may be contaminated by human and animal pathogens, and, in addition, soil may be the reservoir of other agents, such as fungi. Soil and water may contain the infective agent or its intermediate host, such as the water snail in which the agent of schistosomiasis develops. Dust and air may be vehicles for the indirect transmission (sometimes mistaken for direct) of an agent from person to person or animal to person. They may also disseminate agents present in soil and water. Large droplets of infective material fall rapidly to the ground whereas smaller droplets evaporate rapidly and leave droplet nuclei (aerosols) that may stay in suspension in the air for a long time and easily penetrate to the pulmonary alveoli. Toxic insecticides and other poisonous chemicals may be dispersed in the environment.

The environment may cause either a cluster of cases, when several persons are infected simultaneously, a situation that is relatively easy to recognize, or a number of sporadic cases, when the persons concerned are dispersed; this makes contact tracing difficult. The

Table 38. Epidemic diseases transmitted by the environment

	Disease			
Source	Bacterial, chlamydial (C) or rickettsial (R)	Parasitic	Viral	Mycotic
Water	Cholera *Campylobacter* enteritis Enteritis due to *Escherichia coli*[a] Leptospirosis Melioidosis Paratyphoid[a] Salmonellosis[a] Shigellosis[a] Tularaemia Typhoid fever[a] Yersiniosis[a]	Amoebiasis[a] Dracontiasis Giardiasis[a] Meningo-encephalitis due to *Naegleria* and *Acanthamoeba* Schistosomiasis Toxoplasmosis	Adenovirus 3 infection[a] Conjunctivitis, inclusion Viral hepatitis A Viral hepatitis non-A, non-B Acute viral gastroenteropathy	— —
Soil	Leptospirosis Melioidosis Tetanus	—	—	Coccidioidomycosis Cryptococcosis Histoplasmosis Sporotrichosis
Dust	Anthrax, inhalation Botulism, infant Melioidosis Meningococcal meningitis Q fever (R) Streptococcal infection[a]	— —	—	Lymphocytic choriomeningitis Coccidioidomycosis Cryptococcosis Histoplasmosis Sporotrichosis, pulmonary
Air (aerosols)	Legionnaires' disease Ornithosis (C) Plague, pulmonary[a] Q fever (R)		Influenza[a] Rabies Smallpox[b]	
Air (droplet spread)	Meningococcal meningitis Pertussis[a] Plague, pneumonic[a] Pneumonia due to *Mycoplasma pneumoniae*[a] Pneumonia due to *Streptococcus pneumoniae*[a]	—	Pneumonitis, viral[a] Haemorrhagic conjunctivitis[a] Enteroviral vesicular stomatitis with exanthem[a] Enteroviral vesicular pharyngitis[a] Gammaherpes-viral mononucleosis[a] Measles[a] Mumps[a] Epidemic myalgia[a] Rubella[a] Varicella[a]	—

[a] Person-to-person transmission is also possible.
[b] Now considered to have been eradicated.

contamination may be immediately obvious or its effects may be delayed, sometimes for a relatively long period; contact tracing is then again difficult.

The various modes of transmission are summarized in Table 39.

Table 39. Modes of transmission of diseases from the environment to man

Reservoir	Direct transmission	Indirect transmission
Soil	Contact	Dust Water Animals Food and drinks
Water	Drinking Bathing	Soil Animals Food and drinks
Air	Inhalation	Dust Aerosols Air-conditioning

Statistical analysis. The association of a disease with an epidemiological factor may be fortuitous or may result from a cause-effect relationship. The hypotheses of causation must be tested for chances of error. Statistical methods may indicate the probability of an error, or the validity of the hypothesis if the calculations show that it is "statistically significant", i.e., the probability of error P is less than 5% ($P < 0.05$). Statistical methods are discussed in Annex 2.

5.3 Laboratory data

5.3.1 Laboratory methods

The value of laboratory examinations depends on the proper collection, storage, and shipment of specimens and their examination by suitable methods in competent laboratories.

A number of different methods are used in laboratories to demonstrate an etiological agent: visualization, isolation, cultivation and characterization of the agent itself, or the use of serological tests to demonstrate an immunological host response.

Visualization of the agent. In the classical techniques, smears of pathological material are stained, e.g., with Gram stain for bacteria and Giemsa for parasites. New techniques have recently been developed that show the agent or its antigens by using a specific serum coupled with a fluorescent dye (immunofluorescence (IF)) or an enzyme reacting on a substrate to produce a colour (enzyme immunoassay (EIA) or enzyme-linked immunosorbent assay (ELISA)). These new techniques may be used for almost all agents— bacterial, rickettsial, chlamydial, viral, and parasitic—provided that a monospecific or group-specific serum is available to react with the agent concerned. These new techniques represent a considerable advance, particularly for viruses. Techniques using precipitation in agar gel, such as counterimmunoelectrophoresis (CIE), may be used for certain diseases if an antigenic extract can be prepared from the causative agent and if sufficiently potent specific antisera are available. Histopathological and cytological techniques may show specific lesions caused in organs by the agent and can sometimes be used to visualize the agent itself. Biochemical reactions in body fluids (blood and cerebrospinal fluid) have a diagnostic value in some diseases, as in the chemical examination of cerebrospinal fluid.

Visualization methods have the great advantage that the results are available in a few hours. The general indications for the use of these techniques are summarized in Table 40.

Table 40. Use of visualization and other techniques for laboratory examinations

	Techniques					
	Direct microscopy				Histopatho-	
Agent	Gram stain	Giemsa stain	IF[a]	EIA and ELISA[b]	logical and cytological	Bio- chemical
Parasitic		+	+	+	+	+
Mycotic		+	+	+	+	+
Bacterial	+	+	+	+	+	+
Mycoplasmal		+	+	+		+
Rickettsial		+	+	+	+	+
Chlamydial		+	+	+	+	+
Viral			+	+	+[c]	+

[a] Immunofluorescence.
[b] EIA: enzyme immunoassay; ELISA: enzyme-linked immunosorbent assay.
[c] Electron microscopy in certain diseases.

Isolation of the agent. Some pathogenic bacteria may be isolated on standard culture media but many organisms, e.g., certain cultivable parasites, require special media that are not available in all laboratories. In particular, when no specific agent is suspected, a laboratory will have to use a battery of selective enrichment media to eliminate saprophytes. The same applies to mycotic and mycoplasmal agents.

Rickettsiae, chlamydiae and viruses require living cells in which to develop so that animals and/or cell-culture systems have to be inoculated. Here again, several of these substrates will be required when there is no indication as to the identity of the agent, which is often the case at the beginning of an epidemic.

Although isolation techniques are expensive and time-consuming— they take approximately 1–3 weeks—they have to be used if it is necessary to ascertain the exact nature of the agent. They may also provide evidence of the appearance of a new "variant" of an agent, with unusual biological properties; in this case, visualization techniques based on previously applicable specific sera may have failed to identify the agent. Such a variant may also require different therapy and methods of prevention, as compared with those normally used.

Serological tests. As a rule, when direct visualization methods and/or isolation show that a causative agent is present in an individual, serological tests must be carried out to confirm this result. Such tests show that specific antibodies appeared at the time of the illness and thus prove that it was that agent that caused the infection and not one accidentally present at the time (a "passenger" agent) or the agent of a chronic infection. Furthermore, the possibility of visualizing or isolating an agent that is present transiently during the acute phase may be small, whereas antibodies, being constantly present soon after infection, are easier to detect. If no particular etiological agent is suspected, the laboratory will have to test the sera with a large battery of different antigens; if these are not available locally, it will have to call on the services of a WHO collaborating centre.

The serological methods that may be used include the following:

—agglutination (mainly for bacterial agents);
—complement fixation;
—haemagglutination inhibition (mainly for viruses);
—neutralization;
—immune electron microscopy;
—immunofluorescence;
—enzyme immunoassay.

The laboratory may indicate to the investigator which serological methods should be preferred in terms of sensitivity versus specificity. Since, in certain diseases, the antibodies (immunoglobulin G) may persist at a high titre for some time, the laboratory tests must show that they appeared or increased considerably during the disease. It is recommended, therefore, that two serum specimens (paired sera) be tested—one collected soon after disease onset and one at least 7 days later. To confirm that a particular agent is present, the results of such tests should show that the appropriate antibodies appeared (seroconversion) or increased in titre by a factor of at least four. A smaller increase might be due to unavoidable test-to-test variation. However, in some diseases a high antibody titre in a single specimen indicates a recent infection. Tests have now been developed to detect immuno-globulin M (IgM) instead of immunoglobulin G (IgG), as the former disappears more quickly after the disease and a single serum specimen can give a significant result. The use of serological methods is summarized in Table 41.

Table 41. Serological evidence of recent infection

Specimen	Result
Single serum	Presence of IgM specific for the incriminated agent (non-specific reactions must be eliminated)
	High titre of specific undifferentiated (IgM + IgG) antibodies, if higher than the long-lasting immunity level for the disease concerned
Paired sera[a]	Fourfold increase in titre (IgM + IgG) with specific antigen

[a] The first sample should be collected soon after disease onset, the second at least 7 days later.

5.3.2 Significance of results

Multiple positive results obtained by visualization of an agent, cultivation and/or serological tests on collected specimens are not always significant in terms of the etiological role of that agent in the outbreak. Negative results do not always mean that the hypothesis as to the responsibility of an agent can be eliminated; they may be the consequence of inappropriate techniques. Both positive and negative results must be interpreted with caution, bearing in mind the possible causes of error listed in Table 42.

Statistical methods may be able to show whether the presence of a certain agent or its antibodies in affected and unaffected population groups is a factor that can be significantly associated with an outbreak (Annex 2).

5.4 Identifying the source of the outbreak

The role of the EHS coordinator is to reach a conclusion about the source of the outbreak on which control measures can be based. If the approach shown in Fig. 7 is followed, the collection and analysis

Table 42. Causes of error in the interpretation of laboratory results

False positive results	False negative results
Visualization methods	
Saprophyte present	Inappropriate sampling
Non-specific staining	Inappropriate dye
	Need for electron microscopy
	Scarcity of agent in specimen
Isolation methods	
Trivial agent easier to detect than causative agent or withstands storage conditions of specimen better[a]	Inappropriate sampling: specimen inadequate or sample taken at wrong time
Concurrent endemic infection (e.g., malaria, schistosomiasis)	Damage to agent by storage conditions: heat, freezing-thawing cycles
Only one of two concurrent agents is isolated	Inappropriate laboratory techniques
Concurrent pathogen in an outbreak primarily caused by a toxic agent	"New" agent requiring unusual conditions for isolation
Contamination of specimens or reagents	Presence of immune complexes
Serological methods	
Presence of antibodies to endemic disease or trivial agent	Sample taken at wrong time
Antibodies cross-react with antigenically related agent	Inappropriate techniques: lack of specificity and sensitivity
Non-specific reaction	Inappropriate antigen battery
Previous immunization	Presence of immune complexes
For IgM antibodies: Excess of IgG Presence of rheumatoid factors	

[a] Saprophytes may become pathogenic in immunocompromised or undernourished individuals.

of the clinical data should yield a list of possible agents that might have caused the observed syndrome. Analysis of the epidemiological data, in turn, should lead to hypotheses as to the conditions that favoured the outbreak, the mode of transmission of the disease and the likelihood that it will spread, and these hypotheses can be evaluated by statistical analysis. The results of laboratory examinations should enable the etiological agent to be identified, either definitely or with some degree of probability. These data are summarized in Table 43.

Table 43. Data required as basis for control measures

Clinical data	Epidemiological data	Laboratory data

Features of:
  mild cases
  severe cases
Sequelae rate
Death rate
	Incidence:
	  in time
	  in place
	  in population groups
	  (attack rates by sex,
	  age, occupation, etc.)
	Mode of transmission:
	  person-to-person
	  common source of
	  infection
	  common source of
	  infection followed
	  by person-to-person
	  transmission
	Communicable period
		Confirmatory diagnosis
		of cases:
		  isolation of agent
		  serological survey
		Infection rate
		Apparent/inapparent
		  case rate
		Immune status of
		  population at risk

The investigator may nevertheless be faced by difficulties in reaching the correct conclusion at this stage. The laboratory results may arrive late, and the "art" for the epidemiologist is to identify the source of the outbreak quickly and correctly, on the basis of the clinical and epidemiological data alone, while remembering that laboratory examinations are necessary, not only in determining the etiology, but also in finding subclinical cases that can nevertheless spread the disease.

Several new epidemic diseases have emerged during the last 20 years, for a variety of reasons:

—the causative agent, although well known for many years, has recently been introduced into a new receptive population, or its pathogenicity has changed because more virulent strains have been selected, resistant or mutant strains developed, or immuno-compromised hosts became available;

—the causative agent, although present in the environment, did not affect the human population until man interfered with its ecology, e.g., Lassa, Marburg and Ebola viruses, the agent of haemorrhagic fever with renal syndrome (Korean haemorrhagic fever) ("Hantaan virus"), and Legionella bacteria;

—the true causative agent (or agents) is still unknown, e.g., Guillain-Barré syndrome, Kawasaki syndrome, Reye's syndrome, etc.;

—natural disasters have introduced a new specific pathogen into the environment, heightened the susceptibility of the population to infection, or intensified the transmission of local pathogens.

In such circumstances, an outbreak must be investigated in a particularly methodical way, especially in establishing its characteristics, such as the incubation period, period of communicability, portals of entry, routes of excretion, statistical significance of associated factors and recommended methods for laboratory diagnosis. Socioeconomic development may also create other new epidemic diseases. Fortunately, however, some epidemic diseases, e.g., smallpox, can be eradicated, or brought under control, e.g., measles, if man is the only reservoir of the infectious agent.

BIBLIOGRAPHY

ACHA, P. N. & SZYFRES, B. *Zoonoses and communicable diseases common to man and animals*. Washington, DC, Pan American Health Organization, 1980 (Scientific Publication No. 35A).

BENENSON, A. S., ed. *Control of communicable diseases in man*, 14th ed. Washington, DC, American Public Health Association, 1985.

EVANS, A. S. *Viral infections of humans: epidemiology and control*. New York & London, Plenum Medical Book Company, 1976.

EVANS, A. S. & FELDMAN, H. *Bacterial infections of humans: epidemiology and control*. New York & London, Plenum Medical Book Company, 1982.

South-East Asia Region meeting on research in viral haemorrhagic fevers in the Eastern Mediterranean, South-East Asian, and Western Pacific Regions. WHO Regional Office for South-East Asia, unpublished document, SEA/Haem. Fever/37, 1980.

The management of emergencies caused by "unusual" diseases. Unpublished WHO document, WHO/SMM/80.16.

WHO Technical Report Series, No. 598, 1976 (*Microbiological aspects of food hygiene*: report of a WHO Expert Committee with the participation of FAO).

WHO Technical Report Series, No. 639, 1979 (*Human viruses in water, wastewater and soil*: report of a WHO Scientific Group).

WHO Technical Report Series, No. 642, 1980 (*Viral respiratory diseases*: report of a WHO Scientific Group).

WHO Technical Report Series, No. 682, 1982 (*Bacterial and viral zoonoses*: report of a WHO Expert Committee with the participation of FAO).

WHO Technical Report Series, No. 719, 1985 (*Arthropod-borne and rodent-borne viral diseases*: report of a WHO Scientific Group).

6. General measures for the control of outbreaks

An outbreak of communicable disease may be controlled by:

—eliminating or reducing the source of infection;
—interrupting transmission;
—protecting persons at risk.

It may take some time before the exact nature of the causative agent is known and this will delay the application of specific control measures, such as the immunization of persons at risk or the treatment of carriers. In an emergency, therefore, the first step must be to try to interrupt transmission, since the epidemiological investigations will quickly provide some indication of the possible mode of transmission involved. This may be:

—person-to-person transmission, whether direct or indirect;
—common-source infection;
—a combination of both.

General protective measures to be taken in various types of outbreak are described below; specific additional protective measures applicable once the causative agent has been determined are given for each disease in Annex 3.

In emergency conditions, control measures may require a degree of improvisation whenever the necessary equipment is not immediately available; this is not difficult when the principles to be followed are well understood.

6.1 Protective measures in outbreaks of diseases with person-to-person transmission

Protective measures may be necessary in respect of patients, their contacts and the community.

6.1.1 Patients

The health personnel participating in medical care, evacuation, specimen collection, laboratory examination, post-mortems, and field operations during epidemiological investigations will all require protection. Immune personnel (after immunization or natural

107

infection) should be employed if possible. However, when the agent is unknown or if there is no vaccine, general precautions are indicated which must be adapted to the degree of contagiousness of the disease; they should be reliable but not excessive, so as to avoid waste of time and money.

General precautions. The most effective general precaution is careful *hand-washing* after any contact with a patient, or with a suspected case. Protective measures may be divided into four categories, depending on the degree of communicability of the disease and its mode of transmission, as determined by the epidemiological investigations (Table 44). Nursing techniques and the facilities required to achieve the necessary level of protection are described briefly in Annex 4 and decontamination procedures in Annex 7. Appropriate protective measures for specific diseases are indicated in Annex 3.

Duration of precautions or isolation. The infective or contagious period is known for most communicable diseases. (See Table 32, which indicates the number of days during which precautions or isolation should be maintained in order to avoid direct or indirect transmission of the disease to other persons. This period is fixed by law in many countries.) When the agent is unknown, the period of contagiousness can be determined from the data on infective contacts collected during the epidemiological investigations, which may fit one of a number of different patterns (see Fig. 6).

Medical care. Even if strict isolation is necessary, the best possible medical care should be given to patients, who are often critically ill. The premises used for isolation should be equipped with at least minimal intensive care facilities.

Supportive care plays an important role in addition to specific therapy. Sedative and analgesic drugs are necessary to combat fever and pain or to control nausea and vomiting. Rehydration, relief of respiratory distress, or treatment of circulatory shock may be essential, depending on the disease. Such treatment may require serial monitoring of vital functions, e.g., blood and pulse pressure, erythrocyte volume fraction, central venous pressure, urine specific gravity and electrolytes, as well as electrocardiographic monitoring, blood-gas analysis, etc.

Medical evacuation. The precautions to be taken during the medical evacuation of acutely ill patients should be in line with those indicated in Table 44 for the protection of personnel. Moving a patient over long distances may be contraindicated if he or she is severely ill, particularly during the acute period of viral haemorrhagic fevers. Medical evacuation should therefore preferably be considered at the onset of symptoms, i.e., during the prodromal phase. Equipment for medical evacuation is described in Annex 4.

Table 44. General precautions to be taken in outbreaks of diseases with person-to-person transmission

Contagiousness of patients	Route of transmission	Type of protective measures	Diseases[a]
Moderate	Direct or indirect contact with one or several of: faeces, urine, oral secretions, mucocutaneous discharges, blood and articles contaminated by any of these	A. *Standard precautions* Hand-washing, gloves, gown, mask, safe disposal of contaminated articles, only authorized visitors admitted	Most infectious diseases (except for those requiring types B, C and D precautions) according to route(s) of transmission, including varicella and hepatitis B or unspecified hepatitis
High	Direct contact with persons and with faeces and oral secretions	B. *Enteric isolation* Private room, contact precautions, visitors admitted under control	Cholera (in non-endemic areas), gastroenteritis in children caused by *Escherichia coli*, rotavirus, hepatitis A or unspecified hepatitis, *Salmonella*, *Shigella*, *Staphylococcus*, *Yersinia enterocolitica*, typhoid fever
	Direct contact with persons or oral secretions and droplets	C. *Respiratory isolation* Private room, masks, contact precautions, visitors admitted under control	Diphtheria, measles, meningococcal meningitis, meningococcal bacteraemia, rubella, staphylococcal pneumonia, tularaemia, pertussis
Very high	Direct contact with persons, and airborne (infective aerosols, droplet nuclei)	D. *Strict isolation* Private room, special devices constituting a microbiological barrier in a high-security ward, no visitors	Anthrax (pulmonary), disseminated zoster, plague (pneumonic), rabies, suspected smallpox, vaccinia (generalized), viral haemorrhagic fever (Crimean-Congo, Ebola, Lassa, Marburg—possibly yet undescribed viral diseases)

[a] This list is indicative only and may be subject to change, depending on local circumstances.

Disinfection. Safe disposal of excreta, vomit, urine, secretions, discharges, dressings and bedding is recommended, and may be mandatory, depending on the mode of transmission of the disease; this may be achieved by using disinfectants (Annex 7) or by incineration. If contaminated material is to be transported, the double-bagging procedure must be used (see Annex 4).

Terminal disinfection of bedding and bedrooms is required only for a limited number of diseases, as mentioned in Annex 3. Whenever corpses may be a source of infection, they should be wrapped in fabric soaked with a disinfectant such as formaldehyde, further insulated by a plastic sheet and sealed in a plastic bag. Direct contact with corpses during funerals—which is a tradition in certain countries—must be avoided or at least kept to a minimum, and maximum use must be made of disinfection.

6.1.2 Contacts

Persons who are in contact with an infectious patient during the contagious period may be at risk of becoming infected and therefore of becoming in their turn a source of infection. However, the magnitude of this risk is not the same for all diseases and for all persons, and must therefore be assessed and preventive measures adapted accordingly.

Assessment of the risk of infection. The following factors influence the risk of infection:

—the time of contact, and in particular whether it falls within the period of contagiousness;
—the degree of contagiousness of the disease;
—the closeness of contact and the routes of transmission to which the person may have been exposed;
—the specific and non-specific immunity of the person concerned.

During control operations, the time of contact and the closeness of contact are the essential factors in determining the measures to be taken. Two types of contact may be distinguished:

1. a *"close contact"* is a person who has had occasional face-to-face contact, has given personal care without protection measures, or has shared the same meal or room during the period of communicability, or handled the patient's belongings (if indirect transmission is involved);

2. a *"possible contact"* is a person who may have been exposed either:

—at some distance away from a highly contagious case during the period of communicability in circumstances not satisfying the above criteria, e.g, in public transport, in the next bed in a hospital, or in the same workplace; or

—through close contact with a patient, probably, but not certainly, outside the period of communicability, particularly if there is some doubt about its duration.

Quarantine. This is used to restrict the contacts of a well person who has been exposed to a patient with an infectious disease during the communicability period. Quarantine must be adapted to the risk to which the person concerned was exposed and the risk that he represents for the community. The restrictions imposed should not be excessive from either the humanitarian or economic point of view. The four types of quarantine that may be used, depending on the communicability of the disease and the closeness of contact, are indicated in Table 45.

Even when a person has been in close contact with a highly contagious patient, it may be advisable to begin with type 1 quarantine, followed by type 2 when the incubation period is nearly over, and by type 3 or 4 if symptoms appear.

A large number of contacts may have to be dealt with in a few days. They should therefore be divided into "possible contact" and "close contact" groups, which should be dealt with separately. Each group should be divided into cohorts depending on the expected time of onset of the disease concerned; this will be determined by the range of incubation periods following the infective contact (see Fig. 6). When there are numerous contacts, cohorts should be separated physically so as to avoid introducing new suspects into a group that

Table 45. Types of quarantine

Type of contact	Type of quarantine	Requirements
Possible contact (or probable infectious contact, during the incubation period)	1. Self-surveillance	The person is asked to stay at home, to restrict contacts to a limited number of known persons, and to change to type-2 quarantine if any premonitory symptom develops (e.g., fever)
Possible contact (as above)	2. Medical surveillance	The person reports daily to a medical centre or is visited daily by a physician
Close contact, (moderately communicable disease)	3. Standard isolation	Enteric or respiratory isolation (see Table 44) in private room (specialized medical personnel)
Close contact, (highly communicable disease)	4. Strict isolation	Admission to special isolation quarters with equipment for microbiological barrier nursing

has already completed part of the quarantine period and would then be obliged to begin the whole period again.

6.1.3 The community

The protection of patients and the isolation of their contacts in quarantine will considerably decrease the risk for the community. However, as it may not be possible to identify all patients and contacts, other methods also have to be considered.

Mass immunization. Emergency mass immunization is possible for a limited number of diseases (see section 6.3), but there will inevitably be some delay before a large enough part of the population is protected by the vaccine; other methods may therefore be necessary during the interim period.

Restrictions on mass gatherings. Such restrictions may be indicated, including the closure of schools and even of public places, but their effectiveness is generally limited.

Restrictions on travel. These may involve the establishment of a *cordon sanitaire* in order to isolate the epidemic focus or to prevent the entry of infectious persons into a country. There is, however, more justification for a *cordon sanitaire* when immunization is possible and the aim is to make sure that unimmunized persons do not travel and thereby carry the disease to other places. Before a *cordon sanitaire* around an epidemic focus can be established, it is first necessary to define the boundaries of both the infected and the receptive areas. This is expensive, and requires close cooperation between the health services, the police, and the army, without which the measure may be ineffective. Furthermore, considerable economic loss and inconvenience may be caused to individuals.

Strengthening of epidemiological surveillance. This has proved to be both more efficient and less expensive than the *cordon sanitaire*. Case finding, contact tracing, and prevention of transmission should all be strengthened in any group in which suspected cases have appeared.

Community participation. Keeping the community informed will reduce the risk of panic. If the community can be induced to participate in the control measures, this will contribute considerably to their effectiveness.

6.2 Control of outbreaks caused by a common source of infection

Whenever an outbreak is caused by a common source of infection—whether by arthropods, rodents, direct contact with vertebrate animals, food, water, air, soil or a combination of any of these—control methods should be based on source reduction and interruption of transmission. The assistance of a specialist entomologist, mammalogist, veterinarian or sanitary engineer may be required.

6.2.1 Mosquito-borne diseases

Mosquitos capable of transmitting diseases to man belong to several species and their control raises technical problems that require the assistance of a specialized team. They constitute the most important group of insect vectors, transmitting malaria, filariasis and a number of arboviruses, including those causing outbreaks of yellow fever, dengue and dengue haemorrhagic fever, Japanese encephalitis, New World equine encephalitides, and several dengue-like fevers. Only the females bite man. They lay their eggs in impounded water, selected according to the preference of the species. The time necessary for the eggs to hatch and for the larvae they produce to become pupae and adults is reduced at higher temperatures. If it is to be cost-effective, mosquito control requires methodical planning of strategy, logistics, and field operations. It should be noted that a patient with a mosquito-borne disease, e.g., dengue or yellow fever in *Aedes aegypti*-infested areas or malaria in *Anopheles*-infested areas, should not be moved into an area where such mosquitos are present; such movement may be subject to local health regulations.

Strategy. The choice of the methods to be used in field operations will be affected by the factors listed in Table 46. The final choice will depend on a comparison of the different methods in terms of their cost-effectiveness.

Logistics. This requires a consideration of the following:

—the availability of local stockpiles of insecticides and spraying equipment;
—funding for personnel, transport, insecticides, equipment and supplies;
—manpower, including suitably trained local staff (supervisors, spraymen, drivers and mechanics);
—the supply of selected insecticides and spraying equipment (see Annex 6);
—protective clothing for spraymen;
—safety instructions for the handling of insecticides and guidance on the management of insecticide poisoning (see Annex 6);
—arrangements for aerial spraying;
—the provision of adequate and appropriate transport.

Of these, the last is vital for successful emergency vector control operations, and interdepartmental agreements should exist on the

Table 46. Factors affecting the choice of mosquito control methods

Factor	Implications for choice of method
Affected area: size, number of households, vegetation, wind	Affects selection of spraying technique and equipment
Responsible vector species	Affects selection of insecticide (efficacy/resistance, cost, availability)
Breeding habits	Determine practicability of larval control by environmental and/or chemical methods
Host choice	Determines sites for application of control measures by defining contact between mosquito, viraemic vertebrate hosts and man
Feeding habits	May affect the choice of indoor as opposed to outdoor spraying
Resting habits	If largely indoors, the use of residual contact insecticides applied indoors may be indicated; if outdoors, then aerosol formulations should be applied by aerial spray
Flight range	Determines size of area where vector-control measures will be required.

rapid transfer of vehicles from one department to another in emergencies. Sufficient spare parts should be kept in store to maintain existing vehicles in a roadworthy condition, and workshop facilities should be available, staffed by an adequate number of competent mechanics to keep the vehicles on the road. The transport available should include vehicles for carrying spraymen and a 5-tonne truck should be on call for transporting heavy equipment and large quantities of insecticides and stores. Four-wheel-drive vehicles may be necessary and covered pick-ups capable of carrying 0.5–1.5-tonne loads may be required for general use. Minibuses may be suitable in some circumstances for carrying spraymen.

Field operations. In emergency situations, the methods used for the control of mosquitos will vary according to the mosquito species concerned (for details see Annex 6). They include insecticide spraying, personal protection, source reduction and environmental management.

The spraying of insecticides to which the vectors are susceptible is used in emergency measures, mainly to control the mosquito vectors of malaria and epidemic arboviral diseases, and can rapidly reduce the density of the man-biting segment of the vector population and thus quickly stop or drastically reduce transmission to man. The methods of application are described in Annex 6.

Well maintained bed-nets and mesh screens fitted to doors and windows can give good personal protection against mosquitos. Long sleeves and trousers are recommended. Repellents have only a temporary effect.

The cooperation of the population in source reduction in the affected area should be enlisted, through public notices, the media, and government officials, and in assisting personnel carrying out preliminary geographical reconnaissance and spraying operations. The local population should also be encouraged to carry out communal or individual activities to reduce vector breeding sites. *Aedes aegypti* mosquitos can breed very successfully in small containers present in urban and domestic refuse, e.g., tyres, tins, jars and flowerpots, and among agricultural debris, e.g., split cocoa pods and coconut husks.

Environmental management constitutes an important means of controlling mosquito vectors, both in an emergency and long-term. Open drains and ditches frequently provide breeding sites for large numbers of certain mosquito species. Drains and ditches should be kept in good order so as to ensure gravitational flow and the disposal of unwanted water and effluent. Soak-pits require sealed covers, and latrines should have well-fitting lids. Flooding of pastures may be reduced by appropriate drainage. Small pools of water scattered in and around villages can be eliminated by filling them in. A sanitary engineer should be consulted.

6.2.2 Diseases transmitted by other arthropods

Information on the identification of other arthropods of medical importance, control methods, and the insecticides and equipment required, is given in Annex 6.

6.2.3 Rodent-borne diseases

Rodents may be reservoirs of a number of epidemic diseases, including leptospirosis, plague, tularaemia, yersiniosis, lymphocytic choriomeningitis, Lassa fever, Junin and Machupo haemorrhagic fever, and haemorrhagic fever with renal syndrome. Certain rodent-borne diseases may be passed from rodents to man by "direct" transmission, others through arthropod vectors. "Direct" transmission occurs as a result of contamination of food and water by rodent urine and can thus also be regarded as indirect.

The results of the epidemiological investigation will determine which procedure(s)—environmental improvement, rodent-proofing, and domestic rodent extermination by rodenticides—are to be used and in which order. Table 47 gives some information on these methods and further details on the use of rodenticides are given in Annex 6.

In an outbreak of plague, the first step in control operations is to use insecticides to kill rat fleas before using rodenticides to kill the rats.

Table 47. Control of domestic rodent populations

Method	Procedures required
Environmental improvement	Storage of food in rodent-proof containers
	Inspecting and periodically moving stacks of food, hay, etc.
	Collecting food wastes
	Locating dumps well away from inhabited areas
	Eliminating nesting sites, such as piles of debris
	Improving warehousing to eliminate rat harbourages
Rodent-proofing	Finding and stopping all openings in buildings through which rodents can enter, particularly spaces under doors and where pipes pass through walls; sealing cracks in walls
	Sealing of sewage systems and conduits for electric cables
	Fitting collars around the trunks of trees to prevent access for nesting
Extermination	Using poisoned baits (anticoagulants and acute poisons, with suitable precautions to avoid accidents to children and domestic animals) (see Annex 6)
	Trapping (break-back traps)
	Gassing with fumigants

6.2.4 Zoonoses

Different routes of transmission to man are possible, as follows:

—direct;
—through arthropods and rodents;
—through food and the environment.

Direct transmission is mainly an occupational risk of veterinary personnel, farmers, and hunters, and may be more frequent in areas of poor hygiene. Control measures for outbreaks resulting from direct contact with animals vary, depending on the diseases and circumstances, as shown in Table 48.

6.2.5 Food-borne diseases

Food-borne diseases may be divided into intoxications (food poisoning) and infections (Table 37). Outbreaks are most frequently caused by *Salmonella, Clostridium perfringens, Staphylococcus aureus, Bacillus cereus, Campylobacter, Escherichia coli, Clostridium botulinum,* and *Yersinia enterocolitica.* However, in many cases, the origin of food-

Table 48. Control measures for major zoonoses transmitted
directly to man[a]

Disease	Measures applicable to man	Measures applicable to animals
Anthrax	Precautions against contact with infected animals (goats, cattle, sheep) and their products and contaminated environment; strict isolation of pulmonary anthrax	Vaccination, placing of herds under quarantine, antibiotic treatment of sick animals, protection of environment
Brucellosis	Precautions against occupational risks, pasteurization of milk, antibiotic treatment	Serological testing of livestock Bovines, goats, sheep: slaughter of sick animals, vaccination of others Swine: slaughter of sick animals, placing of herds under quarantine
Campylobacter enteritis	Precautions against contact with infected poultry, thorough cooking of foodstuffs, pasteurization of milk	Hygiene of flocks
Cercopithecid herpesvirus 1 disease (simian B disease)	Precautions in handling recently caught Old World monkeys	Quarantine of laboratory monkeys
Echinococcosis[b]	Precautions against contact with infected dogs	Prevention of access by dogs to raw viscera of sheep
Haemorrhagic fevers (HF):		
Ebola and Marburg virus diseases	Precautions in handling recently caught monkeys in Africa; human immune plasma seems of value	Quarantine of laboratory monkeys
Junin HF	Specific immune globulin given during the first week; a vaccine is under development	Use of herbicides in shrub-covered areas to eliminate field rodents
Lassa fever	Human immune plasma of high antibody content and antiviral drugs	Control of multimammate rat (*Mastomys natalensis*)
Machupo HF	Human hyperimmune serum or globulin	Elimination of domestic and peridomestic rats (*Calomys*)
Lymphocytic choriomeningitis	Control mouse population in houses; avoid hamsters as pets; laboratory precautions	No control possible; surveillance of colonies of laboratory mice

Table 48 (continued)

Disease	Measures applicable to man	Measures applicable to animals
Ornithosis	No vaccine, chemo-prophylaxis based on tetracyclines	Quarantine and mass treatment of fowl in infected farms
Monkeypox	Prevention of contact with infected animals	Quarantine of primates
Q fever	Formalin-inactivated vaccine for occupation-ally exposed groups, pasteurization of milk	Incineration of placentas and fetal membranes of cattle and sheep
Rabies	Immune globulin and post-exposure immuniz-ation; pre-exposure im-munization for exposed professional groups	Vaccination of dogs, cats and cattle
Rat-bite fever	Disinfection of bites	Control of rat population
Salmonellosis	Prevention of contact with infected pets such as dogs, monkeys, hamsters; hygiene measures for farm-workers	Hygiene in farming
Tanapox virus disease	Prevention of contact with infected animals	Quarantine of primates
Toxoplasmosis	Prevention of contact, es-pecially in pregnancy, with raw meat and cat faeces; fly and cockroach control	No control possible; cats should not be kept on farms
Tularaemia	In contaminated areas, education of hunters in handling animals, pro-tective clothing against ticks, thorough cooking of meat, disinfection of water, laboratory pre-cautions (aerosols); treat-ment with antibiotics, immunization	Control of sheep ticks by acaricide applied by dip-ping or spraying
Yaba pox virus disease.	Prevention of contact with infected animals.	Quarantine of animals.
Yersiniosis	Control of pets and peri-domestic rodents, limi-tation of numbers of birds and fowls in public places	Potential carriers: rats, mice, hares, guinea-pigs, cats, dogs, sheep, swine, fowl, pigeons; no control possible

[a] See also Annex 3 under the individual diseases.
[b] Long incubation period (several months).

borne outbreaks remains unknown and viral agents, including hepatitis A virus, may be more frequently involved than indicated by present data. In addition, food may be contaminated by a large number of toxic chemicals (including pesticides) and their identification and the treatment of those affected require the services of a toxicologist.

Outbreaks of food-borne diseases usually constitute an emergency because of the threat that they pose to the life of the individual or to the community, irrespective of the number of cases. The measures to be taken when an outbreak occurs are either general, if the agent is unknown, or specific, if it has been identified. The occurrence of an outbreak should serve to stimulate improvements in food sanitation so as to ensure that a repetition is avoided.

General measures. These include:

(1) Elimination of ingested food:

—by gastric lavage (contraindicated in convulsing patients);
—by inducing vomiting (a portion of vomit should be kept for analysis).

(2) Symptomatic and supportive treatment, including:

—support of respiratory and cardiovascular functions (mouth-to-mouth respiration is to be avoided because vomited material may contain toxic substances);
—fluid and electrolyte replacement, if necessary, to correct acidosis. An oral glucose-electrolyte solution may be given if vomiting and diarrhoea are moderate.[1] If vomiting and diarrhoea cause large water losses, small doses of intravenous infusions may be necessary, but the quantity should be monitored to avoid pulmonary oedema.

(3) Nursing with appropriate precautions (if a contagious agent is suspected) in the handling of faeces and contaminated clothing and bed linen, and in the disinfection of faeces and contaminated articles.

(4) Prevention of extension of the outbreak by:

—withdrawal of suspect food; indiscriminate measures, such as the banning of international trade, may be more detrimental than effective;
—identification and treatment of contacts if person-to-person transmission can occur;
—identification of infected food handlers;
—identification of faulty practices in the processing and storage of food;
—re-establishment of good food sanitation.

---

[1] One level teaspoon of table salt, 1 level teaspoon of baking soda, and 8 level teaspoons of sugar per litre. Oral rehydration salts can also be used.

Specific measures. These may be taken where the agent has been identified, and are outlined below for various situations.

(1) *Bacterial food poisoning:*

—cholera, non-cholera vibrios and *Vibrio parahaemolyticus*: rehydration, supportive treatment and administration of tetracycline;
—enterotoxigenic *Escherichia coli*: rehydration; the value of antibiotics is uncertain;
—staphylococcal: rapid replacement of fluids by intravenous infusion;
—botulism: hospitalization is required, and trivalent botulinal antitoxin (types A, B and E) or a specific antitoxin (the type-E toxin is associated with seafood) should be used; sensitization to horse serum should be checked before administration, or the Besredka method used;[1]
—*Clostridium perfringens* food poisoning: supportive measures.

(2) *Non-bacterial food poisoning:*

—poisoning by mushrooms, poisonous plants, fish (*Ciguatera*), shellfish, and chemicals: supportive treatment together with specific therapy where it exists;
—pesticide poisoning, without a history of direct exposure: may be caused by contamination of vegetables, drinking-water or fish. Treatment will depend on the type of pesticide concerned, as follows. Organophosphorus compounds: atropine and reactivators (oximes) are required to combat the cholinesterase inhibition. Carbamate pesticides: these also inhibit cholinesterase but symptoms usually disappear rapidly and atropine is often not necessary; oximes should not be given. Toxic organochlorine compounds (endrin, aldrin, dieldrin): anticonvulsant treatment is required.

(3) *Infections:*

—bacterial infections with systemic symptoms: antibiotics;
—viral infections: symptomatic and supportive treatment only; antibiotics are not indicated. Viral hepatitis A requires prophylactic treatment of contacts of patients and persons known to have consumed the food concerned.

Food sanitation. The objective of food sanitation is to eliminate the risk of contamination by microorganisms at different stages in food production and processing, shown in Table 49. Health education is an important component of food sanitation, even in industrialized countries.

---

[1] The prescribed serum is injected in three doses, the first of 0.1 ml, the second, after 15 minutes, of 0.25 ml, and the remainder after a further 15 minutes. This method avoids possible allergic shock caused by sensitization to animal serum, and should be used even if the serum has been purified.

Table 49. Food sanitation

Type of production or stage in food production	Action to be taken or hazard to be prevented
Agricultural products (fruits, vegetables), meat, poultry, fish and other seafood, milk and cheese, eggs	Improvement of environmental sanitation, surveillance of zoonoses and animal-rearing methods
Processing: Thermal (sterilization, pasteurization, cooking)	Food being processed should be maintained at the necessary temperature for the appropriate length of time (pasteurization is either at 63–66 °C for at least 30 minutes, or not less than 72 °C for at least 15 seconds); the staphylococcus toxin is heat-stable
Salting and smoking	Always a risk of contamination
Freezing	Organisms are not destroyed by freezing and may multiply when thawing occurs
Handling	Improvement of hygiene and checking of carrier status of food handlers; cleanliness of utensils and surfaces
Preservation	Ineffective additives, and incorrect duration and temperature of storage may permit the development of microbes
Distribution	Contamination during transport and while on sale

6.2.6 Diseases with an environmental source of infection

A list of possible diseases has been given in Table 38. Whereas the control of diseases whose source is soil, dust or air poses specific problems to which it may be possible to find a local solution, water-borne diseases can usually be dealt with by the general methods summarized here. Certain other aspects of the control of diseases with an environmental source of infection are also dealt with, namely the disposal of solid wastes, housing and methods of dealing with the corpses of disease victims.

Drinking-water. Whenever drinking-water is incriminated in epidemic emergencies, simultaneous domestic water disinfection and protection of the community water-supply system are required.

The easiest way of disinfecting domestic drinking-water is to bring it to a "rolling boil" for 5 minutes. Filtration at home is not reliable (filters must be cleaned and boiled at frequent intervals). Addition of bleaching powder (chloride of lime) is not satisfactory because it has a low content of "available chlorine", produces an insoluble material, and is unstable on storage. High-strength hypochlorite materials available in granular form are preferable, while liquid chlorine is more suitable for water supplies in larger communities. On average, the quantity required to disinfect 1 m^3 (1000 litres) of drinking-water, for any one of these products, is:

Product	Quantity per 1000 l of water
Bleaching powder (25–35%)	2.3 g
High-strength calcium hypochlorite (70%)	1 g
Liquid bleach (5% sodium hypochlorite)	14 ml

Larger quantities can be used for the initial disinfection of wells and reservoirs. Test kits are available for determining residual free chlorine.

The measures to be used for protecting a community water-supply system are indicated in Table 50; the assistance of a sanitary engineer will be required in implementing them. Where it is suspected that tankers, wells, or reservoirs are contaminated, one of the following products should be used for disinfection:

Table 50. Protection of community water supplies

Water-supply system	Protection measures
Rural:	
Wells	Impervious concrete apron to exclude surface water; parapet, or eduction pipe sealed to prevent entry of animals; sides of well sealed water-tight for 3 m below ground level; correct operation of chlorine diffuser apparatus; surrounding area free from liquid wastes and privies (no human or animal faeces to be deposited within a protection perimeter of radius at least 30 m)
Springs	Ditch around spring to divert surface water; protection of collection structure from users; drainage below the outlet pipes; animals excluded from spring area; prevention of faecal contamination (as above)
Ponds, irrigation canals	Infiltration gallery in bed of pond properly constructed; extension of collecting well 1 m above ground; collecting well sealed water-tight throughout; inlet and outlet pipes properly fitted; correct operation of chlorine diffuser apparatus; prevention of faecal contamination
Urban:	
Waterworks and pumping stations	Correct operation of plant components; correct dosage of residual free chlorine; bacterial analyses
Reservoirs and mains	Inspection for clogging; bacterial analyses; prevention of animal access; prevention of back-siphoning
Water tankers	Disinfection before bringing into service (see p. 122)

	Quantity
Product	*per 100 l of water*
Bleaching powder (25–35 %)	10 g
High-strength calcium hypochlorite (70 %)	4.3 g
Liquid bleach (5 % sodium hypochlorite)	60 ml

After 12 hours, chlorinated drinking-water may be reintroduced into the system.

Simple devices for the chlorination of drinking-water in rural areas are available, as are portable powered hypochlorinators, which may be used in emergencies for urban water supplies.

Recreational water. The use of recreational water should be discouraged during epidemics.

Latrines. A number of different types of latrine are available for use in rural settings; the defects that may have to be remedied are listed in Table 51.

Disposal of liquid wastes. In rural areas, roadside cesspools for household waste liquids, including urine and latrine washing water, act as storage tanks until they are emptied, creating pools at the roadside in which animals wallow and where flies and mosquitos abound. Soak-pits filled with rough filter media are frequently non-operational because of rapid clogging; during epidemics, such places should be disinfected. Liquid wastes in roadside earth ditches and open drains should not be allowed to remain stagnant and the effluent should be chlorinated at the discharge point in watercourses during epidemics.

Table 51. Possible defects in latrines

Type of latrine	Possible defects
Conservancy	Absence of seat cover; bucket chamber not fly-proof; absence of drains and soakpit for wash wastes; no disinfection of buckets; spillages in transport of night soil; unsanitary intermediate depot; unsanitary disposal site; location less than 6 m from dwellings and less than 30 m from wells, springs, streams, ponds
Pit-type and bore-hole	Defective cover for the floor slab opening; inadequate fly control; lack of impervious ring at top of cavity to prevent emergence of larvae; defective lining of walls; liability to surface flooding; incorrect location (see above)
Septic tank	Cracks in the concrete tank; lack of flush water; inadequacy of absorption surface at effluent discharge point in ground; presence of flies

In urban areas, any defects in existing sewerage facilities should be remedied, including:

—breaks, blockages, and overflows in mains;
—inadequate storm overflows;
—defective treatment of sewage effluents before discharge into watercourses.

The use of raw sewage for farming is hazardous unless it has been treated in an oxidation pond. It should not be used in the cultivation of green vegetables that are eaten raw. Raw sewage discharged into a watercourse, a lake or the sea during epidemics creates risk zones that require chlorination. The use of discharge areas as recreational water should be prohibited during epidemics.

Solid wastes. These include animal droppings, stable manure, animal carcasses, and human faeces which may be deposited along roadsides in areas with poor sanitation, creating high-risk areas during epidemics because of the pullulation of flies and rodents and the danger of water pollution during rains and floods.

Solid wastes should ideally be collected and incinerated, especially in an emergency. Collection points should be sprayed with insecticides once a day. Particular attention should be given to cleanliness around eating-houses, markets and hospitals. Refuse dumps in backyards should be sprayed daily with insecticides. Disposal sites should be located at least 1 km away from inhabited areas and wastes should be covered by at least 60 cm of packed earth. Seepage water and surface run-off from refuse-disposal sites should be prevented from reaching watercourses.

Housing. The minimum requirements for sanitary conditions in housing should include the monitoring of tapwater and household sanitary privies. Overcrowding is another undesirable factor, since it leads to person-to-person transmission by the faecal-oral route, and droplet and aerosol transmission. Housing should be located away from polluted areas. The kitchen, cooking methods and health habits are key factors in preserving family health. Elimination of houseflies, use of mosquito screens and mosquito nets, and rat-proofing will protect against vector-borne diseases.

Other sources of infection. During epidemics, the dead may be a source of infection. For example, the handling and disposal of the bodies of cholera victims require special precautions. After the body orifices have been plugged with cotton wool soaked in an antiseptic, the corpses should be wrapped in shrouds dipped in antiseptic, such as hypochlorite. If possible, they should be placed in plastic bags. Those concerned with funerals should wash their hands before and after, and wear protective clothing, including masks and gloves if available. Similar precautions are applicable to other diseases where transmission is by direct contact, e.g., pulmonary plague, pulmonary anthrax, and certain haemorrhagic fevers.

6.3 Immunization and chemoprophylaxis

Immunization is normally intended as a prophylactic measure and those at risk should be immunized well in advance of exposure, since immunity takes at least 7 days to develop and for some diseases a series of injections is necessary. However, even with these limitations, immunization may be helpful in combating epidemics. In an emergency, the methods used to conduct a mass immunization campaign will be different from those employed under normal circumstances. For some diseases, passive immunization or chemoprophylaxis is also available for populations at risk.

6.3.1 Emergency immunization

Strategy. The following should be considered in deciding how to conduct an emergency mass immunization campaign.

— *The population to be immunized*: this may be children only (the vaccine dose required may then be lower) or adults only (occupational disease). Generally, all age groups in the infected area and surrounding areas will require immunization unless otherwise indicated by seroepidemiological investigations. This has the advantage of avoiding the need to investigate individual immunization status and simplifies the recording procedure. It also makes it easier to calculate the doses needed and to choose the location of immunization centres and itineraries.
— *The choice of vaccine*: different preparations may be available, and the choice will be determined by cost, mode of delivery (oral, bifurcated needle, subcutaneous) and thermostability.
— *Access to the population*: mobile teams may be required in rural areas, operating at designated points or by means of door-to-door visits on established itineraries; alternatively, immunizations may be carried out by health personnel at fixed centres in towns; a combination of both methods may be necessary if rural and urban areas are involved.
— *The definition of priority zones*: it will be necessary to decide whether immunization should be started at the centre of the epidemic focus and proceed outwards to the periphery or vice versa, and whether the populations of large cities at some distance away should also be immunized, such decisions being based on the results of epidemiological investigations.
— *The time schedule for completing the immunization campaign*: the aim should be to complete immunization as rapidly as possible and the logistics should be planned accordingly.

Logistics. In mounting the operations, the supplies, etc., shown in Table 52 will be necessary.

Evaluation. Problems may easily occur under emergency conditions. Attention should therefore be paid to the following:

—*the effectiveness of the cold chain*: the WHO Expanded Programme on Immunization has selected chemical indicators for monitoring the temperature of vaccines during shipment or storage and has recommended approved devices for cold storage;[1]

—*the potency of the vaccines*: this should be tested by the manufacturer and checked at the immunization points whenever there have been problems with the cold chain (freezing and thawing of live vaccines is detrimental to their potency; unopened vaccine ampoules put back into refrigeration at the end of a session should be the first to be used the next day);

—*the final evaluation of the efficacy of immunization*: this may be seen from the incidence curve of the epidemic; other parameters of immunization efficacy include the percentage coverage, the frequency of conversion, and antibody titres in samples of the population before and after immunization;

—*cost-benefit calculations*: these may provide useful information for public health administrators, and the costs may be compared with the estimated costs of regular preventive mass immunization.

Contraindications to immunization. These may be either general (persons with chronic pulmonary, cardiac, neurological or renal diseases), or specific to each vaccine. Live vaccines are generally contraindicated for immunocompromised persons and for pregnant women; this is particularly true of rubella vaccine for the latter because of the risk of malformation of the fetus. Killed vaccines have fewer contraindications. Live vaccines with a high egg protein content in the substrate may cause allergic reactions, e.g., urticaria, asthma, serum sickness, and anaphylactic shock. Children may require a lower dosage of vaccine, or a less reactogenic preparation. In an emergency, when medical examination of each individual person is not feasible, it will have to be decided whether such risks are ethically admissible.

6.3.2 Specific indications for immunization

These are shown in Table 53. Not all vaccines are able to interrupt rapidly the course of an outbreak. However, even if protection is delayed, such vaccines may protect the population at risk from a possible extension of the outbreak and prevent recurrences.

---

[1] *Chemical indicators for monitoring the cold chain. A review of laboratory tests and field trials.* Unpublished WHO document, EPI/CCIS/81.10.

Table 52. Requirements for emergency immunization operations

Item	Requirements
Vaccine	—vials of 20, 50 or 100 doses according to the population density and injection equipment (50- and 100-dose vials are more appropriate for jet injectors) —supplies ordered in advance and distributed to peripheral depots —quantities calculated to allow for admissible wastage —cold chain from central supply to immunization points, if necessary
Injection equipment: Syringes	—disposable individual syringes (rapid but expensive procedure; must not be reused) —reusable glass syringes (multidose syringes requiring a new needle for each individual are not recommended as reflux may occur and cause transmission of viral hepatitis B) —sterilization of reusable syringes in water brought to a "rolling boil" for 20 minutes (a hepatitis hazard may still remain if sterilization is not properly supervised); autoclaving for 25 minutes at 120 °C eliminates viral hepatitis if the operation is carried out correctly (no air left in the autoclave, no close packing of syringes); these operations are time-consuming
Injectors	—these save considerable time and reduce the strain on personnel since a vaccination rate of more than 1000 vaccinations per hour can be achieved with one injector. The model used should take 50- or 100-dose vials. The apparatus should be carefully disinfected in accordance with the manufacturer's instructions. Spare parts most frequently needed should be stock-piled. A supervisor should frequently check that injectors are functioning properly and are being correctly handled
Bifurcated needles	—since sterilization by flaming carries a risk of transmission of viral hepatitis B, autoclaving is necessary
Transport	—as for mosquito control, where appropriate (see p. 113).
Personnel	—auxiliary personnel (may be trained on the spot to assist professionals but will require close supervision)
Community participation	—cooperation by the population (easily obtained in an emergency). The media can be used to motivate the population and explain the procedures to be followed. Officials, auxiliaries and volunteers can be motivated and mobilized for immunization and community sanitation purposes

Table 53. Specific indications for immunization

Disease	Type of vaccine	Indications for use and time taken to develop immunity
Adenoviral respiratory disease	Live adenovirus types 4 and 7, attenuated, oral	Previous outbreaks have occurred among military recruits in USA
Cholera	Inactivated bacterial suspension	No value in stopping an outbreak (personal protection only, of 6 months duration)
Dengue[a]	Live attenuated tetravalent (in preparation)	
Diphtheria	Inactivated toxin, subcutaneous	Close contacts: erythromycin is preferred; other contacts: immunization
Diseases caused by arboviruses, such as eastern and western encephalomyelitis, Venezuelan equine encephalitis, Omsk haemorrhagic fever[a]	Experimental	No use in outbreaks, restricted to professionals at permanent risk
Influenza	Inactivated; should contain antigens to most recent variants of type A and B viruses; a pandemic may require a live virus vaccine	Priority groups: patients with chronic diseases or immunodeficiencies; key personnel in public services and industries
Japanese encephalitis	Mouse-brain, inactivated, subcutaneous, two doses (for children); inactivated hamster-cell culture (used in China)	Children; slow rise in immunity
Measles	Live attenuated	After 6 months of age; provides protection after a week
Meningitis, meningococcal	Meningococcal polysaccharide vaccines; serogroup A: 2 doses, 3 months apart, for children 3 months to 2 years of age, single dose for older children; serogroup C: poorly immunogenic in children less than 2 years of age	Effective in 5 days; should be complemented by chemoprophylaxis for household contacts
Mumps	Live attenuated, prepared in chicken fibroblast cell culture; one dose	Effective in 5–7 days; children 1 year of age and all males with no history of mumps

Table 53 (*continued*)

Disease	Type of vaccine	Indications for use and time taken to develop immunity
Pertussis	Suspension of killed bacteria adsorbed on aluminium salts; 3 doses 1 month apart, booster 1 year later and at ages 3 and 6 years	All children from 2 to 3 months of age, immunity develops slowly and is not complete; chemoprophylaxis with erythromycin has not been shown to be effective for family contacts
Plague	Killed bacteria, 2 or 3 doses and booster doses	Mainly for individual protection; rodent and flea control is preferred for stopping outbreaks; antibiotics effective in man
Pneumonia due to *Streptococcus pneumoniae*	Polyvalent pneumococcal polysaccharide vaccine; less effective in children under 2 years of age	Outbreaks in closed population groups; short-term prophylaxis with antibiotics for close contacts
Poliomyelitis	Trivalent live oral vaccine	The oral vaccine, which acts rapidly by competition in the intestinal tract, is preferred to the formalin-inactivated vaccine, which does not give immediate protection
Q fever	Inactivated chick-embryo yolk-sack	Restricted to those engaged in hazardous occupations
Rabies	Inactivated vaccine prepared on human diploid cells or duck embryo, or animal brain (sheep, rat)	Subjects bitten by suspected rabid animal; administer rabies immune globulin when indicated; pre-exposure immunization of persons at high occupational risk
Rocky Mountain spotted fever	Inactivated chick-embryo yolk-sac	Mainly for persons at high occupational risk in laboratories
Rubella	Live attenuated	Children over 1 year of age; contraindicated in pregnant women
Smallpox[b]	Live vaccinia virus	Contraindicated if skin lesions present; the disease has now been eradicated; any suspected case should be notified to WHO for confirmation before vaccination is considered
Tetanus[a]	Inactivated toxin (toxoid), booster doses	Patients with even minimal injuries contaminated by earth, or bites from cattle or horses

Table 53 (*continued*)

Disease	Type of vaccine	Indications for use and time taken to develop immunity
Tick-borne encephalitis	Mouse-brain, inactivated (used in Austria and USSR)	Persons at high risk
Tuberculosis	Live bacilli, BCG strain	Ineffective in emergencies, slow increase in immunity
Tularaemia[a]	Live attenuated vaccine (used in USA and USSR)	Persons at occupational risk
Typhoid fever	Inactivated bacilli; 2 subcutaneous doses several weeks apart, boosters every 3–5 years	No value in stopping an outbreak rapidly
Typhus[a]	Egg-yolk, inactivated; a live vaccine is under study	To supplement application of residual insecticide

[a] No person-to-person transmission.
[b] Considered to have been eradicated.

6.3.3 *Specific indications for passive immunization*

The administration of antibodies derived from immunized persons or animals has only limited and specific indications during epidemics, as shown in Table 54. A number of different products are available: human immune plasma, human standard or specific immunoglobulins, of which only certain preparations can be given intravenously, and purified antitoxins of animal origin (these may cause anaphylactic shock in persons sensitized to animal proteins unless injection is performed according to the Besredka method (see p. 120)). Specific immunoglobulins are often available only in limited quantities, and none is really suitable for large population groups but they may be considered for the protection of highly exposed persons, such as medical personnel or investigators during outbreaks, or for the treatment of patients, provided that they can be administered early in the course of the disease.

6.3.4 *Indications for chemoprophylaxis*

Chemoprophylaxis may sometimes be used during epidemics to protect persons who have been in contact with the source of infection or with an infected person. Some indications for chemoprophylaxis are given in Table 55.

Table 54. Indications for passive immunization in emergencies

Disease	Type of immune preparation	Indications for use or tests required
Botulism	Trivalent botulinal antitoxin (types A, B and E), or the specific antitoxin required	Before administration, check for sensitization to horse serum[a]
Diphtheria	Antitoxin	Before administration, check for hypersensitivity[a]
Pertussis	Human immune globulin, special pertussis hyper-immune globulin	Value not proven
Rabies	Rabies immune globulin, injected locally and intramuscularly	Must be complemented by vaccination; check for sensitization if immune globulin of animal origin is used[a]
Tetanus	Equine or bovine tetanus antitoxin or human immune globulin (special preparation for intravenous administration)	Check for sensitization to animal serum; [a] start active immunization with adsorbed toxoid and administer antibiotics
Varicella	Human varicella-zoster immune globulin	Give within 3–4 days of exposure; limited supplies, restricted to special medical indications
Viral haemor-rhagic fevers (Lassa, Ebola, Marburg, Junin and Machupo), tick-borne encephalitis	Immune plasma from convalescents, free from residual virus (immune globulin for Junin and Machupo HF)	Limited quantities (available through WHO); efficacy still doubtful (it should preferably be administered in the first 4 days)
Viral hepatitis A	Human immune globulin with a specific titre of at least 100 IU	Should be given to household contacts within 2 weeks of exposure; travellers at risk
Viral hepatitis B	Human hepatitis B immune globulin	Household contacts

[a] Besredka desensitization method (see p. 120) recommended before antitoxin of animal origin is injected.

6.4 International Health Regulations

The International Health Regulations constitute a formal international agreement by which most Member States of WHO are bound without reservation. The Regulations originally covered six communicable diseases of international concern often referred to as the "quarantinable diseases": smallpox, cholera, yellow fever, plague, relapsing fever due to *Borrelia recurrentis*, and typhus fever due to

Table 55. Indications for chemoprophylaxis

Disease	Indications and drugs used
Cholera	Tetracycline or furazolidone for household contacts
Conjunctivitis, bacterial	Erythromycin ophthalmic ointment (no effect on viral conjunctivitis)
Diphtheria	Erythromycin (and first dose of vaccine)
Influenza	Amantadine (effective only for type A) for contacts suffering from chronic diseases
Malaria	See Annex 3 (p. 193)
Meningitis, meningococcal	For household or close community contacts: sulfadiazine, *only if the meningococcal strain is shown to be non-resistant* (0.5 g for children, 1.0 g for adults, every 12 hours for 4 days); rifampicin is contraindicated so as not to develop resistance to treatment of leprosy; immunization should be initiated in all cases (against serogroups A and C)
Plague	Contacts of pneumonic plague should be given 15 mg of tetracycline per kg of body weight daily for 1 week
Trypanosomiasis, African	Pentamidine isothionate in a single 250-mg dose protects an adult for 3–6 months; however, pentamidine-resistant strains have developed; not recommended in areas where there is a risk of infection by *Trypanosoma brucei rhodesiense*, and a risk of administering a subcurative dose to individuals already infected

Rickettsia prowazekii. Each health administration was required to notify the Organization by telegram or telex within 24 hours of having been informed that the first case of a disease subject to the Regulations had occurred in its territory. This list was revised in 1969, when only smallpox, plague, cholera and yellow fever were kept "under the Regulations". At the same time typhus and relapsing fever, together with viral influenza, paralytic poliomyelitis, and malaria, were placed under "international surveillance". In addition to their responsibilities under the International Health Regulations, Member States have an obligation to report outbreaks of communicable disease.

In 1980 the World Health Assembly declared that smallpox had been eradicated and it was therefore removed from the Regulations.

The International Health Regulations have the aim of ensuring maximum security against the international spread of disease combined with the minimum of interference with international trade and traffic. Cholera is an example of a disease for which quarantine measures were ineffective and caused considerable economic losses as a result of interference with such trade and traffic. To avoid such situations, every attempt is made to have health administrations interpret the International Health Regulations on a sound epidemiological basis. In the case of cholera, the requirement of a vaccination certificate cannot be justified on epidemiological grounds and this requirement was deleted from the International Health Regulations in 1973.

BIBLIOGRAPHY

Appropriate uses of human immunoglobulin in clinical practice: Memorandum from an IUIS/WHO meeting. *Bulletin of the World Health Organization*, **60**: 43–47 (1982).

ASSAR, M. *Guide to sanitation in natural disasters*. Geneva, World Health Organization, 1971.

BAILEY, J. *Guide to hygiene and sanitation in aviation*. Geneva, World Health Organization, 1977.

Chemical indicators for monitoring the cold-chain. A review of laboratory tests and field trials. Unpublished WHO document, EPI/CCIS/81.10.

Disaster prevention and mitigation. Vol. 8. Sanitation aspects. New York, United Nations, 1982.

DUNSMORE, D. J. *Safety measures for use in outbreaks of communicable disease*. Geneva, World Health Organization, 1986.

Emergency health management after natural disaster. Washington, DC, Pan American Health Organization, 1981 (Scientific Publication No. 407).

FEACHEM, R. G. ET AL. *Sanitation and disease: health aspects of excreta and wastewater management*. Baltimore, Johns Hopkins University Press, 1982.

Guidelines for drinking-water quality. Vol. 3. Drinking-water quality control in small-community supplies. Geneva, World Health Organization, 1985.

Guidelines for the management of accidents involving microorganisms: a WHO Memorandum. *Bulletin of the World Health Organization*, **58**: 245–246 (1980).

Treatment and prevention of acute diarrhoea: guidelines for the trainers of health workers. Geneva, World Health Organization, 1985.

Health services organization in the event of disaster. Washington, DC, Pan American Health Organization, 1983 (Scientific Publication No. 443).

Manual of the international statistical classification of diseases, injuries, and causes of death. Geneva, World Health Organization, 1977.

Manual on personal and community protection against malaria. Geneva, World Health Organization, 1974 (WHO Offset Publication No. 10).

RAJAGOPALAN, S. & SHIFFMAN, M. A. *Guide to simple sanitary measures for the control of enteric diseases*. Geneva, World Health Organization, 1974.

Technician's handbook for compression refrigerators. Unpublished WHO document.

User's handbook for compression refrigerators. Unpublished WHO document.

User's handbook for gas and electric operated absorption refrigerators. Unpublished WHO document.

User's handbook for kerosene and electric operated absorption refrigerators. Unpublished WHO document.

User's handbook for vaccine cold stores. Unpublished WHO document.

Vector control in international health. Geneva, World Health Organization, 1972.

WHO emergency health kit. Geneva, World Health Organization, 1984.

7. Follow-up of control measures

The efficacy of control measures should be assessed day by day during the outbreak, a final assessment being made after it has ended. This will provide a logical basis for postepidemic surveillance and preventive measures aimed at avoiding the repetition of similar outbreaks. As soon as the pressure of events has decreased, a review of all the facts will be most useful, and an account of the experience acquired should be published for the benefit of others.

7.1 Evaluation of control measures

7.1.1 Indicators

One of the functions of the emergency health service advisory committee is to choose the indicators that will be used to assess the success of control measures. These indicators provide a measure of the efficacy of both control measures and medical care.

Indicators of the efficacy of control measures. A critical appraisal is necessary in order to reach a correct conclusion as to the efficacy of control measures. The most obvious indication that an outbreak is subsiding is a fall in the daily attack rate, but caution must be exercised in interpreting its fluctuations. Thus a decrease in the daily attack rate may mean that:

—the control measures are beginning to have an effect;
—all the receptive population at risk has been affected;
—reporting is uneven;
—the source of the contagious agent has been reduced by a natural phenomenon, e.g., migration of the animal reservoir or vector, a decline in mosquito activity following a fall in temperature, temporary competition by another non-infective vector or reservoir species, and many others, all of which will permit a resurgence of the outbreak at a later stage if the actual cause has not been eliminated.

No general rule can be laid down as to when it is safe to say that an outbreak has ended, but the following criteria may be applied:

—*Diseases transmitted directly from person to person*: when the longest incubation period (or twice the mean incubation period) has elapsed without any further case having occurred, provided that no healthy carrier is involved.

—*Diseases having a common source*: when the infectious material has been brought under control.

—*Arthropod-borne diseases*: when no further case has occurred during a period equal to the sum of the viraemic period in man or other vertebrate reservoir, the "extrinsic" incubation period in the insect vector, and the "intrinsic" incubation period in man; however, for some diseases, the insect vector may remain infected long after the incubation period has elapsed, or even for life.

On the other hand, even with effective control measures, a continuing increase in daily attack rates may occur if the disease has a long incubation period or if reporting of cases has improved.

Some diseases can recur annually as epidemics in the same population (influenza has provided many examples of this) until a high level of immunity has been achieved.

Indicators other than the attack rate may also be of value, e.g., the density of mosquitos or rodents, if these are the sole agent of transmission of the disease to man.

Indicators of the efficacy of medical care. The efficacy of medical care may be assessed by the decrease in:

—the duration of hospitalization;
—the proportion of complications or sequelae;
—the case-fatality rate.

7.1.2 Cost-effectiveness

It is often impossible to calculate the expenses involved in respect of the many sectors of human activity affected during an epidemic. As a general rule, the direct and indirect expenses associated with an outbreak greatly exceed those under normal conditions. It is reasonable to assume that preparedness for epidemics will substantially reduce these excess costs. The estimated cost of an outbreak may be compared with that of the preventive measures by which it could have been avoided. Above all, avoidance of human suffering must be the primary consideration.

7.2 Postepidemic measures

At the end of an outbreak, further epidemiological investigations are necessary in order to determine the origin and impact of the disease and to select appropriate indicators for use in prospective surveillance and the prevention of recurrences.

Two types of epidemiological investigation are shown in Table 56.

Table 56. Postepidemic investigations

Type	Objectives
Serological survey	To define infected areas, infection rates in different population groups and their susceptibility rates, and identify risk groups still remaining
Ecological and/or socioeconomic survey	To determine the sources, vehicles, reservoirs and vectors involved in the outbreak, the triggering factor(s) and the effect of, e.g., climatic, economic or social conditions

Awareness of the conditions that led to the outbreak will enable the emergency health services to introduce or to improve the following:

—surveillance and early warning systems;
—preparedness for epidemics and contingency plans;
—preventive immunization of population groups at risk;
—sanitation in the affected and related sectors, e.g., foodstuffs, the environment, animal husbandry, vector control, water supply.

The cost/benefit ratio of such activities may be compared with the expenses incurred in repeated outbreaks when it is necessary to justify requests for funds to carry them out.

7.3 Sharing of experience

Although only a few agents are often the cause of "classical" epidemics, some particular feature of the circumstances that led to the occurrence of an outbreak may be of interest. The interest is even greater when the outbreak has been caused by an unusual agent. All public health officers will benefit if the experience acquired is shared by the publication of an account of the outbreak.

7.3.1 Final report

The information indicated in Table 57 should be included in the final report, which should be submitted to the public health authorities and remain confidential until it has been given official clearance. This point should not be neglected by consultants from outside the country concerned.

7.3.2 Publication

Publication of the experience acquired is of considerable value. WHO endeavours to give the widest possible publicity to reports on epidemics in its periodicals (*Bulletin of the World Health Organization, World health forum, WHO Chronicle, Weekly epidemiological record,* and regional publications), which are translated into various

Table 57. Information to be included in the final report on an epidemic

Section	Contents
1. Background	Geographical location Climatic conditions Demographic status (population pyramid) Socioeconomic situation Organization and operation of health services Surveillance and early warning systems Preparedness for epidemics Normal disease prevalence

2. Historical data	Previous occurrence of epidemics of the same
	   disease, locally or elsewhere
	Occurrence of related diseases, if any:
	   —in the same area
	   —in other areas
	Discovery of the first cases of the present outbreak

3. Methodology of
   investigations
	Case definition
	Questionnaire used in epidemiological
	   investigations
	Survey teams
	Health centres survey
	Household survey
	Retrospective survey
	Prospective surveillance
	Collection of laboratory specimens
	Laboratory techniques

4. Analysis of data	Clinical data:
	   —frequency of signs and symptoms
	   —course of disease
	   —differential diagnosis
	   —death or sequelae rates
	
	Epidemiological data:
	   —mode of occurrence
	     —in time
	     —by place
	     —by population groups
	   —overt/subclinical rates
	
	Mode(s) of transmission:
	   —source(s) of infection
	   —route(s) of excretion and portal(s) of entry
	   —factors influencing transmission
	
	Laboratory data:
	   —isolation of suspected agent(s)
	   —serological confirmation
	   —significance of results
	
	Interpretation of data:
	   —comprehensive picture of the outbreak
	   —hypotheses as to cause(s)
	   —formulating and testing hypotheses of caus-
	     ation by statistical analysis (see Annex 2)

Table 57 (*continued*)

Section	Contents
5. Control measures	Definition of strategies and methodology
	Implementation:
	—constraints
	—results
	Evaluation:
	—significance of results
	—cost/effectiveness
	Preventive measures

languages. The WHO regional offices and the Division of Communicable Diseases at headquarters, or other relevant divisions, may also provide any documentation that public health officers may require to complete their reports.

7.3.3 International cooperation

WHO encourages the establishment of close international cooperation in the field of emergencies caused by epidemics. In the post-epidemic phase, such cooperation may concern, e.g., the exchange of epidemiological information, experts, teachers, and equipment, the holding of joint conferences or workshops, and the undertaking of joint prevention or elimination programmes, and may operate not only at governmental level but also between institutions. The eradication of smallpox is the best example of the benefits of such cooperation under the aegis of WHO.

BIBLIOGRAPHY

Ebola haemorrhagic fever in Sudan, 1976: Report of a WHO/International Study Team. *Bulletin of the World Health Organization*, **56**: 247–270 (1978).
Ebola haemorrhagic fever in Zaire, 1976: Report of an International Commission. *Bulletin of the World Health Organization*, **56**: 271–293 (1978).

ANNEX 1

Explanation of epidemiological terms[1]

Carrier
    An infected person or animal, which may be a source of infection but without showing any symptoms (incubatory carrier, convalescent carrier, transient carrier, chronic carrier).

Contagious (communicable) period
    The period during which an infected person or animal, whether or not showing symptoms, can transmit a disease.

Contact
    A person or animal that has been exposed to possible transmission of an infectious or parasitic agent by a patient, a sick animal or a carrier, or by contamination of the environment (including foods).

Contamination
    The presence of an infectious or parasitic agent on body surfaces and inanimate supports, such as water, food, soil, air, dust and fomites.

Disease occurrence rates
    Different rates may be utilized to quantify the occurrence of a disease in a population. They are calculated as fractions, in the form:

$$\frac{\text{Number of cases}}{\text{Number of persons in the population investigated}[2]}$$

and expressed as rates per hundreds, thousands, or millions as convenient. The following rates should be used as appropriate:

(a) Clinical incidence (attack) rate

$$\frac{\text{Number of new cases}}{\text{Population considered at risk}}$$

---

[1] For an explanation of the term "epidemic", see p. 3.
[2] This may be the entire population or a specific group (by age, sex, occupation, residence, etc.).

where the numerator is the number of overt cases (fitting the case definition) appearing during a specified period of time; the nature and extent of the population at risk should be defied.

(b) Infection rate

$$\frac{\text{Number of new infections}}{\text{Population considered at risk}}$$

where the numerator is the number of overt (laboratory-proved) and silent infections (diagnosed only by laboratory tests) appearing during a specified period of time; the nature and extent of the population at risk should be defined.

(c) Case–fatality ratio

$$\frac{\text{Number of deaths}}{\text{Number of cases}}$$

It should be stated whether the numerator is the number of etiologically confirmed deaths, or of presumptive deaths; the completeness of case detection (hospitalized cases, non-hospitalized cases, severe forms, mild forms, inapparent infections, all inclusive) should be specified.

(d) Prevalence rate

$$\frac{\text{Number of persons affected}}{\text{Number of persons examined}}$$

where the numerator may include only those clinically affected or, in addition, inapparent infections, at a given time (i.e., the date of the survey).

(e) Morbidity rate[1]

$$\frac{\text{Number of persons with overt disease}}{\text{Population under surveillance}}$$

where the numerator generally covers confirmed and suspected cases over a period of 1 year and the population concerned may be the entire population or a particular group.

(f) Mortality rate

$$\frac{\text{Number of deaths}}{\text{Population under surveillance}}$$

where the deaths concerned are those directly or indirectly attributed to an agent, and the population may be the entire population or a particular group.

---

[1] This term may be a source of confusion when indiscriminately used to refer to incidence or prevalence and should preferably be avoided.

Endemic (enzootic for animals)
(Of a disease) continually present in a given area or community. Endemicity may be low or high, or even evidenced by only a few sporadic cases.
An *endemic area* is the limited zone in which a disease is known to occur constantly.

Epidemic (epizootic) focus
The limited area in which an outbreak has been occurring.

Fomites
Inanimate objects or materials, e.g., clothing, toilet articles, dressings, bedding, on which infectious agents may be carried.

Immunity
Resistance to a second infection by a particular agent (homotypic immunity) or by an antigenically related agent (heterotypic immunity).

Inapparent (subclinical) infection
Infection without clinical signs and symptoms in man or animal, detectable only by laboratory techniques, such as isolation of the agent, characterization of the antigen, and/or serological tests.

Infected area
The area in which, whether temporarily or permanently, an infectious or parasitic agent may be transmitted to man or animals.

Infection
The entry and multiplication or development in the body of an infectious (bacterial, chlamydial, fungal, rickettsial, viral) or parasitic agent (protozoal, helminthic).
Portals of entry include the respiratory tract, digestive tract, genital tract, skin (including injections) and conjunctivae.
Routes of excretion include, in addition to the above, excreta (stools, urine, vomitus), secretions (oral, nasal, sputum, saliva, tears, semen, vaginal secretions) and blood.

Outbreak
The occurrence of an epidemic disease at a particular time and place.

Pandemic
A worldwide epidemic.

Reservoir
Human beings, animals, plants, soil, water or any other substance in or upon which an infectious or parasitic agent is normally or

occasionally found or multiplies in such a manner that it can be transmitted to a receptive person or animal.

Sporadic occurrence

The occurrence of a few cases of a disease without any relationship in time and with or without a relationship to a focus.

Transmission

The mechanism whereby an infectious or parasitic agent is transferred from an infected person or animal or a contaminated object to a receptive host (person or animal).

Transmission may be *direct*, by contact with the source of an infectious or parasitic agent, or *indirect* when it takes place through the intermediary, e.g., of an insect vector, air (when the agent is in suspension, e.g., in aerosols), dust, fomites, water or soil.

Vector

Arthropods of the class Insecta (mosquitos, flies, sandflies, fleas, lice, and other species), Arachnida (ticks and mites), or Crustacea (cyclops, crabs and crayfish), or vertebrate animals, e.g., rodents, that may transfer an infectious or parasitic agent from a reservoir to a receptive person or animal. The first two classes, namely Insecta and Arachnida, are commonly referred to as insects.

Zoonosis

An infectious or parasitic disease of animals, which may be transmitted to man. A zoonosis may be enzootic, epizootic or sporadic, and transmission may be direct or indirect.

ANNEX 2

Procedures for assembling epidemiological data and formulating and testing hypotheses of causation

A2.1 Compilation of data

Unless the number of cases is very small, about 12 or fewer, it is difficult to assemble case data directly from forms A, B, and C (see Tables 25, 26, and 29). Some method of summarizing the most important facts is needed if patterns of occurrence are to be demonstrated. If an electronic computer is available, individual case data can be coded on form A and entered on to a computer tape or disk, for later retrieval. Even where computer facilities and personnel are immediately available, the investigator will probably need and want to update, change and re-examine the data and compilations frequently, and the use of a computer must be supplemented by less formal methods. If a computer is not available, other compilation approaches are essential.

A2.1.1 Line-listing of cases and preparation of hand-sorted cards

The first step in summarizing data is to prepare a line-listing of all cases so as to provide a permanent record. For this purpose, the most important data are selected and presented simply and clearly so as to facilitate compilation. Exactly what is "most important" will differ according to the nature and circumstances of the outbreak and the objectives of the investigation. It will always be necessary to list age, sex, locality and date of onset of disease, but there may be other details of equal importance. An *example* (not a universal model) of a line-listing of cases is shown in Table A2.1.

Cases are listed as they are reported, in numerical, not chronological, order. If numbers have previously been assigned to cases, an additional column must be provided in which they can be recorded. Many items of valuable information on forms A, B, and C are not indicated in this summary. Depending on the purpose, the line-listing may have to be extended or other lists created.

143

Table A2.1. Line-listing of cases in a dysentery epidemic

Serial No.	Age (years)	Sex	Village	Occupation	Water supply	Date of onset	Signs/symptoms							Laboratory tests[a]			Severity	Diagnostic level[b]
							Diarrhoea	Fever	Bloody stool	Vomiting	Abdominal pain	Death	None	Faecal exudate	Agent isolation			
001	18	M	G	Farming	Pond	3/9	+	+	+		+	+		+		S	P
002	2	M	C	—	Pond	5/9	+	+	+	+	+	+		+	Sh. dys.	S	C
003	30	F	D	Weaving	Shallow well	18/8	+		+		+		+			S	S
004	25	M	A	Fishing	Deep well	2/9	+	+					+	−		M	S
005	0.5	F	F	—	Pond	6/9	+	+	+					−	−	S	S
etc.																	

[a] If no tests are performed, insert + in the "None" column.
Faecal exudate: if examined, record result as + or −.
Agent isolation: if attempted, record result as − or give name of agent.
[b] C = confirmed; P = presumptive; S = suspect.

If there are a large number of cases, preparing tabular summaries directly from the line-listing may be both tedious and prone to error. It is advisable, therefore, to prepare hand-sorted cards. Standard index cards measuring 8 cm × 12 cm are readily available and will conveniently hold 9 items of information; larger cards may be used if there are more than 9 items. One card is made out for each case, and the data from the line-listing are transferred to cards, as shown in Fig. A2.1 for the first case in Table A2.1.

The hand-sorted cards may be used to make any tabulations desired. For example, the cards may be sorted into two piles by sex, and the male and female subsets then further subdivided by age-group. After the subset cards have been counted and recorded in a

Fig. A2.1. Hand-sorted cards

A. Model for hand-sorted card set

Age	Locality	Sex
Date of onset	Serial No.	Severity
Occupation	Water supply	Diagnostic level

B. Hand-sorted card for first case

18	Village G	M
3/9	001	S
Farming	Pond	P

WHO 851020

table, the cards can be reassembled and used for other tabulations. When all the tabulations needed at a particular time have been made, the cards can be put back into numerical order so that any individual case can be located when required.

As new cases are reported, they are added to the line-listing and additional hand-sorted cards are prepared. Similarly, if new or revised information is received on cases already recorded, changes can be made in both records. New and revised tabulations may then be made as the investigation progresses.

A2.1.2 Incidence (attack) rates by personal characteristics

Tables of incidence rates should be prepared for all the subgroups considered to be relevant to the disease under investigation and the circumstances of the outbreak. Table A2.2 shows a simple *example*, based on a hypothetical epidemic of dysentery.

It will be seen from Table A2.2A that attack rates for males greatly exceeded those for females, and that the disease occurred most

Table A2.2. Attack rates in a hypothetical epidemic of dysentery

A. By age and sex

Age (years)	Males			Females		
	Population	Cases	Rate per 1000	Population	Cases	Rate per 1000
≤10	1500	5	3.3	1400	4	2.9
10–19	1200	20	16.7	1200	5	4.2
20–39	1000	30	30.0	800	8	10.0
≥40	1000	10	10.0	800	2	2.5
Total	4700	65	13.8	4200	19	4.5

B. By occupation in males aged 10 years or over

Occupation	Estimated population	Cases	Rate per 1000
Farmers	1800	15	8.3
Fishermen	900	40	44.4
Artisans	200	1	5.0
Schoolchildren	100	1	10.0
Others	200	3	15.0
Total	3200	60	18.8

frequently among young adults. Table A2.2B shows the attack rates for the various occupational groups and demonstrates that the epidemic was concentrated among fishermen.

The age groups used in Table A2.2 are suitable because preliminary examination of the case data indicated that there were only a few cases among children and very old people. If cases had been concentrated among the very young or the elderly, different age-groups would obviously have been selected. In this example it was necessary to estimate the size of the different occupational groups, and in practice sufficiently detailed census data will rarely be available; the best information available locally may therefore have to be used. Finally, in epidemics of other diseases, very different personal characteristics may have to be used in the analysis.

Table A2.2 includes all cases reported in the investigation, regardless of the degree of certainty with which they were diagnosed. By definition, a "confirmed" case implies a reliable diagnosis whereas "suspect" cases imply some degree of doubt as to its correctness. If there are enough cases, each of the three diagnostic levels—confirmed, presumptive, and suspect—can be tabulated separately. If the distribution of the cases by age, sex, place, time and other characteristics is dissimilar (because the "suspect" group includes cases of some other diseases), analysis should be limited to the confirmed or presumptive cases; if all groups appear to be similar, data can be combined, as in Table A2.2.

A2.1.3 Incidence (attack) rates by place

To examine whether the cases among fishermen were concentrated in certain fishing villages, the hand-sorted cards are sorted by locality, and tables similar to Table A2.2 prepared to show distribution by place. However, the analysis should be carried one step further. If all the cases of dysentery among fishermen were found in villages A and B, this may mean either that there are no fishermen in villages C and D, or that fishermen in those villages were unaffected. In order to decide which of these alternatives is correct, population counts must be made in places not affected by the disease in order to determine whether they had zero attack rates or merely contained no persons in the occupational group concerned.

The location of cases can readily be seen by preparing a "spot map", as shown in Fig. A2.2, again based on the hypothetical dysentery outbreak used as an example in Table A2.1. A spot is used to indicate one or more cases and, in this instance, distinctive symbols are used to differentiate between fishermen and others. Other spot maps could be prepared, with other symbols, to show sex or age distribution, onset during particular periods of time, etc.

Fig. A2.2. Spot map showing occurrence of dysentery cases in villages of subdistrict

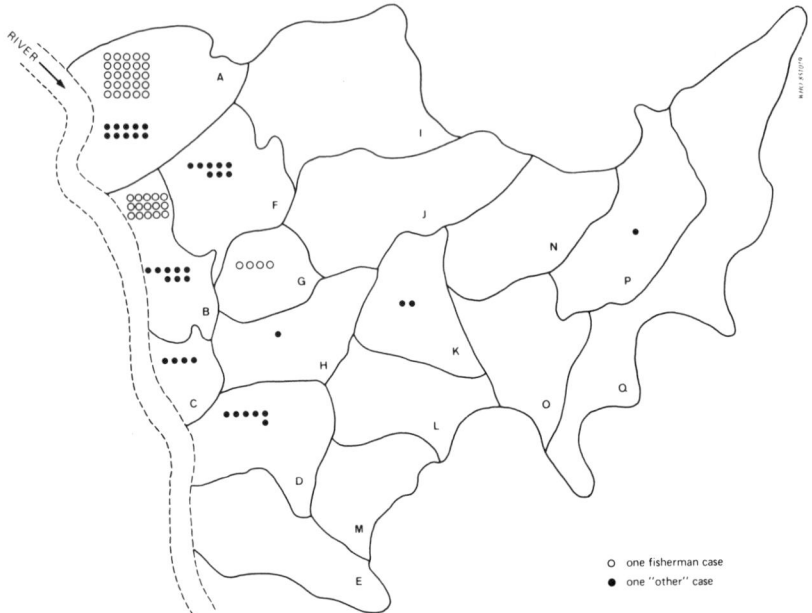

A2.1.4 Distribution of cases in time

The third and equally important epidemiological characteristic is time distribution of cases. The hand-sorted cards may again be used to put the cases into chronological order, and tables similar to Table A2.2 can be prepared to show attack rates during various time intervals. Graphs, however, are even more effective for showing the distribution of cases in time.

The simplest and most useful graph for this purpose is a histogram in which each case is represented by a box on graph paper with the horizontal axis indicating a convenient time unit (a single day, two days, one week, etc.). This may be used as a "working" graph, begun with the first case reports and kept up to date as new cases are notified. Fig. A2.3, based on the same dysentery cases as those recorded in Table A2.1, shows cases where the onset occurred during the 1-month period that included the epidemic.

Fig. A2.3 shows three types of case: those in fishermen, those in the families of fishermen, and those in other persons. Many other characteristics of cases can be shown on a graph, e.g., the degree of diagnostic certainty of the cases (confirmed, presumptive, suspect); occurrence in different areas; occurrence by age, sex, and ethnic or occupational group; severity (survival, sequelae, death); the introduc-

Fig. A2.3. Dysentery cases in subdistrict (18 August–17 September 1982)

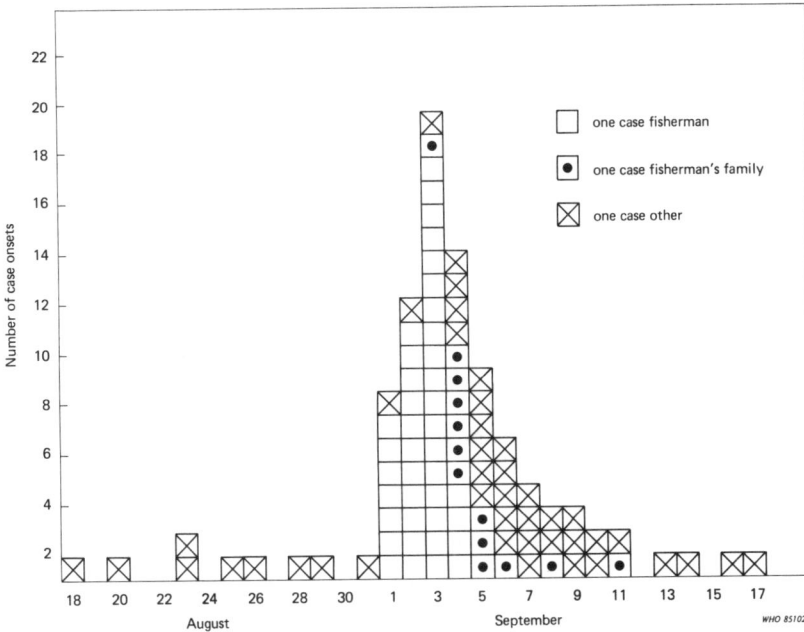

tion of control measures, etc.; however, if too many details are shown, clarity will be lost.

Examination of Fig. A2.3 reveals a number of important facts: (1) endemic cases of dysentery had been reported in this district almost every day; (2) the epidemic began suddenly on 1 September and ended on about 11 September; (3) the earliest epidemic cases were among fishermen, but cases followed quickly in their families and other members of the communities. This information will be useful in developing hypotheses as to the origin and development of the epidemic.

A.2.2. Formulating and testing hypotheses of causation

The control of an epidemic requires a plan of attack, and such a plan must be based on the most plausible explanation of the origin and continuation of the epidemic—a hypothesis of causation. In the absence of such a hypothesis, control activities may be disorganized or misdirected; they may not be given the appropriate order of priority, and it may be difficult to evaluate their effectiveness if targets have not been established. It must be emphasized, however, that a hypothesis is merely a tentative explanation based on currently available information, to be rejected or modified, as necessary, as additional information is accumulated, or changed if the pattern of transmission changes. The officer in charge of control activities must therefore continuously re-examine the hypothesis, and must be prepared to adapt activities to changes in views as to the nature of the outbreak.

A hypothesis of causation is formulated on the basis of all the information available on the outbreak: clinical features, laboratory diagnostic studies, epidemiological patterns, the results of environmental and ecological surveys and assessments (including vector and reservoir studies), and whatever additional information an experienced and imaginative investigator may be able to gather about the movements of people, changes in activities, imports, environmental and climatic disturbances, etc. The main point of interest, however, is always the diagnosis of the disease involved. If this can be established with certainty, standard works of reference can be consulted and the possible sources and transmission mechanisms identified. The next step in hypothesis formulation is epidemiological analysis.

A2.2.1 Determining the mode of transmission

For certain diseases, the mechanism of transmission is known; for example, it can safely be assumed that an outbreak of yellow fever is being propagated by infected mosquitos, and that measles is being transmitted by the respiratory route, person-to-person. Even with such diseases, however, further information may be necessary, e.g., with yellow fever it may be essential to know the focal distribution and particularly to explain the origin of the first focus, while with measles it may be necessary to determine the origin and pattern of spread. For other diseases, such as dysentery, both common-source contamination and person-to-person transmission are of major importance, and their specific role in any particular epidemic must be elucidated. With a disease of unknown etiology, as was the case with Lassa fever at the time of its first appearance, no guidance for the investigation is initially available.

Descriptive data of the type described above are used to obtain tentative answers to questions concerning origin and propagation. The recommended procedure is to examine each table, graph or map separately at first, for two purposes—to interpret its possible meaning, and to identify any missing information or additional detail that should be sought. In yellow fever, for example, the presence of a sex differential in reported cases will suggest differing exposures of men and women; this in turn suggests that information on occupation should be obtained, and hence possibly on the localities where those concerned were employed. In measles, separate tabulation of cases by immunization status means that age-specific immunization records will have to be obtained (in order to calculate attack rates for immunized and unimmunized children), together with information on attendances at school or other gathering places (in order to search for foci of transmission), and on contacts (in order to trace chains of transmission and, for control purposes, as a guide to an emergency immunization programme).

Where a disease may be propagated either by common-source exposure of large numbers of people or by person-to-person spread, first priority in an investigation must be given to determining which pattern best explains the known cases. The distribution of case onsets over time may provide the first and best clue while the shape of the epidemic curve may also be helpful. Fig. A2.4 shows a number of

Fig. A2.4. Typical shapes of epidemic curves

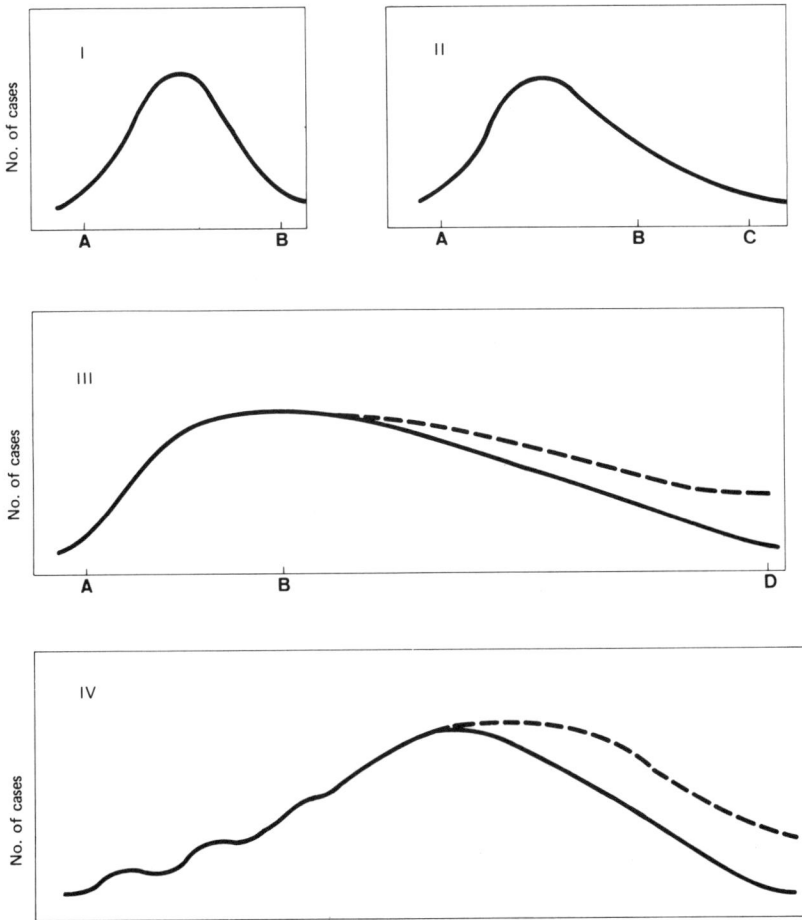

WHO 851018

typical (and stylized) curve patterns characteristic of various types of exposure. In all such curves the number of cases is shown on the vertical axis and the passage of time (measured in hours, days, or weeks) on the horizontal axis.

Curve I represents a simple common-source epidemic. Since all the cases are the consequence of a single exposure over a particular period of time, e.g., to toxin-contaminated food (with the case onsets extending over a period of hours) or as a result of the temporary pollution of a community water supply (over a period of days for dysentery or of weeks for hepatitis A), they must all have had their onset during a period of time (A–B) which lies within the usual *range* of incubation periods for the disease concerned. For example, in typhoid fever, where the great majority of cases have incubation periods of 7–21 days, the interval between A and B should not be more than 15 days if all exposures occurred on the same day. In actual practice, however, when a hypothesis of causation is being formulated, it is necessary to reason backwards in time from current observations. When a curve resembling Curve I is plotted for a disease diagnosed as typhoid fever, if the interval A–B is 15 days or less it may be hypothesized that one brief common exposure *could* account for all cases.

For a disease such as typhoid fever, common-source cases often pass the infection on to contacts by person-to-person transmission, so that a limited number of secondary cases may develop. The epidemic will then continue for an additional period of time (B–C in Curve II). The time represented by B is, of course, unknown but if the first 75–80% of the cases in a typhoid epidemic occurred within the above-mentioned period of 15 days, common-source exposure followed by secondary spread may be hypothesized.

Curve III shows a somewhat different situation, namely that of an epidemic continuing for a longer period of time (A–D) and ending either at the pre-epidemic level of endemicity or at some higher level. If such an epidemic began with common-source exposure, *either* it was followed by uncontrolled person-to-person transmission completely obscuring the time point B *or* the common source of exposure was continuously present over a long period of time. A curve of this shape is not very helpful in hypothesis formulation and clues must be sought elsewhere.

Finally, Curve IV shows the slower, gradual build-up of cases in an epidemic that does not originate from a common source of exposure. A wave-like pattern may sometimes be seen early in the course of the outbreak, with the "waves" representing successive "generations" of transmission; the interval between two crests is the average incubation period. An epidemic curve such as this may be found with enteric and respiratory diseases and with vector-borne diseases in which man serves as the reservoir.

A2.2.2 Estimating the date of common-source exposure

If it has been decided that an epidemic probably resulted from common-source exposure, the next stage is to estimate when that exposure could have taken place. The procedure is a simple one, and is illustrated in Fig. A2.5, which shows the distribution of cases in a typhoid fever epidemic with 81 cases; the epidemic began on 24 March and ended on 4 April, its total duration being 12 days. As this is within the usual range of typhoid incubation periods (15 days), a common-source outbreak can be hypothesized. The "minimum-maximum" method of estimation shows that, if all cases had been exposed on the same day, the first two cases must have become infected not less than 7 days earlier (the minimum incubation period), i.e., before 17 March. The last case must then have been the one with the longest incubation period (21 days) and therefore could not have been infected earlier than 14 March. A single common exposure some time between 14 and 17 March could thus account for all the cases. The hypothesis that exposure took place at some time during this limited period provides valuable guidance in searching for the event that caused the exposure.

An alternative method is to make use of the *average* incubation period. Taking the date of onset of the median case (41st in chronological order in this outbreak of 81 cases), and counting back 14 days (the average incubation period of this disease), 15 March is found to be the approximate date of the common exposure.

Fig. A2.5. Estimating date(s) of possible exposure in a common-source outbreak

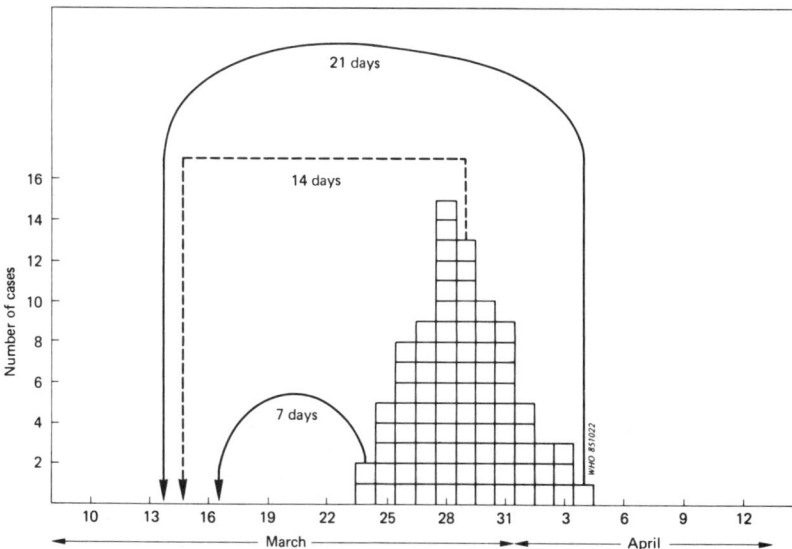

Occasionally it is possible to find cases among people who have visited the area of the epidemic for a brief period of time and then gone away, so that the onset of the disease takes place in an area in which no other case has occurred. Epidemics originating at fairs or festivals may produce many such cases. The interval between the brief exposure and the onset of the disease reflects the incubation period, and the date(s) on which the person concerned resided in the epidemic (or suspect) area define(s) the period during which infection took place.

If an epidemic curve resembles Curve II in Fig. A2.4, the problem of estimating the date(s) of common exposure is more complicated because the time point B is unknown. It may be possible, however, to identify common-source cases by careful examination of contact histories. If the second and subsequent cases in individual households are separated from the first by the length of an incubation period, they may be assumed to be contact cases. The first case in every household may then be plotted on a separate graph, and the date of common exposure estimated from this. In the dysentery epidemic described in Section A2.1.2 and plotted in Fig. A2.3 this procedure was followed and cases were divided into three categories: fishermen, the families of fishermen, and others in the villages. The entire outbreak, shown in Fig. A2.3, lasted for 11 days—too long for it to be entirely common-source in character, since the incubation period for dysentery has a range of only 1–7 days and is most commonly 1–3 days. The onset of cases among fishermen, however, occurred only over a period of 4 days (from 1 to 4 September) and they could therefore have been exposed to a common source. The estimated date of that exposure would be some time between 28 and 31 August, and most probably on the latter date.

A2.2.3 Case–control studies to identify specific causes

A hypothesis of causation may be adequate as a basis for control activities even when derived only from analysis of descriptive data and a comparison of attack rates among identifiable population subgroups, as shown previously. For example, if yellow fever is occurring *only* among adult male wood-cutters in a South American forest, and not among other groups, it is reasonable to conclude that mosquito transmission is occurring only in the forest. Sometimes, however, differences in attack rates are not sufficient to determine the source of exposure precisely because it is not clear how to subdivide a particular group into relevant subgroups. A simple case–control study may then be helpful.

Thus the dysentery outbreak referred to in section A2.1.2 affected 40 of the 900 people who claimed to be fishermen. A brief inquiry may reveal that only 100 were fishing during the suspect period of 28–31 August, including all those who became ill. Further subdivision of this group by place or activity may not be feasible, and another epidemiological approach—a case–control study—is needed to identify a possible specific exposure. If a questionnaire is drawn up covering food and water consumption each day during the suspect period, it will be possible to obtain and compare information on these (or other) exposures from cases and non-cases (the "controls") among those who were fishing. A possible (somewhat oversimplified) result of such an investigation is shown in Table A2.3.

If feasible, as many as possible of the cases should be interviewed; if there are very many cases, a representative sample should be selected for interview, together with at least as many controls. The numbers need not be equal, however. For Table A2.3 it was assumed that all the men concerned could answer all the questions; if not, the percentages of respondents who answered "yes" would have to be calculated. The table shows only one activity in which a substantially greater proportion of cases than controls had engaged, namely drinking pond water at place B. If it is confirmed statistically that the difference between these proportions is unlikely to have occurred merely by chance (see Section A2.2.4) it can be hypothesized that this pond was the source of infection.

Table A2.3. Activities indulged in by cases and controls among fisher-men between 28 and 31 August[a]

Activity	Cases		Controls	
	No.	%	No.	%
Brought food from home	32	80.0	39	70.9
Purchased food at place A	36	90.0	50	90.9
Purchased food at place B	30	75.0	45	81.8
Ate fish caught in river	31	77.5	41	74.5
Drank river water	39	97.5	55	100.0
Drank pond water at place B	35	87.5	17	30.9
Drank well-water at place A	33	82.5	48	87.2

[a] 40 cases and 55 controls.

Many other case–control inquiries can be made, limited only by the experience, skill, and imagination of the investigator. The basic principle is that the study is started by selecting a case group and a control group that *are comparable and had an equal chance of being exposed*. Questions are then asked about exposures relevant to the disease and the circumstances. The proportions of "cases" and "non-cases" that experienced the exposure are compared and statistically significant differences noted.

A2.2.4 Statistical assessment

When attack rates or proportions (in case–control studies) are being compared, the objective is to determine whether there are real differences between various population groups of interest. Since differences may occur by chance alone, it is necessary to have some method of estimating the probability that the differences *could* have occurred by chance or, conversely, that they are *unlikely* to have occurred by chance and are therefore likely to be real. The method used is the calculation of statistical probability, commonly referred to as "statistical significance".

Two approaches are available, the most frequently used being the direct calculation of the statistical probability that differences as great as those found could have occurred by chance. The result is expressed as a probability proportion—the number of times out of 100 or 1000 that a difference of the magnitude observed could have occurred by chance. This is written, e.g., as "$P = 0.13$", "$P = 0.03$" or "$P = 0.003$", meaning respectively 13 times out of 100, 3 times out of 100, and 3 times out of 1000. It has become the convention to consider $P = 0.05$ as the point that separates differences that are unlikely to be chance variations ("statistically significant", and therefore possibly meaningful) from those that might easily have occurred by chance (and are therefore "not statistically significant"). That is, a "P-value" of 0.05 or less (a chance event expected to occur 5 times in every 100 or less frequently) suggests a real difference, while one greater than 0.05 provides no strong evidence that the difference found is other than a chance happening. This arbitrary dividing line should not be treated as an absolute, however, and values above it should not cause a hypothesis to be rejected out of hand nor should one below it cause a hypothesis to be accepted blindly. Instead, the statistical evidence should be weighed together with all other information, and a conclusion reached accordingly.

For an epidemic control officer who is not well trained in statistical methodology a simpler but very useful approach is available. If the conventional 0.05 level of probability is accepted as a reasonable dividing line between differences that are likely to be chance variations (values above 0.05) and those that are likely to be meaningful (values of 0.05 or lower), simple formulae can be used to show whether two rates or two proportions differ "significantly". These are given in section A2.3, together with guidelines for their use and interpretation.

Although the question is not discussed at length in this manual, the disease control officer is often interested in determining the prevalence of some characteristic in a population, e.g., he may wish to determine the prevalence of amoebic cysts, of BCG immunization scars, or of households with vessels in which mosquitos are breeding. After selecting a representative sample of people or households, and making the necessary investigations, he calculates the rate. The rate obtained in the sample is obviously only an *estimate* of the true rate in the entire population, and will vary from sample to sample. Furthermore, the precision of the estimate will depend on the size of the sample, just as 10 tosses of a coin may easily produce 4, 5, or 6 "heads", but 100 tosses are likely to produce close to 50% "heads". Some statistical method of assessing the precision of a rate found by such an investigation is therefore necessary. The statistical calculation of "confidence intervals" provides a range of values that define the upper and lower limits within which the true population prevalence may confidently be expected to lie. A simple procedure for calculating a confidence interval is described in section A2.3.

A2.3 Statistical analysis

Most investigations conducted by an epidemiologist are concerned with the rate of occurrence of a particular phenomenon in a group of individuals under observation. It is helpful to distinguish between surveys to determine the rate of phenomenon X in population Y and descriptive epidemiological studies designed to discover whether there is a difference between the rates of occurrence of phenomenon X in populations Y and Z. In the first instance the statistical approach is to define a "confidence interval" for the rate, in the second, to determine whether the difference in the observed rates is likely to be a chance occurrence or not. Each of these approaches will be examined in turn.

Much of the work that a statistician does when analysing rates can be understood by any epidemiologist willing to study and make use of two concepts: the standard normal score and a statistical value often called Pearson's chi-squared statistic.

One-rate studies will be considered first here. The statistical formulae to be used in two-sample studies are given on pp. 160–163.

A2.3.1 Confidence intervals

Suppose the specific question to be answered is: "What is the rate of infection among all adult males exposed to virus X?". Since it is not feasible to study all such males, a representative sample of those exposed to the virus is selected, and the rate of infection in that sample is determined. It would be naive to assume that the rate found in this particular group is exactly equal to that for *all* exposed adult males. Instead, the statistician usually defines a 95% confidence interval to indicate the range within which the true overall rate is likely to lie.

If the true (but unknown) overall rate is called R, and the observed rate r, the confidence interval is given by the following formula:

$$R = r \pm (1.96) \sqrt{\frac{r(1-r)}{n}}$$

where n is the number of men in the sample.

For example, if 100 exposed men constitute the study group, and 30 become infected, then $r = 0.3$ and $n = 100$. The 95% confidence interval is then:

$$0.3 \pm (1.96) \sqrt{\frac{(0.3)(0.7)}{100}}$$

$$= 0.3 \pm (1.96)(0.046)$$

$$= 0.3 \pm 0.090.$$

The lower boundary, therefore, is $0.3 - 0.090 = 0.210$ and the upper boundary is $0.3 + 0.090 = 0.390$. The statistical interpretation is that 95 out of 100 confidence intervals established in this fashion will include the true value for R, the rate in the entire population of adult males. In non-statistical terminology, the epidemiologist interprets this result to mean that, while 30% is the best estimate of the infection rate among all men, he is confident that the true proportion of infected men in the community lies between 21% and 39%.

It should be noted that the confidence interval depends markedly on the size of the sample studied. If n were only 50 instead of 100 as above, the result would be 0.3 ± 0.127 (i.e., 0.173–0.427), and if it were 500 the result would be 0.3 ± 0.040 (i.e., 0.26–0.34). A large sample provides a far better estimate than a small one.

It is also important to note that the figure of 1.96 used in the formula is a standard normal score. The use of this value (for a 95% confidence interval) is a common convention, but is *not always* appropriate. If n is small and the rate is either very high or very low, a much more complicated formula is required and the assistance of a statistician may be needed. A quick rule of thumb is that 1.96 can safely be used if the sample contains at least 5 people who have experienced the phenomenon under study (i.e., were infected in this example) and 5 who have not experienced it (i.e., were not infected).

A2.3.2 Significance test

It is useful to distinguish between "single-group" studies and "multiple-group" studies. In a single-group study, the rate in the study group is compared with some rate established from information available before the study begins. In a multiple-group study, the rates for the two or more groups included in the study are compared with each other.

In both single- and multiple-group studies, the individuals included in the study are thought of as a sample taken from some larger population. The rate observed in a study group is considered to be an estimate of the actual rate for the entire population having similar characteristics and exposures. The epidemiologist therefore asks: "Is the difference between the observed rate and the 'established' rate for the entire population (or between the two observed rates) a real difference, or could it be merely a chance variation?" In other words, a "significance test for the difference between rates" must be made.

Single-group studies. Suppose that it is known that the rate of phenomenon X is 60% (i.e., the proportion is 0.6) in a general population. This rate has been found and confirmed in a number of settings. A need then arises to determine the rate of phenomenon X (which might, for example, be the malaria parasite rate) in some subpopulation of interest (the study population). A sample of 2000 persons from this study population is examined and a rate for malaria parasitaemia is obtained. This observed rate can be expected to differ somewhat from 60%. Does the difference between the observed rate and 60% indicate that the rate for the entire study population is different from 60%, or does it merely reflect the kind of variability that can be expected as the result of chance?

The appropriate test of significance in this problem is the calculation of Pearson's chi-squared statistic. The symbol used is χ_p^2 and the calculation is as follows.

Step 1. Calculate how many persons in the sample could be expected to have malaria parasites, on the assumption that the rate is the same in the study population as it is for the general population. In the example given, this expected number, E, will be equal to 1200 (0.6 times 2000).

Step 2. Determine the difference between the number of persons "expected" to have malaria parasites and the number actually observed. Then, ignoring the direction of the difference (i.e., whether it is negative or positive), reduce this figure by 0.5, and call the result D. In the example, suppose that 1300 of the 2000 people examined had malaria parasites. The difference between the expected and observed figures is 100; if this is reduced by 0.5, a value for D of 99.5 is obtained.

Step 3. Now calculate Pearson's chi-squared statistic from the formula:

$$\chi_p^2 = \frac{n(D^2)}{E(n-E)}$$

where n is the total number of people in the sample.
In the example given, $n = 2000$, $E = 1200$ and $D = 99.5$, so that

$$\chi_p^2 = \frac{2000\,(99.5)\,(99.5)}{1200\,(2000-1200)} = 20.626.$$

Step 4. Compare the resulting value of χ_p^2 with the number 3.84. A sample can be expected to yield a value of χ_p^2 as large as 3.84 by chance 5 times out of 100, if the true rate in the study population is equal to that in the general population. Since the value for the sample exceeds 3.84, it can therefore be concluded that there is a real difference between the rate for the study population and that for the general population. In statistical terminology, since the value exceeds 3.84, the result is statistically significant at the 0.05 level.

Again, it is important to note the effect of sample size on the result. If the sample had included only 200 people instead of 2000, and *the same percentages had been obtained* (i.e., $n = 200$, $E = 120$, observed value = 130, and $D = 9.5$), χ_p^2 would have been 1.89. This would have been "not statistically significant at the 0.05 level". It is possible to estimate in advance the size of the sample needed to demonstrate an expected possible result, but the assistance of a statistician may be required.

It must also be emphasized that the entire procedure described is appropriate only when the sample size is large enough for both E and $n - E$ to be greater than or equal to 5. If this is not the case, a more complicated analysis will be required and a statistician should be consulted.

Two-sample studies (unmatched). In studying the rate of occurrence of phenomenon X in population Y, it may be essential to compare rates for X between subgroups within that population (as in the dysentery epidemic discussed in section A2.1), e.g., for males as compared with females, exposed with unexposed persons, people over 40 years of age with those 40 years old or younger, etc. Once again, even if the rates are identical for all groups within population Y, it would not be reasonable to expect the rates actually found in the study groups to be identical. It is again necessary to be able to determine when differences in the observed rates reflect real differences in subpopulation rates and when they are likely to be due simply to chance. If members of the two subgroups are chosen independently of each other (i.e., without matching) the analysis involves calculation of χ_p^2 for a 2×2 table. (For "matched pairs", see p. 162.)

The case–control study described in section A2.2.3 may be taken as an example. The 40 dysentery cases and 55 controls were questioned about food and water consumption while they were fishing, and it was found that the two groups had differed considerably in the extent to which they had drunk pond water at place B. Cases and controls had not been matched. The results were displayed as percentages in Table A2.3, but for chi-squared analysis a different arrangement is required, as shown below:

Did you drink pond water?	Cases	Controls	Total
Yes	35 = a	17 = b	52
No	5 = c	38 = d	43
Total	40	55	95

The observed rates for drinking pond water—87.5% for cases and 30.9% for controls—seem to be very different, but do they indicate a real difference between these groups, or could they have been due to chance? To find out, Pearson's chi-squared statistic is calculated, as follows:

Step 1. Find the product $a \times d$ ($35 \times 38 = 1330$) and the product $b \times c$ ($17 \times 5 = 85$).

Step 2. Subtract the smaller product from the larger ($1330 - 85 = 1245$) and call the difference P_1.

Step 3. Find the product of all subtotals ($40 \times 55 \times 52 \times 43 = 4\,919\,200$) and call it P_2.

Step 4. Calculate Pearson's chi-squared statistic from the following formula:

$$\chi_p^2 = \frac{n(P_1 - n/2)^2}{P_2}$$

where n equals the total number in the study.
In the example, $P_1 = 1245$, $P_2 = 4\,919\,200$ and $n = 95$, so that:

$$\chi_p^2 = \frac{95(1245 - 95/2)^2}{4\,919\,200} = \frac{95(1197.5)^2}{4\,919\,200} = \frac{136\,230\,000}{4\,919\,200} = 27.694.$$

Step 5. Compare the value of χ_p^2 with the number 3.84. When the subpopulation or group rates are equal, samples of the size used can be expected to result in values of χ_p^2 as large as 3.84 by chance about 5 times out of 100. Since the value calculated is well above 3.84, it is concluded that the difference observed is unlikely to have occurred by chance alone and that the cases and controls really did differ in the extent to which they drank pond water at place B. In statistical terminology, a significant difference has been found between cases and controls at the 0.05 level of significance. The conclusion would have been quite different if the case–control differences for the characteristic "brought food from home", as shown in Table A2.3 had been tested. There the record showed that 32 out of 40 cases (80.0%) had brought food from home and 39 out of 55 controls (70.9%) did so. Calculating Pearson's chi-squared statistic as above gives a value of χ_p^2 equal to 0.589. Since this is below 3.84, it can be concluded that the difference between cases and controls could well be a chance variation.

It must be emphasized that the analysis just described is *not appropriate* if the number of people observed is small and rates are extremely high or extremely low. A rule of thumb is that, in the combined group of cases and controls (or males and females, etc.), at least 10 persons must be observed to exhibit the phenomenon and at least 10 persons must be observed not to do so. If these figures are not reached, other and more complicated statistical procedures will be needed, and the help of a statistican must be sought.[1]

Two-sample studies (paired data). In the preceding section, Pearson's chi-squared statistic was used on the assumption that the groups being compared were independent of one another. If males were compared with females or cases with controls, for example, it was assumed that each group represented all the components of its subpopulation. Sometimes, and particularly with relatively small samples in case–control studies, this assumption cannot be made. For example, in the analysis of the dysentery outbreak, it was assumed that the fishermen were a fairly homogeneous group and that the 40 cases and 55 controls were reasonably representative. If, however, the cases in a different outbreak occurred among members of three socially isolated clans, which had distinctive customs and habits and, furthermore, if different age groups traditionally lived and worked separately from each other, it could not be assumed that the 40 cases and the 55 controls selected at random would adequately represent the subgroups. To overcome the danger that cases and controls might come from different subgroups, and might therefore have different exposure histories simply because of that fact, the procedure known as matching can be employed, whereby for each case identified as belonging to a particular clan and age group, a control belonging to the same clan and age group would be selected. There would then be 80 subjects in the study, representing not two independent groups— cases and controls—but arranged as 40 pairs of subjects, the members of each pair differing from each other only in that one is a case and the other a control. In this situation, Pearson's chi-squared statistic is inappropriate. Instead, McNemar's chi-squared test for correlated proportions may be used. The symbol χ_M^2 will be used for the corresponding statistic.

Suppose that there are 40 case–control pairs in a study constructed as just described. When each pair is questioned about drinking pond water, four results are possible:

(a) both drank pond water;
(b) the case drank pond water, but the control did not;
(c) the control drank pond water, but the case did not;
(d) neither drank pond water.

The answers to the questions may be tabulated as follows:

---

[1] The analyses descried in this Annex and the formulae used have been developed by Professor Dale E. Mattson, for use in the restricted circumstances described. For a detailed discussion of the general use of Pearson's chi-squared test, see: Mattson, D. E., *Statistics: difficult concepts, understandable explanations*, Chicago, Bolchazy Carducci Publishers, 1984 (chapter 9, lesson 3).

		Control	
		Yes, drank pond water	No, did not drink pond water
Case	Yes	24 = a	11 = b
	No	3 = c	2 = d

The calculation of χ^2_M depends only on the number of pairs with differing outcomes for cases and controls, i.e., cells b and c. The steps are as follows:

Step 1. Count the number of pairs in which the case exhibits the phenomenon in question (drinking pond water) and the control does not. Call the result b. In the example, $b = 11$.

Step 2. Count the number of pairs in which the control exhibits the phenomenon and the case does not. Call the result c. In the example $c = 3$.

Step 3. Subtract b from c or c from b, depending on which is the smaller. In the example, since c is the smaller, it is subtracted from b $(11 - 3 = 8)$. Call the result P_1.

Step 4. Add b and c to obtain P_2. In the example, $P_2 = 11 + 3 = 14$.

Step 5. Calculate χ^2_M from the following formula:

$$\chi^2_M = \frac{(P_1 - 1)^2}{P_2}$$

In the example:

$$\chi^2_M = \frac{(8 - 1)^2}{14} = \frac{7^2}{14} = \frac{49}{14} = 3.5$$

Step 6. Compare χ^2_M with the number 3.84. Once again, if the calculated value of χ^2_M is equal to or greater than 3.84, it can be concluded that the rates for the subpopulation represented by cases and for that represented by controls are different. In the example, even though 35 cases had drunk pond water and only 27 controls had done so, the value of χ^2_M is less than 3.84 and it is therefore concluded that the difference could have been a chance variation (although it is a borderline result). In statistical terminology, the difference in rates (of drinking pond water) is not significant at the 0.05 level.

Once again, the analysis just described does not apply to all situations. It is appropriate only when sample sizes and rates are large enough to result in a value for P_2 of at least 10. If P_2 is less than 10, the solution is much more complicated and an epidemiologist without statistical training will need to seek the advice of a statistician.

BIBLIOGRAPHY

Guidelines on studies in environmental epidemiology. Geneva, World Health Organization, 1983 (Environmental Health Criteria No. 27).

MATTSON, D. E. *Statistics: difficult concepts, understandable explanations.* Chicago, Bolchazy Carducci Publishers, 1984.

Diseases that may cause epidemics[1]

Acquired immunodeficiency syndrome (AIDS)

Generalized lymphadenopathy of at least 3 months' duration involving two or more extrainguinal sites, afebrile or with prolonged intermittent fever, ending with severe opportunistic infections (*Pneumocystis carinii* pneumonia (see p. 203), disseminated *Mycobacterium avium* intracellular infection, Kaposi's sarcoma). Associated with a retrovirus. Laboratory: reactive hyperplasia of lymph nodes, abnormal T-lymphocyte helper/suppressor ratio. Incubation: possibly long. Transmission: sexual, blood and blood products, factors VIII and IX. Occurrence: first described in the United States of America in 1981, later identified in equatorial Africa and the Caribbean; in developed countries, clusters in homosexual males and intravenous drug addicts; cases have been described in female sexual partners of males with AIDS, children of infected mothers, and persons with haemophilia; in equatorial Africa, AIDS is acquired mainly through heterosexual contact. Control: investigation of contacts; same precautions for hospital and laboratory personnel as for viral hepatitis B. Reference: WHO Technical Report Series, No. 736, 1986 (Sixth report of the WHO Expert Committee on Venereal Diseases and Treponematoses).

Acute bacterial conjunctivitis (ICD 372.0)

Hyperaemia of the palpebral and bulbar conjunctivae of one or both eyes, photophobia, mucopurulent discharge. Caused by different bacteria: *Haemophilus influenzae* biotype III (Koch-Weeks bacillus), pneumococci, *H. influenzae* biotype I, *Moraxella lacunata*, staphylococci, streptococci, *Pseudomonas aeruginosa* and *Corynebacterium diphtheriae*. Differential diagnosis: gonococcal ophthalmia in the first 3 weeks of life. Laboratory: microscopic examination of a smear of discharge and isolation on appropriate culture media. Incubation: 1–3 days. Transmission: direct contact with discharges through contaminated fingers, possibly by droplets from the throat, indirect

---

[1] Where possible, the appropriate ICD code is given, taken from: *International Classification of Diseases*, 9th rev., Geneva, World Health Organization, 1977.

through soiled toilet articles, optical instruments, and flies. Occurrence: frequently epidemic, particularly in warm climates or communities with poor sanitation. Control: local application of sulfonamides or antibiotics; personal hygiene; vector control (flies, eye gnats). Safe disposal of ocular secretions during acute phase.

Acute schistosomiasis (ICD 120)

General malaise, spiking fever at night, profuse sweating, abdominal pain, myalgia, arthralgia, diarrhoea, dry cough, loss of weight, hepatomegaly, splenomegaly, urticaria, swollen eyelids; syndrome may last for 3-4 months. Complication: chronic stage (see Schistosomiasis, urinary and intestinal). Caused by: maturation, migration and early oviposition of *Schistosoma haematobium, S. mansoni,* and *S. japonicum.* Differential diagnosis: malaria, typhoid fever, salmonellosis, bacillary dysentery. Laboratory: high erythrocyte sedimentation rate, eosinophilia, microscopic detection of eggs in the stool or urine sediment, serological tests. Incubation period: 4-6 weeks after cercarial penetration in the skin (see Swimmers' itch). Transmission: contact with infested water by bathing or drinking. Occurrence: possible clustering of cases among tourists visiting endemic schistosomiasis zones. Control: treatment with antischistosomal drugs (praziquantel) should be delayed to avoid massive liberation of antigens. Reference: STUIVER, P. C. Acute schistosomiasis (Katayama fever). *British medical journal,* **288**: 221–222 (1984).

Acute viral gastroenteropathy (ICD 008.8)

Sudden onset, low-grade fever, nausea, vomiting, diarrhoea, abdominal cramps, headache, myalgia. Endemic forms are caused by rotaviruses (see Rotaviral enteritis), astroviruses, coronaviruses, adenoviruses, caliciviruses, and other small round viruses. Epidemics have been caused by Norwalk virus and related agents. Evidence is inconclusive for enteroviruses. Laboratory: immune electron microscopy and enzyme-linked immunosorbent assay (ELISA) for rotaviruses. Incubation: 48 hours or less. Transmission: direct by faecal-oral route or indirect via food and water. Occurrence: worldwide, greater in areas where hygiene is poor; predominantly in the United States of America for Norwalk virus (food-borne or water-borne outbreaks, sometimes with sharp onset; contagion has also occurred in swimming-pools). Control: no specific treatment; rehydration in severe cases; investigation of contacts and source of infection. Excreta precautions, enteric isolation for children during acute phase. Reference: WHO SCIENTIFIC WORKING GROUP. Rotavirus and other viral diarrhoeas. *Bulletin of the World Health Organization,* **58**: 183–198 (1980).

Acute viral pharyngitis (ICD 462)

Sore throat, mild fever, local pain, difficulty in talking and swallowing, cervical lymphadenopathy (may be the initial stage of a systemic infection or bronchitis). Caused by viruses such as influenza viruses, parainfluenza viruses, respiratory syncytial virus, adenoviruses, cytomegalovirus, human (gamma) herpesvirus 4 ("Epstein-Barr virus"), other herpesviruses, measles virus, mumps virus, arboviruses, Lassa fever virus, Ebola virus, or bacteria or agents such as *Mycoplasma pneumoniae*. Incubation: a few days. Transmission: droplets, occasionally aerosols, articles freshly soiled with pharyngeal discharges; asymptomatic carriers are frequent. Occurrence: worldwide. Control: no specific treatment. Secretion precautions.

Acute viral rhinitis (ICD 460)
Rhinitis with nasal watery discharge, mild fever. Caused by rhinoviruses, coronaviruses, respiratory syncytial virus, parainfluenza viruses, adenoviruses and certain enteroviruses. Complications: sinusitis, otitis, tracheitis, bronchitis. Incubation: 12–72 hours. Occurrence: worldwide, explosive outbreaks. Treatment: symptomatic. Secretion precautions.

Adenoviral conjunctivitis (ICD 077.3)
Sudden onset, unilateral or bilateral inflammation of conjunctivae, oedema of the lids, pain, photophobia, occasionally low-grade fever, headache, malaise, duration about 2 weeks. Complication: petechial haemorrhages of the cornea. Caused by type 8 adenovirus and occasionally other serotypes. Laboratory diagnosis: isolation of virus from eye swabs or conjunctival scrapings inoculated in cell culture; serological tests. Incubation: 5–12 days. Transmission: direct or indirect contact with eye secretions. Occurrence: worldwide, sporadic cases or explosive outbreaks which can originate in eye clinics; household spread; dust has been incriminated. Control: no specific treatment, rigorous asepsis in eye clinics (hand-washing), personal toilet articles, disinfection of conjunctival and nasal discharges and articles soiled therewith. Precautions: ocular secretions.

Adenoviral respiratory disease
See Pneumonitis, viral

Amoebiasis (ICD 006.9)
Acute form with fever, chills, tenesmus, blood and mucus in stools, or mild and recurrent afebrile forms. Complications: liver abscess, intestinal perforation. Fatalities linked to complications. Caused by *Entamoeba histolytica*, a protozoon. Differential diagnosis: shigellosis, balantidiasis, giardiasis, strongyloidiasis. Laboratory: microscopic demonstration of trophozoites and cysts in fresh faecal specimens on repeated examinations. Incubation: 2–4 weeks or longer. Transmission: faecal–oral, contaminated water, drinks (milk) and raw vegetables (cysts), food handlers, flies, asymptomatic carriers. Occurrence: all ages, prevalent in warm climates and under poor sanitary conditions, clusters of cases. Control: specific treatment, excretion precautions, investigation of source and contacts, protection and disinfection of water (boiling is preferred, since chlorination may be insufficient), cooking of vegetables, fly control. Precautions: excreta.

Reference: WHO SCIENTIFIC WORKING GROUP. Parasite-related diarrhoeas. *Bulletin of the World Health Organization*, **58**: 819–830 (1980).

Angiostrongyliasis (ICD 128.8)

Onset with low-grade fever, severe headache, stiffness of the back
and neck, various paraesthesias, temporary facial paralysis. Not lethal;
infection may be asymptomatic. Caused by a nematode (lung worm)
of rats, *Angiostrongylus cantonensis*. Differential diagnosis: tuberculous
meningitis, coccidioidal meningitis, aseptic meningitis, cerebral
cysticercosis, hydatidosis, gnathostomiasis. Laboratory: eosinophils,
and possibly the worm, in the cerebrospinal fluid. Transmission:
ingestion of insufficiently cooked snails, prawns, fish, vegetables.
No direct transmission. Occurrence: endemic in Australia, Egypt, East
Asia, Pacific islands and Madagascar. Control: boiling of incriminated
food.

Anthrax, cutaneous (ICD 022.0)

Itching of the exposed skin surface, appearance of a papular lesion,
which becomes vesicular and gives a depressed black eschar in 2–6
days, surrounded by moderate oedema and sometimes secondary
vesicles. Complications: if untreated, septicaemia; see also Anthrax,
intestinal and pulmonary. Caused by *Bacillus anthracis*. Differential
diagnosis: orf (contagious pustular dermatitis). Laboratory: demonstration of bacillus in local lesion or discharges by microscopic
examination after Gram staining; blood culture. Incubation period:
2–5 days. Transmission: common-source infection, contact of skin
with infected animal tissues or products made from them, or
contaminated soil. Occurrence: worldwide, sporadic or clusters of
cases as occupational hazard in farmers, veterinarians, workers in
agriculture-related industries (manufacture of animal feeding stuffs),
campers. Control: treatment with penicillin or tetracyclines, isolation
of discharges; disinfection of discharges and soiled articles by autoclaving to destroy spores, terminal cleaning; immunization of those
at occupational risk; prompt immunization of all animals at risk;
carcasses should be burned or buried deeply with anhydrous calcium
oxide. Precautions: skin discharges.

Anthrax, intestinal (ICD 022.2)

Fever, signs of septicaemia, abdominal symptoms, gastroenteritis
with vomiting and blood in the stools. Mortality is high.
Transmission: ingestion of contaminated undercooked meat.
Occurrence: rare, discrete foci, especially in developing countries.

Anthrax, pulmonary (ICD 022.1)

Onset: mild fever and non-specific symptoms, resembling common
upper respiratory tract infection, followed in 3–5 days by acute
respiratory distress, shock and death. Caused by *Bacillus anthracis*.

Laboratory: microscopic examination of sputum, isolation of agent by culture or animal inoculation (maximum containment laboratory). Incubation: 2–7 days, usually 2–5. Transmission: inhalation of spores. Occurrence: in foci of zoonotic anthrax, all climates, occupational hazard in agricultural workers, laboratory infections; may cause major outbreaks and nosocomial infections. Control: tetracyclines, **STRICT ISOLATION**, investigation of contacts and source of infection, terminal disinfection.

Argentine and Bolivian haemorrhagic fevers
See Junin and Machupo haemorrhagic fevers.

Arthropod-borne viral encephalitides (ICD 062/063)
Sudden onset, high fever, headache, meningeal signs, tremors, convulsions in infants, spastic paralysis (occasionally flaccid, as in Far Eastern tick-borne encephalitis), stupor, disorientation, coma. Other cases begin with an initial influenza- or dengue-like stage, followed by nervous system symptoms 4–10 days after apparent recovery. Mild cases do not proceed beyond the stage of aseptic meningitis. Severe infections may leave sequelae. Fatality rate: 0.5–60%. Caused by viruses belonging to different genera: Japanese encephalitis virus in the western Pacific, south-east Asia and India; Murray Valley encephalitis virus in Australia and Papua New Guinea; western equine encephalomyelitis virus in the USA and Canada; eastern equine encephalomyelitis virus, St Louis virus and California encephalitis viruses in the Americas; Rocio virus in Brazil; tick-borne encephalitis virus complex and Far Eastern tick-borne encephalitis in Europe, West Nile virus in Africa, south-west Asia, Europe and India. Differential diagnosis: non-paralytic poliomyelitis, rabies, mumps meningoencephalitis, lymphocytic choriomeningitis, aseptic meningitis due to enteroviruses, herpesviral encephalitis, postvaccinal or postinfection encephalitides, bacterial, protozoal, leptospiral, and mycotic meningitides. Laboratory: mild leukocytosis ($50–100/mm^3$) in cerebrospinal fluid; sometimes isolation of virus from brain tissue of fatal cases, rarely from blood; serological tests. Incubation: 5–15 days. Transmission by bites of mosquitos and ticks infected on animals (e.g., birds, rodents); no person-to-person transmission. Central European tick-borne encephalitis may also be transmitted by milk from infected goats or sheep. Occurrence: worldwide but greater in warm climates or in summer and limited to certain specific foci; sporadic or epidemic in all age groups but certain viruses predominantly affect children. Control: no specific treatment; protection against vectors; vaccination for Japanese encephalitis and restricted to laboratory workers for some of the other diseases. No isolation. References: MONATH, T. P. Arthropod-borne encephalitides in the Americas. *Bulletin of the World Health Organization,* **57**: 513–533 (1979); WHO Technical Report Series, No. 719, 1985 (*Arthropod-borne and rodent-borne viral diseases*: report of a WHO Scientific Group).

Arthropod-borne viral fever (ICD 066)

Signs and symptoms are similar to those of dengue (dengue-like fevers): sudden onset, fever, headache, muscular and joint pains, vomiting, and occasionally rash and lymphadenopathy. Usually not lethal. Caused by about 80 viruses belonging to several genera. Differential diagnosis: most frequently, influenza and malaria. Laboratory: isolation of virus from blood during the first 3–5 days; serological tests (IgM in single serum or IgG elevation in paired sera). Incubation: 2–15 days, usually 3–6. Transmission: by different arthropods: mosquitos, ticks, *Phlebotomus* (sandflies) and *Culicoides* (gnats). No direct person-to-person transmission. Occurrence: in all types of climate, depending on viruses prevalent locally, their vertebrate reservoirs and arthropod vectors; explosive outbreaks possible. Control: no specific drug, identification of vector and appropriate vector-control measures. See also dengue fever. Isolation under bed-net during the first few days when domestic mosquitos may be vectors. Reference: WHO Technical Report Series, No. 719, 1985 (*Arthropod-borne and rodent-borne viral diseases*: report of a WHO Scientific Group).

Aseptic viral meningitis

See Meningitis, viral.

Balantidiasis (ICD 007.0)

Diarrhoea, abdominal pains, vomiting, tenesmus, mucus and blood in stools. Fatality rate low. Caused by *Balantidium coli*, a protozoon. Incubation: unknown, perhaps a few days. Transmission: ingestion of cysts from contaminated swine, contaminated water, meat, vegetables, flies, soiled hands of food handlers. Occurrence: worldwide, rare except under poor sanitary conditions, water-borne epidemics possible. Control: metronidazole and tetracyclines, excreta precautions, protection against water and food contamination, fly control.

Bartonellosis (ICD 088.0)

There are two forms: Oroya fever, with severe anaemia and generalized lymphadenopathy, and verruga peruana, with muscular and joint pains, disseminated haemangioma-like dermal or deep-seated nodular lesions. Fatality rate of untreated Oroya fever: 10–40 %; verruga is rarely fatal. Caused by *Bartonella bacilliformis* within red blood cells. Incubation period: 16–22 days, up to 4 months. Transmitted by bite of sandfly (*Phlebotomus*); man is the reservoir. Occurs only at high altitudes in mountain valleys in south-west Colombia, Ecuador, and Peru. Control: treatment with antibiotics, house spraying with insecticides.

Bornholm disease

See Epidemic myalgia.

Botulism
See Food poisoning.

Boutonneuse fever
See Spotted fever group.

Bronchiolitis (ICD 466.1)
A respiratory disease of infancy; fever, cough, rapid breathing, expiratory wheezing, cyanosis, X-ray shows atelectasis and emphysema. High fatality rate—an infant may die overnight. Caused by respiratory syncytial virus, occasionally by parainfluenza viruses (mainly type 3) and influenza virus. Occurrence: worldwide; epidemics in spring, autumn and winter; nosocomial infections. Laboratory: virus isolation or specific immunofluorescence in nasopharyngeal aspirates. Control: secretion precautions, or respiratory isolation.

Bronchitis (ICD 466.0)
Generally follows an infection of the nasopharynx, slight fever, cough initially dry and becoming mucopurulent. Complication: chronic bronchitis in adults. Caused by viruses (influenza and parainfluenza viruses, respiratory syncytial viruses, adenoviruses, measles virus), *Mycoplasma pneumoniae*, or bacteria (*Haemophilus influenzae* and pneumococci). Laboratory: isolation of agent by cultivation of sputum in bacterial or viral media; serological tests. Incubation: a few days. Transmission: droplets, articles freshly soiled by discharges. Occurrence: worldwide, seasonal, clusters of cases in closed communities. Control: secretion precautions, antibiotics if bacterial pulmonary complications develop.

Brucellosis (ICD 023.9)
Acute or insidious onset, undulant fever, profuse sweating and weakness. Complications: meningitis, pneumonitis and local infections. Fatality rate without treatment, 2 % or less. Caused by different serotypes of a bacterium, *Brucella abortus*. Differential diagnosis: long-term "sweating" fevers, e.g., malaria. Laboratory: isolation of agent from blood or discharges; serological tests on paired sera in laboratories with appropriate expertise and facilities. Incubation: 5–30 days. Transmission: milk or milk products; occupational disease (contact with infected domestic animals), possibly airborne, no person-to-person transmission, laboratory infections. Occurrence: worldwide. Control: search for source of infection (animal or dairy products), tetracyclines. Isolation: not required. Reference: WHO Technical Report Series (Sixth report of the Joint FAO/WHO Expert Committee on Brucellosis) (in press).

Campylobacter enteritis (ICD 027.8)
Fever or normal temperature, malaise, headache, backache, abdominal pains, vomiting, and after 1–3 days profuse diarrhoea,

with liquid foul-smelling stools and blood streaks, which may last from a few days to 3 weeks. Complications: typhoid-like syndrome, septicaemia, endocarditis. Fatality rate does not seem high. Caused by a curved-rod vibrio-like bacillus, *Campylobacter jejuni*. Laboratory: isolation of the organisms by culture on special media. Incubation: 2–11 days. Transmission: direct contact, faecal–oral route (children to parents), contact with infected chickens, undercooked food, milk, water; frequent inapparent infections. Occurrence: probably world-wide, all ages, but especially children, sporadic cases, common-source outbreaks in families and institutions. Control: erythromycin, excretion precautions, search for source of infection and contacts. Reference: WHO SCIENTIFIC WORKING GROUP. Enteric infections due to *Campylobacter, Yersinia, Salmonella* and *Shigella. Bulletin of the World Health Organization*, **58**: 519–537 (1980).

Capillariasis (ICD 128.8)

There are three forms: enteropathy causing malabsorption, ascites, pleural transudate; acute or subacute hepatitis with eosinophilia; and pulmonary form with fever and asthmatic symptoms. Heavy infections may be fatal. Caused by *Capillaria* nematodes. Laboratory: detection of eggs in the sputum or faeces. Incubation period: 3–4 weeks. Contamination by ingesting soil-contaminated food or water; rats, dogs, cats and carnivores are reservoirs. Occurrence: hepatic and pulmonary forms are very rare, but worldwide; intestinal form is epidemic in the Philippines. Control: protect water supplies and food from animal faeces and dirt. Isolation not necessary.

Cercarial dermatitis

See Swimmers' itch.

Cercopithecid herpesvirus 1 disease (ICD 054.3;[1] 323.4[2])

Acute febrile onset followed by neurological symptoms and ascending encephalomyelitis, almost invariably rapidly fatal or leaving sequelae. Caused by *Herpesvirus simiae*. Laboratory: isolation of virus. Incubation period: up to 3 weeks. Transmission by bite of Old World monkeys, exposure of naked skin to saliva or monkey tissues. Occurrence: occupational disease, veterinarians, laboratory workers. Control: quarantine and precautions in handling monkeys.

Chagas' disease

See Trypanosomiasis, American.

Chickenpox

See Varicella.

---

[1] Primary code for underlying disease.
[2] Secondary code referring to the manifestation in the affected organ.

Chikungunya haemorrhagic fever (ICD 065.4)

Infection with Chikungunya virus (an arbovirus belonging to the genus *Alphavirus*) is common in Africa and Asia, with dengue-like symptoms. Haemorrhagic signs, petechiae, haematemesis and melaena have occurred only during epidemics in India and east Asia; there is no shock, and fatality rate is very low. Transmission: *Aedes* mosquitos. Laboratory: isolation of virus from blood, demonstration of antibodies. Control: symptomatic treatment; isolation under bednets during the first few days, protection from *Aedes* mosquitos. References: *Dengue haemorrhagic fever: diagnosis, treatment and control.* Geneva, World Health Organization, 1986; WHO Technical Report Series, No. 721, 1985 (*Viral haemorrhagic fevers*: report of a WHO Expert Committee).

Chlamydial conjunctivitis (ICD 077.0)

In adults: follicular conjunctivitis with minimal discharge, preauricular lymphadenopathy, symptoms sometimes persist for a year or longer. In the newborn: abundant mucopurulent discharge, possible superficial corneal involvement, may be followed by chlamydial pneumonia up to the age of 12 months. Caused by *Chlamydia trachomatis* immunotypes B–K. Differential diagnosis: trachoma caused by *Chlamydia trachomatis* immunotypes A, B and C and characterized by conjunctival follicular inflammation leading to deformity of the eyelids, corneal invasion and blindness, highly endemic in warm climates (trachoma). Laboratory diagnosis: demonstration of intracytoplasmic inclusion bodies in the epithelial cells of conjunctival or genital scrapings by Giemsa staining or immunofluorescence and isolation of the agent. Incubation: 5–12 days. Transmission: in adults, eyes are infected by fingers contaminated with genital secretion (chronic carriers may be asymptomatic); in the newborn, direct contact with the infected birth canal. Occurrence: worldwide; outbreaks in non-chlorinated swimming-pools. Control: adults and children, sulfonamides or antibiotics orally and antibiotic ointments; secretion precautions.

Cholera (ICD 001.0)

Sudden onset, profuse watery stools, occasional vomiting, rapid dehydration, acidosis, circulatory collapse; no fever, except sometimes in children. Untreated, fatality rate may exceed 50% and death may occur within a few hours; treated, the rate is below 1%. Mild cases with only diarrhoea and asymptomatic infections are frequent. Caused by *Vibrio cholerae* O-group 1 (biotypes eltor or classical). Differential diagnosis: non-O-group 1 *V. cholerae* strains, which can cause limited outbreaks of cholera-like disease, sometimes with fever and mucus and blood in stools, but no large epidemics. Laboratory: dark-field or phase-microscopy examination of faeces or vomitus shows characteristic vibrio motility inhibited by specific antiserum;

culture on special media; serological tests showing a rise of antibody in paired sera. Incubation: a few hours to 5 days. Transmission: faecal-oral, water, food, flies. Occurrence: endemoepidemic in Africa, Asia, Eastern Europe and India; imported in the Americas and Western Europe; rare outbreaks associated with air travel. Control: rehydration fluid (oral, intravenous), tetracyclines, trimethoprim-sulfamethoxazole, no isolation (except in non-endemic areas), excretion precautions, disinfection of hands, boiling or chlorination of water, search for source of infection and contacts for chemoprophy-laxis; immunization is inappropriate; notification to WHO (disease subject to the International Health Regulations). References: *A manual for the treatment of acute diarrhoea*, unpublished WHO document, WHO/CDD/SER/80.2; *Guidelines for cholera control*, unpublished WHO document, WHO/CDD/SER/80.4; WHO SCIENTIFIC WORKING GROUP. Cholera and other vibrio-associated diarrhoeas. *Bulletin of the World Health Organization*, **58**: 353-374 (1980).

Clonorchiasis (ICD 121.1)
Heavy infections may initially cause fever, chills, hepatomegaly, diarrhoea, mild jaundice and eosinophilia, followed by chronic inflammation of the biliary tree. Caused by *Clonorchis sinensis*, a trematode worm. Laboratory: demonstration of eggs in faeces or duodenal drainage fluid. Incubation period: about 1 month. Transmission: eating undercooked freshwater fish in endemic zone. Occurrence: South-East Asia; dried or pickled fish may cause imported cases. Control: locate source of infected fish, thorough cooking. Isolation not necessary.

Coccidioidomycosis (ICD 114)
Onset may be asymptomatic or resemble influenza followed by erythema nodosum. Complications: disseminated subcutaneous and visceral lesions, meningitis. Caused by: *Coccidioides immitis*, a fungus. Laboratory: direct examination or culture of sputum, pus, urine or cerebrospinal fluid; skin test with coccidioidin, serological tests. Incubation period: 1-4 weeks. Transmission: inhalation of spores from soil. No person-to-person transmission. Occurrence: arid and semi-arid areas of north, central and tropical South America; outbreaks may occur in endemic areas in large groups of susceptible persons from non-endemic areas. Control: treatment with fungicidal drugs.

Common cold
See Acute viral rhinitis.

Conjunctivitis
See Acute bacterial conjunctivitis, Adenoviral conjunctivitis, Chlamydial conjunctivitis.

Crimean-Congo haemorrhagic fever (ICD 065.0)

Sudden onset, influenza-like initial phase with occasional vomiting and diarrhoea. Acute phase: petechial rash, large purpura areas, bleeding from gums, nose, lungs and uterus, haematemesis, haematuria, melaena, shock. Fatality rate: 2–50%; severe form in Central Asia, mild form in Central Africa. Caused by Congo virus (family Bunyaviridae). Laboratory: safety precautions, isolation of virus from blood and necropsy material and serological tests (containment laboratory). Incubation: 7–12 days. Transmission: by ticks infected by feeding on birds, rodents and domestic animals; person-to-person by contact with blood (hospital and laboratory infections). Occurrence: all ages; limited natural foci in rural areas. Treatment: supportive care; convalescent serum. Control: **STRICT ISOLATION;** protection against ticks (repellents, special clothing); disinfection of bloody discharges. References: AL TIKRITI, S. K. ET AL. Congo-Crimean haemorrhagic fever in Iraq. *Bulletin of the World Health Organization,* **59**: 85–90 (1981); WHO Technical Report Series, No. 721, 1985 (*Viral haemorrhagic fevers*: report of a WHO Expert Committee).

Croup

See Laryngotracheobronchitis.

Cryptococcosis (ICD 117.5)

Usually a subacute or chronic meningoencephalitis preceded by pulmonary infection sometimes by several months. Caused by a fungus: *Cryptococcus neoformans.* Laboratory: microscopic examination of cerebrospinal fluid mixed with Indian ink. Incubation: unknown. Transmission: inhalation of saprophytic fungus in the external environment (soil and pigeon droppings); infection also occurs in domestic animals; no person-to-person transmission. Occurrence: worldwide, usually sporadic, adults. Control: treatment with fungicidal drugs.

Delta agent hepatitis

See Viral hepatitis B.

Dengue fever (ICD 061)

Sudden onset, chills, fever, intense headache, joint and muscle pains, prostration and early erythema in certain cases. On 3rd or 4th day, transient defervescence (saddle-back fever). A macular eruption is frequent, sometimes petechiae appear on feet and legs, lymphadenopathy is also frequent. Fatality rate is usually zero. Complication: dengue haemorrhagic fever. Caused by the four serotypes of dengue virus (an arbovirus, genus *Flavivirus*). Differential diagnosis: other arthropod-borne viral fevers (see p. 170), influenza, typhus, sandfly (phlebotomus) fever and rubella. Laboratory: isolation of virus from blood during the first 3–5 days in laboratories with appropriate expertise; serological tests (IgM in single serum or IgG elevation in paired sera). Incubation: 3–15 days (mean 5–6). Transmission: indirect, from person to person mainly by *Aedes aegypti*, or by other *Aedes* mosquitos according to region. Occurrence: endemic areas in tropical regions (Africa, middle America, Asia); all age groups (frequently mild in children), sharp outbreaks when spreading to new areas or in newly exposed groups, spreading by transport of infected mosquitos or viraemic patients. Control: no specific treatment, symptomatic treatment (aspirin may cause bleeding and is contra-indicated); isolation under bed-nets during 3–5 days; individual protection against mosquitos; *Aedes* control measures in community; notification is optional. Reference: information on outbreaks is published by WHO in the *Weekly epidemiological record*.

Dengue haemorrhagic fever (ICD 065.4)

The haemorrhagic syndrome affects mainly non-Caucasian children 6 months to 12 years old in highly endemic dengue areas, and less frequently adults. In the initial phase, the child may have fever, upper respiratory symptoms, headache, vomiting and abdominal pain. Myalgia and arthralgia, characteristic of classical dengue, are uncommon. This minor illness, during which the child is often not confined to bed, lasts 2–4 days and many children recover without any further symptoms. In some, however, the condition suddenly deteriorates on the 3rd or 4th day when the temperature falls and there is abdominal pain, restlessness, lowering of the pulse pressure, peripheral vascular congestion, cold and clammy extremities, elevated erythrocyte volume fraction resulting from plasma leakage through capillaries, leading to hypovolaemic shock which is reversible for a few hours, petechiae, positive tourniquet test, thrombocytopenia, protracted bleeding time, haematemesis, and melaena resulting from disseminated intravascular coagulopathy. Fatality rate: untreated, 10–20%; treated, as low as 1%. Caused by the four serotypes of dengue virus (genus *Flavivirus*). Laboratory: isolation of virus from blood in early phase; serological tests for IgM in single serum and elevation of IgG in paired sera. Incubation: 6 days (range 3–15). Transmission: indirect, from person to person by several species of *Aedes* mosquitos, mainly *Aedes aegypti*; no direct transmission. Occurrence: mainly tropical zones of South-East Asia, and recent extension to South Pacific islands and the Caribbean (Cuba); still unknown in tropical Africa, in spite of the presence of dengue virus types 1, 2 and 4. Control: treatment of hypovolaemic shock by urgent intravenous rehydration carefully monitored to avoid pulmonary oedema; isolation under bed-nets during first few days; individual protection against mosquitos; space-spraying of insecticides during epidemics and breeding-site reduction; a vaccine is under development. Reference: *Dengue haemorrhagic fever: diagnosis, treatment and control*. Geneva, World Health Organization, 1986.

Diarrhoea due to parasites (ICD 127.9)

In addition to amoebiasis, balantidiasis, fascioliasis, fasciolopsiasis, schistosomiasis, and giardiasis, described elsewhere in this Annex, diarrhoeas may be caused by other parasites, such as intestinal nematodes (roundworms). Abdominal pain and diarrhoea preceded by dermatitis if larvae penetrate through the skin and pulmonitis if they migrate through the lungs to reach the intestine. Occurrence: more frequent in warm climates in areas of poor sanitation, numerous asymptomatic carriers, endemic, highly endemic and epidemic in newcomers (tourists). Transmission may be from person to person except for worms that have a developmental stage in animals or in soil. Agents: *Trichuris trichiura* (whipworm), *Ascaris lumbricoides*, *Ancylostoma duodenale* (hookworm, causing severe iron-deficiency anaemia), *Strongyloides stercoralis* (threadworm). Control: specific treatment, faecal hygiene. Reference: WHO SCIENTIFIC WORKING GROUP. Parasite-related diarrhoeas. *Bulletin of the World Health Organization*, **58**: 819–830 (1980).

Diphtheria (ICD 032.3)

Mild fever, patches of greyish membrane on inflammatory zones in pharynx, tonsillar areas, larynx, or nose; cervical lymphadenopathy, oedema of the neck, toxic status. Complication: obstruction of larynx (croup, crow cough). Fatality rate: 5–10%. Differential diagnosis: Vincent's angina, candidiasis, Lassa fever. Caused by *Corynebacterium diphtheriae*. Laboratory: Gram staining has little presumptive value; inoculation of special media; whenever clinical suspicion is aroused, treatment should be initiated without waiting for laboratory results. Incubation: 2–5 days or longer. Transmission: droplets, articles freshly soiled with discharges. Occurrence: worldwide, less frequent in warm climates (cutaneous diphtheria is more frequent). Control: **STRICT ISOLATION**, diphtheria antitoxin, antibiotics, oxygen, tracheostomy if necessary, active immunization, chemoprophylaxis with erythromycin, surveillance of contacts for 7 days, and search for carriers by throat swabbing and laboratory examination.

Dracontiasis (ICD 125.7)

Fever, nausea, vomiting, diarrhoea, dyspnoea, generalized urticaria and eosinophilia, burning and itching in a lower extremity, usually the foot, and occurrence of a blister where the adult female worm (1 m in length) will appear. Caused by *Dracunculus medinensis*, a nematode worm. Incubation: about 12 months. Transmission: infected crustacea of the genus *Cyclops* in drinking-water or step wells and ponds, no person-to-person transmission. Occurrence: localized foci in warm climates. Control: treatment; filtration or boiling of drinking-water, treatment of water with chlorine.

Ebola and Marburg virus diseases (ICD 078.8)

Sudden onset, fever, general pains, vomiting, watery diarrhoea, rapid dehydration, prostration. On 5th–7th day maculopapular rash (may look like measles with conjunctivitis), pharyngitis, ecchymoses, petechiae, bleeding from the nose and gums, haematemesis, melaena, metrorrhagia, circulatory failure, shock, death between days 7 and 16. Oedemas (facial swelling, pleuritic and pericarditic) are more commonly seen in Marburg disease. Fatality rate: 30% (Marburg disease) to 85% (Ebola disease). Caused by two morphologically similar but antigenically distinct viruses (family Filoviridae). Laboratory: isolation of virus from blood and necropsy specimens; serological tests (in maximum-containment laboratory). Incubation: 2–21 days, usually 3–7. Transmission: unknown animal source (monkeys incriminated for Marburg disease); person-to-person transmission through several generations of cases for Ebola disease, rarely exceeding the second generation for Marburg disease, by face-to-face contact (droplets, aerosols) or contact with blood. Occurrence: probably prevalent in most parts of sub-Saharan Africa, may be asymptomatic; isolated outbreaks may occur abruptly. Control: intensive supportive care, **STRICT ISOLATION**, investigation of contacts, immune plasma and antiviral drugs may be beneficial early in the disease. References. SIMPSON, D. I. H. *Marburg and Ebola virus infections: a guide for their diagnosis, management and control.* Geneva, World Health Organization, 1977 (WHO Offset Publication No. 36); Ebola haemorrhagic fever in Sudan, 1976: report of a WHO/International Study Team. *Bulletin of the World Health Organization*, **56**: 247–270 (1978); Ebola haemorrhagic fever in Zaire, 1976: report of an International Commission. *Bulletin of the World Health Organization*, **56**: 271–293 (1978). WHO Technical Report Series, No. 721, 1985 (*Viral haemorrhagic fevers*: report of a WHO Expert Committee).

Echinococcosis (ICD 112.9)

A disease caused in man by cysts of the larval stage of tapeworms which parasitize dogs and other carnivores.

In *unilocular echinococcosis*, there are a limited number of well-encapsulated cysts, most frequently located in the liver and lungs. They may be well tolerated for a certain time or cause severe symptoms and death. The parasite is *Echinococcus granulosus*, a tapeworm of the dog. Laboratory diagnosis is by microscopic identification of hooklets in cysts, membranes or sputum after rupture, serological tests, intradermal tests and histopathological examination. The incubation period extends from months to years. Transmission to man occurs by ingestion of parasite eggs disseminated by infected dogs or other carnivores in their fur, in food and water. Carnivores are infected by eating viscera of sheep, cattle and pigs infected with cysts. Occurrence: worldwide. Control: no specific treatment, surgical removal of voluminous cysts when feasible, limitation of access of dogs to viscera of grazing animals.

In *alveolar hydatid disease*, there are a large number of poorly circumscribed microvesicles (cysts), mainly in the liver but also in other organs. The prognosis depends on the number and location of the cysts and is generally grave. The parasite is *Echinococcus multilocularis*, a tapeworm of foxes, dogs and cats. Laboratory diagnosis is as above. Long incubation period. Transmission to man by ingestion of infective eggs excreted by carnivores which are infected by eating parasitized voles or mice, or through contact with contaminated water, raw vegetables and wild fruits. Occurrence: worldwide. Control: no specific treatment in man, treatment of domestic dogs and cats, precautions in handling foxes.

Polycystic echinococcosis, in which there is rapid proliferation and growth of cysts, occurs in the Americas and is caused by *Echinococcus vogeli*, transmitted to man by hunting dogs.

Encephalitis, viral (ICD 049)
A general term which includes encephalitides caused by alphaviruses, bunyaviruses and flaviviruses (see Arthropod-borne viral encephalitides) and other viruses such as human alphaherpesviruses 1–3, enteroviruses 70 and 71, mumps virus, and cercopithecid herpesvirus 1 (simian B disease). See also Meningoencephalitis due to miscellaneous infectious agents.

Enteritis due to *Escherichia coli* (ICD 008.0)
Three types of *E. coli* cause somewhat different syndromes. Enteroinvasive strains: fever, mucoid and occasionally bloody diarrhoea, as in shigellosis. Enterotoxigenic strains: profuse watery diarrhoea with or without fever, abdominal cramps, vomiting, acidosis, prostration, dehydration, similar to cholera. Enteropathogenic strains: associated with classical severe outbreaks of acute diarrhoea in newborns in nurseries and in summer. Laboratory: isolation of strains from stools and typing with specific sera; antibiotic sensitivity is important. Incubation: 12–72 hours. Transmission: faecal-oral, person-to-person or common-source by contaminated food-handlers (infection may be asymptomatic), water, food and flies. Occurrence: worldwide, outbreaks in nurseries and institutions, individual or clusters of cases of traveller's diarrhoea. Control: oral or intravenous rehydration, antibiotics; scrupulous hygiene practices in nurseries (hand-washing), strict enteric precautions in hospitals, disinfection of discharges and soiled articles. Reference: WHO SCIENTIFIC WORKING GROUP. *Escherichia coli* diarrhoea. *Bulletin of the World Health Organization*, **58**: 23–36 (1980).

Enteroviral exanthematous fever (ICD 048)

Febrile, rubelliform or morbilliform rash usually confined to the face, neck and chest, exceptionally haemorrhagic or vesicular. The course is generally benign but aseptic meningitis may occur. Caused by certain serotypes of coxsackievirus and echovirus. Laboratory: isolation of virus from blood, stools, throat and vesicles; serological tests on paired sera to show an increase in antibody. Incubation: 3–5 days. Transmission: direct person-to-person by faecal–oral route, or droplets; indirect through food, water, flies, swimming-pools, articles contaminated by discharges. Occurrence: worldwide, higher incidence in summer, all ages, clusters of cases in closed communities. Control: no specific treatment, personal and community hygiene; discharge precautions.

Enteroviral haemorrhagic conjunctivitis (ICD 077.4)

Sudden onset, hyperaemia of conjunctivae, seromucous discharge, subconjunctival haemorrhages, occasionally keratitis and uveitis, ocular signs and symptoms resolve in 1–2 weeks. Complications: lumbosacral radiculomyelitis (poliomyelitis-like) in some cases, mainly in South-East Asia. Caused by enterovirus 70; similar disease may be caused by coxsackievirus A24, adenovirus 11, 4 or 10. Laboratory: electron microscopy of conjunctivitis scrapings, inoculation of cell cultures (virus growth may be difficult); serological tests. Incubation: 1–2 days. Transmission: direct or indirect contact with eye discharges, optical instruments, possibly by droplets from the throat of infected persons. Occurrence: worldwide, all ages; explosive outbreaks in communities with poor hygiene, or clusters that can be traced to contaminated eye clinics. Control: no specific treatment, personal hygiene, appropriate disinfection of optical instruments, infected children should not attend school.

Enteroviral lymphonodular pharyngitis (ICD 074.8)

Pharyngitis characterized by raised, discrete, whitish or yellowish nodules surrounded by a narrow annular erythematic zone. Caused by coxsackievirus A10. Laboratory: cultivation of virus. Incubation period: 5 days. Transmission: droplet spread, nose and throat discharges, faeces of infected person; man is the only reservoir. Infectious period: acute stage, longer for stools. Occurrence: worldwide, outbreaks in children in summer and early autumn in nursery schools. Control: reduce person-to-person contact, disinfection of discharges, faeces and soiled articles.

Enteroviral paralytic encephalomyelitis (ICD 048;[1] 323.4[2])

Enterovirus infections, especially with echoviruses and coxsackieviruses (mainly A7, A9, B2–5) and enterovirus 71, may cause flaccid

---

[1] Primary code for underlying disease.
[2] Secondary code referring to the manifestation in the affected organ.

paralysis mainly in children, which can be severe, but may disappear after 2–3 weeks without sequelae. Differential diagnosis: poliomyelitis, Far Eastern tick-borne encephalitis (caused by a flavivirus transmitted by ticks in Asian USSR and central Europe), in which there may be flaccid paralysis mainly of the shoulder girdle, with sequelae; botulism is afebrile and shows very early symmetrical cranial nerve flaccid paralysis; tick-bite paralysis occurs uncommonly but worldwide and is manifested by a flaccid ascending motor paralysis which disappears when the tick is removed. Control: excreta and secretion precautions until clinical recovery.

Enteroviral vesicular pharyngitis (ICD 074.0)
Sudden onset, fever, malaise, sore throat, greyish papulovesicular pharyngeal lesions on erythematous base and ulcers. Not fatal. Caused by coxsackieviruses, group A, and occasionally other enteroviruses. Incubation: 3–5 days. Transmission: droplets, articles freshly soiled with pharyngeal discharges, and faecal–oral. Occurrence: worldwide, mainly in children. Control: no specific drug, personal hygiene.

Enteroviral vesicular stomatitis with exanthem (ICD 074.3)
Sudden onset of fever, oral vesicular lesions and papules, vesicular lesions persisting for 7–10 days on palms and soles, occasionally on the buttocks. Caused by coxsackieviruses and other enteroviruses. Differential diagnosis: foot and mouth disease. Laboratory: isolation of the virus from lesions and faeces; serological tests on paired sera. Transmission: person-to-person by direct contact with nose and throat discharges, droplet spread, local lesions and faeces, no reliable evidence of common-source infection. Occurrence: worldwide, in summer and early autumn, outbreaks among groups of children. Incubation: 3–5 days. Control: no specific treatment, reduce person-to-person contact and crowding, standard isolation, disinfection of discharges.

Epidemic exanthema with meningitis
See Enteroviral exanthematous fever.

Epidemic keratoconjunctivitis
See Adenoviral conjunctivitis.

Epidemic myalgia (ICD 074.1)
Sudden onset, fever, headache, paroxysmal pain in the chest or in the abdomen, simulating appendicitis in children. No fatalities. Complications: myocarditis, aseptic meningitis. Caused by group B coxsackieviruses. Laboratory: isolation of the virus from faeces and throat washings, concomitant with increase in antibody in paired sera. Incubation: 3–5 days. Transmission: faecal–oral, respiratory droplets,

articles freshly soiled, sewage, flies, asymptomatic carriers. Control: no specific drug (oral poliovirus vaccine may be used to try and stop the spread), personal hygiene, community sanitation, excreta precautions.

Erythema chronicum migrans due to *Borrelia burgdorferi* (ICD 695.9)

Progressive onset with fever, malaise and a red macule or papule expanding into a large annular lesion, sometimes multiple. Complications: polyarthritis, aseptic meningitis, encephalitis, cardiopathy. Caused by a spirochaete (*Borrelia*) and transmitted by *Ixodes* ticks. Differential diagnosis: none, the skin lesion is distinctive. Laboratory: no test available. Incubation: 3–21 days after tick bite. Transmission: tick-borne, no person-to-person transmission. Occurrence: endemic foci in the USA; a similar neurological disease but without rash (tick-borne meningopolyneuritis) exists in eastern Europe. Control: treatment with penicillin or tetracycline.

Erythema infectiosum (ICD 057.0)

Often non-febrile, no constitutional symptoms, erythema on the cheeks and limbs, possibly recurrent. Probably viral. Occurrence: children 4–14 years old; household and school outbreaks. Control: isolation not required.

Espundia

See Leishmaniasis, cutaneous.

Fascioliasis (ICD 121.3)

Abdominal pain (right upper quadrant), eosinophilia, biliary colic, jaundice. Caused by *Fasciola hepatica*, a trematode. Laboratory: eggs in the faeces or duodenal aspirate. Incubation: 10–60 days. Transmission: eating uncooked infested aquatic plants such as watercress. Reservoir: sheep and cattle. Occurrence: worldwide. Control: avoid eating uncooked aquatic plants in endemic areas.

Fasciolopsiasis (ICD 121.4)

Diarrhoea, constipation, vomiting, anorexia, eosinophilia. Massive infections may cause oedemas and intestinal obstruction. Caused by a trematode, *Fasciolopsis buski*. Laboratory: eggs in faeces. Incubation period: about 1 month. Transmission: eating uncooked, infested, aquatic plants. Occurrence: Asia. Control: avoid eating uncooked aquatic plants in endemic areas.

Fifth disease

See Erythema infectiosum.

Filariasis (ICD 125.9)

Early acute manifestations: fever, lymphadenitis, lymphangitis (many infected persons show no clinical symptoms). Complication: elephantiasis. Caused by nematodes *Wuchereria bancrofti* or *Brugia malayi*, which develop in lymphatics. Laboratory: eosinophilia; circulating microfilariae often difficult to see in spite of repeated examinations day and night. Incubation: 3 months or longer. Transmission: by bite of vector mosquito, belonging to *Culex, Aedes, Anopheles* and *Mansonia* genera, depending on local prevalence; no direct person-to-person transmission. Occurrence: warm and humid tropical climates. Control: treatment with diethylcarbamazine, vector control, mass treatment of carriers. Reference: WHO Technical Report Series, No. 702, 1984 (Fourth report of the WHO Expert Committee on Filariasis).

Five-day fever

See Trench fever.

Flea-borne typhus

See Typhus fever due to *Rickettsia typhi*.

Food poisoning

(1) *Bacillus cereus food poisoning (ICD 005.8)*

Sudden onset, vomiting only (heat-stable toxin), or diarrhoea and abdominal cramps (heat-labile toxin). Rarely fatal. Caused by the enterotoxin of *Bacillus cereus*. Laboratory: identification of the agent in stools and in the suspect food (counting of bacteria on selective media). Incubation: vomiting type, 1–6 hours; diarrhoeal type, 6–16 hours. Transmission: rice, vegetables and meat contaminated with spores from soil and kept at ambient temperature after cooking, permitting multiplication of the organism; no person-to-person transmission. Occurrence: mainly in Europe. Control: adequate cooking and preservation of food.

(2) *Botulism*

(a) *Food poisoning (ICD 005.1)*

Acute onset, double vision, dryness of the mouth, sore throat, vomiting, diarrhoea, cranial-nerve paralysis, descending paralysis, and respiratory failure. One-third of patients may die in 3–7 days as a result of respiratory failure. Caused by toxins secreted by different types of *Clostridium botulinum*, a bacterium. Laboratory: demonstration of specific toxin in serum or stool; identification of organisms in suspect food. Incubation: 12–36 hours or several days. Transmission: home-canned vegetables and fruits contaminated by spores contained in soil, preserved or smoked meats and fish. Toxin is destroyed by boiling, but spores are resistant. No person-to-person transmission.

Refrigeration does not necessarily prevent toxin production. Occurrence: worldwide; common-source infection. Control: polyvalent antitoxin or monovalent if the bacillus has been typed, detection of one case and identification of source should encourage a search for other possible cases.

(b) Botulism of infants

Progressive onset, constipation, lethargy and paralytic signs as above, with a wide spectrum of severity; case fatality rate: treated, 3%; untreated much higher. The disease results from colonization of the intestine by *C. botulinum* and production of various toxins. Laboratory: identification of bacillus and/or toxin in faeces or autopsy specimens. Incubation: duration unknown. Transmission: honey has been incriminated, no person-to-person transmission. Occurrence: probably worldwide, not well documented, mainly infants under 1 year of age. Control: as in (*a*) above.

(3) Clostridium perfringens food poisoning (ICD 005.2)

Caused by the toxins of several serotypes of *Clostridium perfringens,* an anaerobic bacillus. Type A: abdominal pain, diarrhoea, benign prognosis. Type C: necrotizing enteritis, severe prognosis. Laboratory: semiquantitative anaerobic culture of stools and suspect food (heavy bacterial contamination is required for clinical disease). Incubation: 6–24 hours, usually 10–12 hours. Transmission: beef, pork, turkey or chicken contaminated with faeces or soil containing spores, which germinate during cooking at moderate temperature and on rewarming; no person-to-person transmission. Occurrence: worldwide; outbreaks originate in food-catering firms and restaurants where cooking and refrigeration are inadequate. Treatment: fluid replacement when indicated. Control: only preventive, with special attention to meat, which should be served as soon as it is cooked, or rapidly refrigerated after cooking, and thoroughly reheated, if necessary.

(4) Staphylococcal food poisoning (ICD 005.0)

Violent onset, severe nausea and vomiting, cramps, watery diarrhoea, prostration, low blood pressure, mild or no fever. Short-duration disease, fatality rare. Caused by enterotoxins secreted by certain strains of *Staphylococcus aureus.* Laboratory: isolation of toxin-producing *Staphylococcus* in vomit, faeces or suspect food; their absence does not rule out this etiology if the outbreak has characteristic features. Incubation: 1–6 hours, usually 2–4 hours. Transmission: wide variety of food processed by *Staphylococcus* carriers (finger and eye infections, nasal secretions, apparently normal skin), ham, pressed meat, milk from cows with infected udders; no person-to-person transmission. Occurrence: worldwide, relatively frequent. Control: symptomatic treatment, investigation of source of infection. Prevention: prompt and correct refrigeration of processed food, exclusion of infected food handlers.

(5) *Vibrio parahaemolyticus food poisoning (ICD 005.4)*

Watery diarrhoea, abdominal cramps with vomiting, fever and headache usually present; occasionally a dysentery-like illness with blood and mucus in stools and high fever. Usually non-fatal. Caused by a bacterium, *Vibrio parahaemolyticus.* Laboratory: isolation of organisms from stools on special media. Incubation: 4–96 hours, usually 12–24 hours. Transmission: raw or insufficiently cooked seafood (the organism can survive at 80 °C for 15 minutes) followed by storage at ambient temperature; no person-to-person transmission. Occurrence: worldwide; sporadic cases or common-source outbreaks. Control: adequate cooking.

(6) *Other agents of food poisoning (ICD 005.9)*

These include chemical contaminants and organic substances that may be present in certain foods, such as mushrooms, fish, shellfish, and various fruits and vegetables. Mushroom poisoning may be caused by muscarine (onset in few minutes to 2 hours, salivation, sweating, vomiting, cramps, diarrhoea, confusion, coma), or phalloidine (onset 6–24 hours, same gastrointestinal symptoms plus oliguria, jaundice, liver damage), both of which have a severe prognosis. Among several agents of fish poisoning, icthyosarcotoxism due to ciguatera results from eating fish containing a toxin produced by a marine dinoflagellate of coral reefs in tropical seas. After $\frac{1}{2}$–4 hours, this may cause a common-source-type outbreak characterized by circumoral tingling, vomiting, diarrhoea, generalized pains, fever, prostration and paralysis. Shellfish poisoning by mussels and clams that have ingested poisonous dinoflagellates may cause similar symptoms, 5–30 minutes after eating. Certain oysters may cause gastrointestinal symptoms, bleeding, and liver disturbances, which appear 24–48 hours after ingestion and have a severe prognosis. Chemical poisoning may result from the presence of toxic insecticides on fruit and vegetables, use of lead-glazed pottery, etc. Reference: HALSTEAD, B. W. & SCHANTZ, E. J. *Paralytic shellfish poisoning.* Geneva, World Health Organization, 1984 (WHO Offset Publication, No. 79).

Gammaherpesviral mononucleosis (ICD 075)

Onset with grippe-like malaise followed by high fever, sore throat (exudative pharyngitis), localized posterior cervical or generalized adenopathy, splenomegaly (50 % of cases), hepatomegaly (20 %), jaundice (5 %), orbital oedema, or typhoidal form without sore throat (10 %). Complications: pneumonitis, meningoencephalitis; hepatic sequelae are unusual. Caused by human (gamma) herpesvirus 4 ("Epstein-Barr virus") (family Herpesviridae). Differential diagnosis: streptococcal pharyngitis, diphtheria, necrotizing ulcerative pharyngitis, rubella, adenovirus infection, hepatitis, toxoplasmosis, cytomegalovirus infection. Laboratory: elevated total white blood cell count by the 2nd – 3rd week with lymphocytosis and atypical lymphocytes (occasionally found in viral hepatitis, measles, rubella); heterophil antibody (Paul-Bunnell-Davidsohn test) appears by the 2nd week of illness (may be absent in children and 10 % of adults). Incubation: 4– 6 weeks. Transmission: direct by oral route (saliva), indirect by blood transfusion; excretion may persist for months. Occurrence: worldwide, during early childhood in areas of poor hygiene, during adolescence in higher socioeconomic groups; not very contagious, outbreaks in closed communities (colleges, universities, military groups). Control: no specific treatment; no isolation; safe disposal of nose and throat discharges.

Gastroenteritis, viral
See Acute viral gastroenteropathy and Rotaviral enteritis.

Giardiasis (ICD 007.1)
Chronic diarrhoea, greasy malodorous stools, abdominal cramps, fatigue. Caused by *Giardia lamblia* a flagellate protozoon. Laboratory: identification of cysts or trophozoites in serial examination of stools. Incubation: 2 weeks (range 1–4 weeks). Transmission: faecal–oral, person-to-person, contaminated water supplies (the cysts withstand chlorination), food, frequent asymptomatic carriers. Occurrence: worldwide, children and adults, localized common-source outbreaks. Control: treatment with mepacrine hydrochloride, investigation of source of infection; control of water supplies; personal hygiene and community sanitation: excreta precautions. Reference: WHO Scientific Working Group. Parasite-related diarrhoeas. *Bulletin of the World Health Organization,* **58**: 819–830 (1980).

Glandular fever
See Gammaherpesviral mononucleosis.

Guillain-Barré syndrome (ICD 357.0)
Progressive ascending symmetrical peripheral paralysis of the limbs which may reach the face and trunk, with sensorial alterations but without febrile syndrome. Recovery without sequelae after a period of 2–3 weeks. Rare complication: respiratory paralysis. Very low fatality rate. Laboratory: no cells in cerebrospinal fluid and high protein content (albuminocytological dissociation). No specific agent, rather a complication of recognized or unrecognized viral infections and immunization with viral vaccines 1–3 weeks earlier. No person-to-person transmission. Occurrence: adults, probably worldwide but not documented everywhere. Control: symptomatic treatment.

Guinea-worm disease
See Dracontiasis.

Haemorrhagic conjunctivitis, epidemic
See Enteroviral haemorrhagic conjunctivitis.

Haemorrhagic fever with renal syndrome (ICD 078.0)
Severe form: sudden onset with fever, headache, lethargy, abdominal and lumbar pain, facial flush, injection of the conjunctiva, petechiae. Proteinuria appears on 3rd–5th day, followed on 5th day by hypotensive phase, confusion, delirium, coma, ecchymoses, haemoptysis, haematemesis, haematuria, steep fall in platelets. Oliguric phase over the next 3–4 days, followed by a diuretic phase with risk of hypotension and shock, pulmonary oedema, severe electrolytic imbalance. Mild form: abrupt onset, after 3–6 days backache and abdominal pain are predominant, proteinuria, oliguria, moderate thrombocytopenia. Case fatality rate: untreated 15%, treated 5%, mild form 0.5%. Inapparent infection exists. Caused by Hantaan virus (family Bunyaviridae). Laboratory: safety precautions, isolation of virus from blood difficult, serological test. Incubation: 7–35 days, usually 14–21. Transmission: rodent excrement, field rats in rural areas, *Rattus norvegicus* in urban areas, laboratory rats; no person-to-person transmission. Occurrence: severe form in east Asia, mild form in Scandinavia and possibly in other parts of the world; seasonal, adults, rural foci. Control: no specific treatment; gown, gloves and mask isolation; disinfection of blood-contaminated discharges: rodent control; no international measures but information desirable. Reference: Haemorrhagic fever with renal syndrome: Memorandum from a WHO meeting. *Bulletin of the World Health Organization*, **61**: 269–275 (1983); WHO Technical Report Series, No. 721, 1985 (*Viral haemorrhagic fevers*: report of a WHO Expert Committee).

Hand, foot and mouth disease
See Enteroviral vesicular stomatitis with exanthem.

Heatstroke—heat exhaustion (ICD 992.0)
Both may mimic outbreaks of infectious disease. Heat stroke: hot, red, dry skin, little sweating (key sign), hard rapid pulse, very high temperature, unconsciousness and convulsions. Heat exhaustion: pale, greyish, clammy skin, weak and slow pulse, low blood pressure and faintness, shock. Treatment of heat stroke: emergency cooling by wrapping in wet cloths or immersing in cool water. Treatment of heat exhaustion: as for syncope, head down, replace lost salt and water orally.

Hepatitis, viral
See Viral hepatitis.

Herpangina
See Enteroviral vesicular pharyngitis.

Herpesviral gingivostomatitis (ICD 054.2)
Deep and painful vesicles and ulcers in the mouth, fever and malaise. Fatality rate low. Complications: keratoconjunctivitis, meningoencephalitis. Caused by type 1 herpesvirus. Incubation: 2–12 days. Transmission: direct contact with pharyngeal secretions; asymptomatic carriers. Occurrence: worldwide, usually an asymptomatic primary infection of young children but outbreaks may occur in closed communities. Control: personal hygiene, drugs being evaluated; secretion precautions.

Histoplasmosis (ICD 115.9)
Pulmonary form of a systemic mycotic infection easily overlooked, fever, malaise, mild respiratory illness, chest pain, cough, dyspnoea, occasionally more severe systemic and pulmonary symptoms, X-rays show pulmonary infiltrates and enlarged hilar lymph nodes. Complications: chronicity. Caused by a fungus, *Histoplasma capsulatum*. Laboratory: Giemsa staining of sputum, histoplasmin reaction, complement-fixation test. Incubation: 5–18 days, usually 10 days. Transmission: airborne, no person-to-person transmission. Occurrence: foci in the Americas, eastern Asia, Europe and Africa (a different variety of the fungus); outbreaks in groups of workers exposed to infected birds and bats or their droppings. Control: amphotericin B.

Icthyosarcotoxism
See Food poisoning, other agents.

Infectious mononucleosis
See Gammaherpesviral mononucleosis.

Influenza (ICD 487.1)
Sudden onset, chills, fever, headache, generalized aches, prostration, coryza, sore throat, severe and protracted cough, duration 2–7 days. Complications: bronchitis, bronchiolitis, pneumonitis, secondary bacterial pneumonia. Caused by influenza viruses A and B. Laboratory: isolation of virus from nasopharyngeal aspirate or throat swabbing, serotyping of strain in WHO collaborating centres; serological tests. Incubation: 24–72 hours. Transmission: droplets, aerosols, nasal discharges. Occurrence: in winter, worldwide, outbreaks of influenza A occur annually, major epidemics at intervals of 2–3 years and pandemics (up to 15–40% attack rate) at intervals of about 10–15 years. Influenza B occurs annually with epidemics at intervals of 4–7 years, with high incidence in closed communities (e.g., nursing homes for the elderly). Control: immunization with

vaccine adapted to current A and B variants in advance of the epidemic season, particularly for personnel of public services, the elderly and immunocompromised persons (with inactivated vaccine); rimantadine as preventive drug after contact or to alleviate infection (ineffective against influenza B); secondary pneumonias require RESPIRATORY ISOLATION or **STRICT ISOLATION**. Notification of epidemics to WHO (disease under surveillance). Reference: periodic information on outbreaks, occurrence of variant strains and recommended composition of vaccines is published in the *Weekly epidemiological record.*

Japanese encephalitis
See Arthropod-borne viral encephalitides.

Junin and Machupo haemorrhagic fevers (ICD 078.7)
The two diseases are very similar although caused by two different arenaviruses. Insidious onset, moderate fever, generalized aches and, after a few days, haemorrhages from the gums and nose, haematemesis, haematuria and melaena. Case-fatality rate varies from 5 % to 30 %; death may result from hypovolaemic shock. Laboratory: safety precautions, isolation of virus and serological tests. Incubation: 7–16 days. Transmission: excreta of infective rodents (*Calomys* spp.) contaminating dust and foodstuffs; a few instances of person-to-person transmission for Machupo haemorrhagic fever. Occurrence: seasonal, mainly in adults in limited rural foci in Argentina and Bolivia. Treatment: immune serum or globulin. Control: rodent control. References: Argentine haemorrhagic fever surveillance. *Weekly epidemiological record*, **57**: 219–220 (1982); WHO Technical Report Series, No. 721, 1985 (*Viral haemorrhagic fevers*: report of a WHO Expert Committee).

Kala azar
See Leishmaniasis, visceral.

Katayama fever
See Acute schistosomiasis.

Kawasaki syndrome
See Mucocutaneous lymph node syndrome.

Keratoconjunctivitis, epidemic
See Adenoviral conjunctivitis.

Korean haemorrhagic fever
See Haemorrhagic fever with renal syndrome.

Kyasanur Forest disease (ICD 065.2)

Clinically similar to Omsk haemorrhagic fever with more frequent meningoencephalitis. Caused by a flavivirus. Incubation: 3–7 days. Transmission: cattle ticks, laboratory infections. Occurrence: only in Mysore State, India. Control: tick repellents, a vaccine is used locally. Reference: WHO Technical Report Series, No. 721, 1985 (*Viral haemorrhagic fevers*: report of a WHO Expert Committee).

Laryngotracheobronchitis (ICD 466.0)

Fever, cough, stridor, respiratory distress. Caused by parainfluenza viruses, respiratory syncytial virus and influenza virus. Incubation: few days to a week. Transmission: oral contact, droplets, articles freshly soiled with respiratory discharges. Occurrence: worldwide, cold season, high incidence in infants and preschool children; sometimes sharp outbreaks. Control: secretion precautions, no specific drug, unless diphtheria is a possibility, oxygen, tracheostomy if necessary.

Lassa fever (ICD 078.8)

Progressive onset with intermittent spiking fever, headache, myalgia, vomiting, diarrhoea, chest and abdominal pain, oropharyngeal ulcers with greyish membranes, cervical adenopathy, swelling of face and neck. During the second week severe cases show oedema, pleural effusion, cardiac and renal failure, haemoconcentration, encephalopathy, haemorrhagic manifestations, and shock. Fatality rate: 36–67%. Mild forms and inapparent infections occur not infrequently in endemic areas. Differential diagnosis: diphtheria, typhoid. Caused by an arenavirus. Laboratory: safety precautions, isolation of virus from blood and the throat during the 1st and 2nd weeks, and from urine during the 2nd–5th weeks; serological tests (maximum-containment laboratory). Incubation: 7–21 days. Transmission: from field and semidomestic rodents (the multimammate rat, *Mastomys natalensis*) to man through contamination of food by urine, or dust; person-to-person contamination through blood, respiratory droplets and aerosols, more frequently by primary cases than by secondary ones. Occurrence: West and Central Africa. Treatment: immune plasma and antiviral drugs are presumed beneficial, intensive supportive care. Control: **STRICT ISOLATION**, surveillance of contacts; rodent control. References: MONATH, T. P. Lassa fever and Marburg virus disease. *WHO Chronicle*, **28**: 212–219 (1974); International symposium on arenaviral infections of public health importance. *Bulletin of the World Health Organization*, **52**: 381–766 (1975); Lassa fever. *Weekly epidemiological record, **49**: 341–343 (1974); WHO Technical Report Series, No. 721, 1985 (*Viral haemorrhagic fevers*: report of a WHO Expert Committee).

Legionnaires' disease (ICD 482.8)
Insidious onset, low-grade fever for 5 days then sudden rise in temperature with chills, diarrhoea, cough, chest or abdominal pain; X-rays show nodular then lobar consolidation; occasional extra-pulmonary manifestations such as diarrhoea, encephalopathy, hepatic and renal dysfunction. Complications: hypoxaemia, renal failure, shock. Fatality rate: 15–20%. Differential diagnosis: other pneumonias. Caused by a bacillus, *Legionella pneumophila* serotype 1. Laboratory: safety precautions, visualization of agent by immuno-fluorescence, cultivation, serological tests by immunofluorescence; IgM antibody remains high for at least 18 months after clinical infection. Incubation: 2–10 days, usually 5–6. Transmission: infected water supplies and air-conditioning systems, dust from excavation works, aerosol spread, no person-to-person transmission yet docu-mented. Occurrence: worldwide, middle and older age groups, sporadic or epidemic, common-source infections. Control: erythromycin intra-venously and rifampicin; gown, secretion precautions; identification of source of exposure and disinfection. Reference: REID, D. ET AL. Illness associated with "package tours": a combined Spanish-Scottish study. *Bulletin of the World Health Organization*, **56**: 117–122 (1978).

Leishmaniasis, cutaneous (ICD 085.9)
Two forms: oriental sore, characterized by single or multiple ulcerating skin lesions, and espundia with same cutaneous lesions and mutilating ulcerative lesions of the nose and pharynx. Oriental sore is caused by *Leishmania tropica*, a protozoan parasite of histiocytes, and espundia by *L. braziliensis* and *L. mexicana*. Laboratory: non-flagellated forms of the parasite may be seen by microscopic examination of stained smears or scrapings from the edges of lesions and this material may be cultivated in special media. Incubation period: from a few days to several months. Infectious period: until healing of lesions. Transmission: bites of phlebotomines (sandflies) infected by feeding on wild rodents and dogs; no direct person-to-person transmission. Occurrence: oriental sore in Africa (except South Africa), south-west Asia, China, India, and the Mediterranean basin; American leishmaniasis is restricted to tropical forests. Control: indoor application of residual insecticides, elimination of breeding sites (rubbish heaps), use of repellents and fine mesh screens; treatment with specific drugs. Reference: WHO Technical Report Series, No. 701, 1984 (*The leishmaniases*: report of a WHO Expert Committee).

Leishmaniasis, visceral (ICD 085.0)
Gradual or sudden onset of fever with continued and irregular course, lymphadenopathy, hepatosplenomegaly, anaemia and leuko-penia. Untreated, usually fatal chronic course. Caused by *Leishmania*

donovani, a protozoan parasite of histiocytes. Laboratory: demonstration of parasite in stained smears of lymph nodes, bone marrow or blood. Incubation: 10 days to 2 years, usually 2–4 months. Transmission: from dogs, cats and rodents to man, or from man to man through the bite of sandflies (phlebotomines). Occurrence: rural areas of tropical and subtropical regions; scattered cases or occasionally limited outbreaks. Control: treatment with specific drugs, vector control, protection from bites of phlebotomines. Reference: WHO Technical Report Series, No. 701, 1984 (*The leishmaniases*: report of a WHO Expert Committee).

Leptospirosis (ICD 100.9)

Abrupt onset, fever, headache, vomiting, muscular aches, conjunctivitis and occasionally rash. Complications (during second phase): jaundice, meningitis, haemorrhages in the skin and mucous membranes; and renal failure. Fatality rate: from low up to 20%. Caused by several serotypes of *Leptospira* (spirochaetes). Differential diagnosis: influenza, other causes of meningitis and hepatitis. Laboratory: isolation of leptospires from blood during the acute illness, from urine after the first week; rising titres in serological tests. Incubation: 4–19 days, usually 10. Transmission: direct contact with infected domestic animals, rodents, wild animals or contaminated water; penetration of leptospires through skin abrasions or mucous membranes. Occurrence: worldwide, urban and rural outbreaks, field workers with hazardous occupations, or recreational hazard. Control: antibiotics, search for source of infection; excretion precautions (urine). Reference: *Guidelines for the control of leptospirosis*, Geneva, World Health Organization, 1982 (Offset Publication, No. 67).

Listeriosis (ICD 027.0)

Sudden onset, fever, headache, nausea, vomiting, signs of meningeal irritation, delirium, coma, occasionally shock. Caused by *Listeria monocytogenes*, a bacterium. Laboratory: cerebrospinal fluid may be turbid (at beginning) or purulent. Incubation: 4 days to 3 weeks. Transmission: largely neonatal or possibly venereal but also by contact with soil contaminated by animal faeces, contaminated food, and inhalation. Occurrence: worldwide, usually sporadic but small epidemics may occur. Control: precautions in handling aborted animal fetuses; antibiotics; secretion precautions.

Lyme disease

See Erythema chronicum migrans due to *Borrelia burgdorferi*.

Lymphocytic choriomeningitis (ICD 049.0)

Onset as for influenza, or directly with meningeal signs and symptoms; possible meningoencephalomyelitis and coma but followed by recovery without sequelae. Caused by lymphocytic choriomeningitis virus. Laboratory: isolation of virus from blood or spinal fluid. Incubation period: 8–13 days for systemic symptoms, 15–21 days for meningeal symptoms. Transmission: food or dust contaminated by urine of infected rodents, usually mice; no person-to-person transmission. Occurrence: worldwide, usually sporadic; hamster pets have caused outbreaks. Control: isolation is not necessary; disinfection of discharges recommended.

Machupo haemorrhagic fever
See Junin and Machupo haemorrhagic fevers.

Malaria (ICD 084.9)
Classical symptoms may be preceded by 2–3 days of low-grade fever and malaise, often misidentified as influenza. Falciparum malaria (caused by *Plasmodium falciparum*), is life-threatening, presents with fever, chills, sweats, and headache and may progress to recurrent attacks or suddenly to disorientation, acute encephalitis, delirium and coma (cerebral malaria) or shock with high case-fatality rate. Malaria caused by *Plasmodium vivax*, *P. ovale* or *P. malariae* is less dangerous, except in the very young; classical attack begins with malaise and shaking chills, followed by rapidly rising temperature with headache and nausea and ending with profuse sweating; attacks recur at fixed or varied intervals; relapses are common for several months. The clinical picture may be atypical in individuals taking inadequate doses of prophylactic drugs or partially immune after long residence in endemic areas. Differential diagnosis: septicaemia, relapsing fever, brucellosis, and several other febrile diseases. Laboratory: repeated thin and thick blood smears; identification of the *Plasmodium* type is useful for prognosis and therapy; double infection is a possibility. Incubation: averaging 12 days for *P. falciparum*, 14 days for *P. vivax* and 30 days for *P. malariae*, but some *P. vivax* strains in the northern hemisphere may have a much longer incubation period (6–9 months). Transmission: man is the reservoir; different species of *Anopheles* mosquito, the great majority of which bite at night, acquire the infection and become infective after a temperature-dependent incubation period; occasional transmission through the placenta or by blood transfusion. Occurrence: in endemic tropical and subtropical areas (see Fig. A3.1); all age groups; commonly increasing attack rate during the rainy season; outbreaks may be explosive in non-immune groups not protected by prophylactic drugs. Control: treatment and prophylaxis require different drugs depending on drug resistance of parasites, particularly *P. falciparum* (see Table A3.1). Chloroquine resistance is widespread, and resistance to sulfadoxine-pyrimethamine is becoming a problem. WHO publishes information periodically in the *Weekly epidemiological record* on areas where resistance has appeared. Other measures include: isolation of patients under bed-nets at night; vector control in

Fig. A3.1. Epidemiological assessment of status of malaria 1984

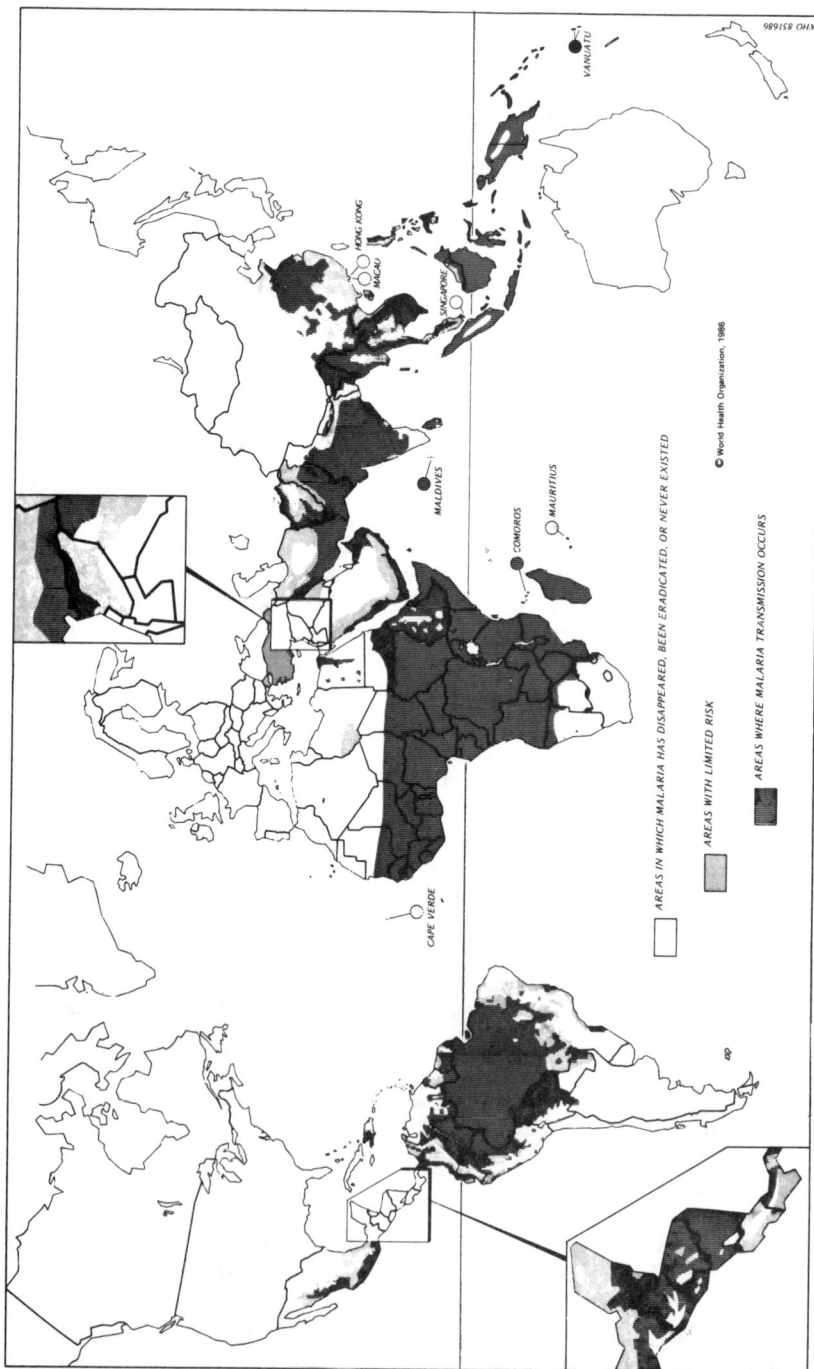

Table A3.1. Treatment and prophylaxis of malaria[a]

	P. vivax, P. ovale, P. malariae, and non-resistant P. falciparum	P. falciparum resistant to chloroquine	P. falciparum resistant to chloroquine and to sulfadoxine-pyrimethamine
Treatment of moderate attack	Chloroquine or amodiaquine,[b] orally	Sulfadoxine-pyrimethamine, orally	Quinine + tetracycline,[c] orally
Treatment of severe attack (P. falciparum)	Quinine (or chloroquine), intravenously	Quinine, intravenously	Quinine, intravenously
Prophylaxis	Chloroquine or amodiaquine, orally (should be continued for 4–6 weeks after exposure)	Amodiaquine[d] orally	Amodiaquine,[d] orally

[a] This table can only give general indications; for further details, including contraindications, see references mentioned in text.

[b] In addition, primaquine is used against hepatic stages of P. vivax.

[c] A new drug, mefloquine, is active against resistant strains but resistance to it may develop; it is not recommended for mass prophylaxis; it is recommended to associate it with sulfadoxine-pyrimethamine for treatment.

[d] Sulfadoxine-pyrimethamine is not recommended for prophylaxis, because of its toxicity; amodiaquine does not offer full protection, and special care should be taken to avoid being bitten by mosquitos. Prompt diagnosis and treatment of breakthroughs are important.

the community e.g., residual spraying, larviciding, source reduction; individual measures, e.g., the screening of openings of dwellings, bednets (may be impregnated with insecticide), staying indoors from dusk to dawn, wearing long-sleeved clothing and trousers after dusk, repeated application of repellents, use of mosquito coils. Notification to national authorities and WHO (disease under surveillance). References: Malaria risk in international travel. *Weekly epidemiological record,* **59**: 221–227, 229–235, 237–240 (1984); Malaria chemoprophylaxis. *Weekly epidemiological record,* **60**: 181–183 (1985); WHO Technical Report Series, No. 711, 1984 (*Advances in malaria chemotherapy*: report of a WHO Scientific Group); WHO Technical Report Series, No. 735, 1986 (WHO Expert Committee on Malaria: 18th report).

Marburg virus disease
See Ebola and Marburg virus diseases.

Measles (ICD 055.9)
Onset with moderate fever, coryza, conjunctivitis, bronchitis, occasionally white Koplik's spots on the buccal mucosa opposite the first and second upper molars (2nd–4th day). On 3rd–7th day: high fever, macular or maculopapular rash spreading rapidly from the face to the trunk and extremities; petechiae and ecchymoses may be present in severe cases. Complications: otitis media, pneumonia

(infants), encephalitis (1 in 2 000 cases) 2 days to 3 weeks after onset of rash. Particularly severe in malnourished children (fatality rate 10%): haemorrhagic (black) measles, mouth sores, dehydration, protein-losing enteropathy, kwashiorkor, skin infection. Congenital malformations in pregnant women. Caused by measles virus, a paramyxovirus. Differential diagnosis: rubella, scarlet fever, roseola infantum, gammaherpesviral mononucleosis, echovirus and coxsackievirus exanthems. Laboratory: the clinical diagnosis is obvious during epidemics; if necessary, serological test for detection of IgM antibody. Incubation: 10 days (range 8–13). Transmission: direct, by droplets and airborne droplet nuclei (aerosols), from 2–4 days before onset of the rash until 4 days after; indirect (unusual) by soiled articles; products of desquamation are not infectious. Occurrence: epidemics every 2 or 3 years in late winter and early spring; mainly affects children between 6 months and 3 years of age in developing countries, older children in developed countries or even nonimmunized young adults; outbreaks may be explosive. Control: no specific treatment, the immunoglobulin is ineffective in complications; **RESPIRATORY ISOLATION** for 7 days after onset of rash; no disinfection; immunization of contacts within 2 days of exposure can protect (if vaccine is contraindicated, immune globulin should be given within 3–4 days of exposure). Prompt immunization at the beginning of an epidemic is essential to limit the spread and immunization should be a requirement for school attendance. Live attenuated vaccine is given in a single injection at 12–15 months of age in developed countries, and at 9 months of age in countries with high incidence. Storage of vaccine at 2–8 °C. Slight fever and malaise may occur in 5–30% of those vaccinated (contraindicated in pregnant women). Reference: Optimal age for measles vaccination in high incidence countries. *Weekly epidemiological record*, **57**: 89–96 (1982).

Melioidosis, pulmonary (ICD 025)

Progressive onset, irregular fever, chest pains, X-rays show pulmonary consolidation with cavitating aspects. Complications: septicaemia (rapidly fatal), abscesses (including brain). Caused by a bacterium, *Pseudomonas pseudomallei* (Whitmore bacillus). Laboratory: Gram staining, isolation of the agent, serological tests. Incubation: from 2 days to several months. Transmission: common-source exposure by contact with soil, dust, water or mud through skin wounds, or ingestion of water contaminated by animal reservoirs; no person-to-person transmission. Occurrence: limited foci in all continents, mainly in warm climates. Control: chloramphenicol, tetracyclines; secretion precautions.

Meningitis due to *Haemophilus influenzae* (ICD 320.0)

Sudden onset, fever, vomiting, lethargy, meningeal irritation. Caused by *Haemophilus influenzae*, a bacillus. Laboratory: isolation of agent from blood or cerebrospinal fluid. Incubation period: 2–4 days.

Infective period: during presence of agent in pharynx; may be prolonged. Transmission: droplets and nasopharyngeal discharges. Occurrence: mainly children below 5 years of age, worldwide, secondary cases in families and day-care centres. Control: isolation not necessary; treatment of patients with antibiotics.

Meningitis, viral (ICD 321.7)

Sudden onset, fever, malaise, headache, vomiting, stiff neck and back; maculopapular, vesicular or petechial rash may occur; may be associated with gastrointestinal and respiratory symptoms. Usually non-fatal, occasionally temporary residual weakness and muscle spasms. Caused by different viruses, most frequently mumps virus, coxsackievirus B, echovirus; less frequently poliovirus, coxsackievirus A, measles virus, herpesvirus, varicella virus, lymphocytic choriomeningitis virus, "Epstein-Barr virus", influenza virus and adenoviruses, but the agent remains unidentified in 33% of cases. Differential diagnosis: postvaccinal meningitis, cryptococcal and other fungal meningitis, chlamydial lymphogranuloma, leptospirosis, listeriosis. See also Meningococcal meningitis and Meningoencephalitis due to miscellaneous infectious agents. Laboratory: cerebrospinal fluid clear with moderate mononuclear pleocytosis (sometimes polymorphonuclear at onset), increased protein, normal sugar and absence of bacteria; the etiological diagnosis is difficult and requires the isolation of the virus from blood, stool or throat washing with a rise of antibody in serum to confirm its pathogenic role. Incubation: varies with the specific agent (2 days to 1 week). Transmission: respiratory and/or faecal-oral. Occurrence: worldwide, occasionally in epidemics, seasonal increase in summer, higher frequency in warm climates. Control: personal, community, and food hygiene, excretion precautions. Prophylaxis: poliovirus vaccination; personal and food hygiene; community sanitation.

Meningococcal bacteraemia (ICD 036.2)

Fever, sudden prostration, petechial rash, ecchymoses, sometimes arthritis, shock; may occur without meningitis. High death rate. Caused by: *Neisseria meningitidis*, the meningococcus. Transmission: see Meningococcal meningitis. RESPIRATORY ISOLATION until 24 hours after start of chemotherapy.

Meningococcal meningitis (ICD 320.5)

Onset sudden with fever, intense headache, vomiting, stiff neck, and frequently petechial rash (rarely vesicles); delirium and coma often appear. Fulminating cases: sudden prostration, ecchymoses, with shock at onset. Fatality rates: untreated, 50%; treated, 10%. Caused by *Neisseria meningitidis*, several antigenic groups. Differential diagnosis: several bacteria may cause a similar disease (except for the rash), but more often sporadic than epidemic: pneumococci,

Haemophilus influenzae, streptococci, *Staphylococcus aureus, Escherichia coli, Salmonella,* members of the *Klebsiella-Enterobacter-Proteus* group, *Pseudomonas aeruginosa, Listeria monocytogenes* and others. See also Meningitis, viral, and Meningoencephalitis due to miscellaneous infectious agents. Laboratory: turbid or purulent cerebrospinal fluid with polymorphonuclear pleocytosis, increased protein; demonstration of meningococci in Gram-stained smear of spinal fluid, isolation of the agent from the cerebrospinal fluid, characterization of group-specific meningococcal polysaccharides. Incubation: 2–10 days, usually 3–4 days. Transmission: direct contact, droplets, discharges from nose and throat, high prevalence of asymptomatic carriers (up to 50%). Contagiousness: as long as meningococci are present in nasopharynx. Occurrence: worldwide, greatest incidence during winter, epidemic waves at irregular intervals, large epidemics in tropical regions during hot dry season. Control: antibiotics (possible resistance to sulfonamides), RESPIRATORY ISOLATION until 24 hours after start of chemotherapy. Prevention: chemoprophylaxis (contacts in closed community), vaccine. References: WHO Technical Report Series, No. 588, 1976 (*Cerebrospinal meningitis control*: report of a WHO Study Group); GALAZKA, A. Meningococcal disease and its control with meningococcal polysaccharide vaccines. *Bulletin of the World Health Organization,* **60**: 1–7 (1982).

Meningoencephalitis due to miscellaneous infectious agents (ICD 323.9)
Postinfectious encephalitis may occur in measles 2 days to 3 weeks after onset of exanthem; while unusual in rubella and varicella, it may occur at the end of the disease or 1–2 weeks after.

Postvaccinal encephalitis may occur, but rarely, after vaccination against smallpox, yellow fever, rabies, whooping cough.

Other diseases: non-paralytic poliomyelitis, lymphocytic choriomeningitis, rabies, herpes, influenza, cat-scratch fever, and certain bacterial, enteroviral, leptospiral, parasitic (trypanosomiasis, cysticercosis, hydatidosis, gnathostomiasis) and mycotic infections.

Simian B virus disease is an ascending encephalomyelitis (only a few cases are known) transmitted by monkey bites, mostly in Africa and India (see Cercopithecid herpesvirus 1 disease).

Primary amoebic meningoencephalitis is characterized by fever, headache, vomiting, nuchal rigidity, somnolence, death in 5–6 days in fulminating forms; aseptic meningitis syndrome may also be seen. Caused by two amoebae, *Acanthamoeba* and *Naegleria.* Incubation: 3–7 days. Transmission: swimming in infected ponds, springs, swimming-pools. Occurrence: rare or undiagnosed, possibly worldwide, in warm season or warm climate. Control: treatment with amphotericin B, miconazole and rifampicin may be successful for *Naegleria* infection.

Monkeypox (ICD 051.9)
Clinically similar to smallpox, but caused by a different virus; case-fatality rate: 16 %. Transmission: animal reservoir not well known, includes monkeys: secondary attack rate of about 10 %. Occurrence: rain-forest areas of West and Central Africa. Control: **STRICT ISOLATION**; see Smallpox and Varicella.

Mononucleosis, infectious
See Gammaherpesviral mononucleosis.

Mucocutaneous lymph node syndrome
A newly identified syndrome, fever lasting 5 days or more, maculopapular rash, bilateral conjunctival injection, oropharyngeal lesions, erythema and indurative oedema of the hands or feet, cervical lymphadenopathy. Complications: meningitis, arthritis, cardiac involvement; case-fatality rate 1 %. Etiology unknown, may be a soluble immunocomplex disorder with a still unknown infectious agent. No usual laboratory test. Transmission: unknown, but not from person to person. Occurrence: outbreaks in children under 5 years of age in Japan and the USA; a few cases reported in Europe. No specific treatment.

Mumps (072.9)
Fever (may be absent), swelling and tenderness of salivary glands, usually the parotid. Complications: orchitis (20 %), aseptic meningitis (frequent) or meningoencephalitis. Fatality: rare. Caused by mumps virus (genus *Paramyxovirus*). Differential diagnosis: in sporadic cases other causes of meningitis or meningoencephalitis are numerous but mumps is a frequent one. Laboratory: isolation of virus from saliva, blood, urine, cerebrospinal fluid; serological tests. Incubation: 2–3 weeks. Transmission: direct by person-to-person contact from 2 days before to 9 days after gland swelling, by droplet spread; about one-third of cases are inapparent but contagious. Occurrence: children, young adults; mainly in winter and spring; clusters of cases in households, schools, barracks, camps. Control: symptomatic treatment; disinfection of articles soiled with saliva; live attenuated vaccine may protect if administered shortly after exposure. **RESPIRATORY ISOLATION** for 9 days.

Murine typhus
See Typhus fever due to *Rickettsia typhi*.

Non-pneumonic Legionnaires' disease (ICD 482.8)
Fever, chills, myalgia, malaise, headache, slight cough, chest pain or constricting sensations, no radiographic evidence of pulmonary disease, duration 2–5 days. Caused by *Legionella pneumophila* serotype 1. Differential diagnosis: influenza. Laboratory: safety

precautions, visualization of agent by immunofluorescence, serological tests by immunofluorescence. Incubation: 5 hours–3 days, usually 1–2 days. Transmission: defective air-conditioning systems, no person-to-person transmission. Occurrence: a very small number of outbreaks have been documented in the USA, might be more widespread. Control: antibiotic treatment.

Omsk haemorrhagic fever (ICD 065.1)
Sudden onset with dengue-like symptoms. Acute phase: meningismus and haemorrhages. Caused by a flavivirus. Incubation: 3–7 days. Transmission: from infected rodents to man by ticks; laboratory infections; no person-to-person transmission. Occurrence: in Siberia, USSR. Control: protection from ticks by protective clothing and repellents; a vaccine is used locally. Reference: WHO Technical Report Series, No. 721, 1985 (*Viral haemorrhagic fevers*: report of a WHO Expert Committee).

Oriental sore
See Leishmaniasis, cutaneous.

Ornithosis (ICD 073)
Sudden onset, fever, headache, myalgia, chills, cough absent or non-productive at beginning, bronchopneumonia, splenomegaly; X-rays as in primary atypical pneumonia. Fatalities: rare. Caused by *Chlamydia psittaci*. Laboratory: safety precautions, isolation of chlamydia from blood or post mortem tissues; serological diagnosis by elevation of antibodies. Incubation: 4–15 days, usually 10 days. Transmission: contact with infected birds, mainly parrots, which may apparently be healthy, inhalation of desiccated droppings in enclosed space, laboratory infections, hospital infections. Occurrence: worldwide. Control: tetracyclines, search for source of infection; secretion precautions. Reference: Ornithosis/psittacosis surveillance. *Weekly epidemiological record*, 57: 1–4 (1982).

Oroya fever
See Bartonellosis.

Paragonimiasis (ICD 121.2)
Pulmonary symptoms and haemoptysis, simulates pulmonary tuberculosis radiologically; the brain, lymph nodes, and other organs may be involved. Caused by trematodes belonging to the genus *Paragonimus*. Laboratory: identification of eggs in sputum by microscope examination, also in faeces. Incubation period: eggs may appear 6 weeks after infestation but symptoms may be considerably delayed. Transmission: ingestion of uncooked freshwater crabs and crayfish in contaminated areas; no person-to-person transmission.

Occurrence: Africa, Pacific coast of South America, Asia; small clusters of cases may occur. Control: food hygiene in endemic areas.

Paratyphoid fever (ICD 002.9)

Sudden onset, fever, diarrhoea, sometimes rose spots on the trunk, enlargement of the spleen. Fatality rate less than in typhoid fever. Caused by *Salmonella paratyphi* A, B and C. Laboratory: isolation of organism from blood and stools; serological tests. Incubation period: 1–10 days (shorter for gastroenteritis than enteric fever). Transmission: faecal-oral, food (meat, milk, eggs), food-handlers, flies, water, asymptomatic carriers. Occurrence: worldwide, all ages, sporadic, outbreaks in closed communities or clusters of cases from common source. Control: antibiotics, excretion precautions, search for source of infection, exclusion of infected persons from food handling. Vaccines have not proved effective.

Pertussis (ICD 033.9)

Insidious onset with cough which becomes characteristically paroxysmic within 1–2 weeks and lasts for 1–2 months. Fatalities occur mainly in infants under 1 year of age and in malnourished children. Differential diagnosis: adenovirus infection. Caused by a bacillus: *Bordetella pertussis*. Laboratory: cultivation of agent from throat swabs. Incubation: 7 days (maximum 21). Transmission: droplets are highly infectious before the paroxysmal cough stage; contagious period from 7 days after exposure to contact to 3 weeks after onset. Occurrence: epidemic, worldwide, mainly in infants and children, rarely in adults. Control: RESPIRATORY ISOLATION, disinfection of secretions; antibiotic treatment has little effect; prevention by vaccine or antibiotics given to contacts.

Phlebotomus fever

See Arthropod-borne viral fever.

Plague, bubonic (ICD 020.0)

Inguinal, axillary or cervical adenitis, rarely without fever. Complications: septicaemic plague (prostration, haemorrhages; 60% fatality rate if untreated—black death), pneumonic plague (highly contagious, lethal in 48 hours). Caused by a bacillus, *Yersinia pestis*. Laboratory: safety precautions, direct Gram staining and culture of fluid from buboes, blood, sputum. Incubation: 2–6 days. Transmission: bites of fleas of wild rodents in rural areas; bites of rat fleas (*Xenopsylla cheopis*), cat fleas and human fleas in urban plague; person-to-person transmission by airborne droplets and fomites in pneumonic plague. Occurrence: sylvatic plague with sporadic cases or small clusters in temperate and warm climates in areas with enzootic wild-rodent plague; urban plague with endemicity or epidemic peaks (domestic rat is a reservoir). Control: treatment with streptomycin, tetracyclines, chloramphenicol; skin precautions for bubonic plague; RESPIRATORY ISOLATION for suspected pneumonia in bubonic plague; disinfection of purulent discharges, sputum; terminal cleaning; strict aseptic precautions for corpses. Contacts: parasite disinfestation with insecticide effective against local fleas and surveillance for 7 days. Community measures: flea control must precede or coincide with anti-rodent measures. Prophylaxis: 3 injections of killed bacteria vaccine and periodic boosters. International measures: notification to WHO (disease subject to the International Health Regulations, which govern movements of ships and aircraft). References: Plague vaccine: Recommendations of the Immunization Practices Advisory Committee (IPAC). *Weekly epidemiological record*, **57**: 332–334 (1982); BAHMANYAR, M. & CAVANAUGH, D. C. *Plague manual.* Geneva, World Health Organization, 1976.

Plague, pneumonic (ICD 020.5)

Sudden onset, high fever, chills, severe headache, cough develops in 24 hours, sputum at first mucoid then rusty or bright red, usually no signs of consolidation. Untreated: death within 48 hours. Differential diagnosis: pneumococcal and other bacterial pneumonias. Caused by *Yersinia pestis*, a bacillus. Laboratory: safety precautions, collection of sputum, Gram staining and culture on ordinary media. Incubation: 2–3 days. Transmission: highly transmissible by respiratory droplets and freshly soiled articles. Occurrence: as a complication of bubonic plague (see above) or as a primary infection. Control: STRICT ISOLATION; treatment: streptomycin, tetracyclines, chloramphenicol. Contacts: identification, isolation for 7 days, and chemoprophylaxis (including medical personnel); notification to WHO (disease subject to the International Health Regulations); other precautions as for bubonic plague.

Pleurodynia

See Epidemic myalgia.

Pneumonia, bacterial (ICD 482.9; 482.4[1])

Fever, varying respiratory symptoms, X-rays showing various types of consolidation. Fatality rate may be high. Most often a complication of viral pulmonary infection. Caused by various bacteria: *Staphylococcus aureus, Klebsiella pneumoniae, Haemophilus influenzae, Streptococcus pyogenes* group A, coliform bacteria, *Pseudomonas* species, *Escherichia coli, Francisella tularensis, Pseudomonas pseudomallei, Brucella abortus* and *Brucella melitensis.* Incubation: 1–3 days. Transmission: respiratory droplet spread, articles freshly soiled with respiratory tract discharges. Occurrence: worldwide. Control: antibiotics, STRICT ISOLATION for staphylo-

---

[1] For pneumonia due to *Staphylococcus.*

coccal infection and group A *Streptococcus*, secretion precautions for others.

Pneumonia due to *Mycoplasma pneumoniae* (ICD 483)

Gradual onset, fever, headache, malaise, paroxysmal cough, pharyngitis which progresses to bronchitis and pneumonia, X-rays show patchy infiltration. Duration: a few days to several weeks. Fatalities: rare. Caused by *Mycoplasma pneumoniae*. Differential diagnosis: pneumonitis caused by bacteria, adenovirus infection, influenza, parainfluenza, measles, Q fever, certain mycoses, tuberculosis. Laboratory: development of cold agglutinins (50 % of cases); cultivation of agent on special media; serological tests. Incubation: 14–21 days. Transmission: aerial route. Occurrence: worldwide, schoolchildren and young adults, occasionally epidemics in institutions and military populations. Control: tetracyclines, secretion precautions.

Pneumonia due to *Streptococcus pneumoniae* (ICD 482.0)

Generally sudden onset, single shaking chill, high fever, pains in the chest, cough, dyspnoea, leukocytosis. After 3 days pulmonary symptoms are evident, rusty sputum, X-rays show a lobar consolidation. Fatality rate: 20–40 % if untreated. Caused by *Streptococcus pneumoniae* (pneumococcus). Laboratory: Gram-positive diplococci in sputum, isolation of pneumococci from blood or sputum. Incubation: 1–3 days. Transmission: respiratory droplets, articles freshly soiled with respiratory discharges. Occurrence: worldwide, outbreaks in institutions (elderly persons), often secondary to viral pulmonary infection. Control: antibiotics, oxygen, secretion precautions, vaccination of high-risk groups (elderly).

Pneumonia due to other agents (ICD 486)

Pneumocystis carinii, a protozoon, endemic in America and Europe, possibly more widely spread, may cause outbreaks of acute or subacute pulmonary disease in infants in hospitals and institutions or opportunistic infections in adults, frequently associated with acquired immunodeficiency syndrome. Often fatal. Laboratory: visualization of the agent in smears of tracheobronchial mucus. Incubation: 1–2 months.

Coccidioides immitis, a fungus, extremely common in arid areas of the Americas, produces an asymptomatic infection or an overt influenza-like illness and progresses to mild limited pulmonary lesions or a generalized granulomatous disease. Highly lethal. Laboratory: microscopic examination and culture of sputum.

Chlamydia trachomatis may cause a distinctive pneumonitis syndrome in infants 4–24 weeks of age with cough, congestion, no fever, diffuse pulmonary involvement on chest X-ray, lasting a month or longer, with no fatalities. Transmission may be perinatal.

Occurrence: may account for up to 30% of pneumonitis in infants admitted to hospitals; may occur in immunosuppressed persons.

Pneumonitis, viral (ICD 480.9)

Diffused interstitial pulmonary lesions, X-rays show increased hilar shadows or, at most, scattered small areas of consolidation. Complications: secondary bacterial pneumonia. May occasionally be fatal. Caused by various viruses: respiratory syncytial virus, and parainfluenza 3 virus in the first 6 months of life (may be responsible for "cot death"), measles virus, varicella virus in young children, adenoviruses types 3, 4 and 7 (acute respiratory disease has been seen in military recruits) and influenza virus at all ages. Laboratory: direct examination of rhinopharyngeal aspirates by immunofluorescence, isolation of agent by cell culture, which should be inoculated at bedside. Incubation: 1–3 days. Transmission: respiratory droplets, articles freshly soiled with respiratory discharges. Occurrence: worldwide, seasonal outbreaks, spreading easily in closed groups (military, nurseries). Control: secretion precautions; influenza and adenovirus vaccines.

Poliomyelitis (ICD 045.9)

Onset with moderate fever, headache, gastrointestinal disturbance, malaise, stiffness of the neck and back. After 2–3 days, sudden occurrence of flaccid asymmetrical paralysis without sensory loss, most commonly of the lower extremities. Minor illness (abortive poliomyelitis), aseptic meningitis, non-paralytic poliomyelitis and inapparent infections are frequent. Complications: lameness, ascending paralysis involving laryngeal and respiratory muscles, bulbar poliomyelitis. Fatality rate: 2–10%, more severe in adults. Caused by poliovirus types 1, 2, 3. Differential diagnosis: postinfectious polyneuritis, coxsackievirus and echovirus infections, tick-bite paralysis (uncommon), Guillain-Barré syndrome; non-paralytic poliomyelitis cannot be distinguished clinically from aseptic meningitis caused by echovirus and coxsackievirus, arboviruses, mumps virus, lymphocytic choriomeningitis virus, herpesvirus and leptospires. Laboratory: lymphocytes in cerebrospinal fluid (may be missing) and slight increase in protein content; isolation of the virus from faeces or oropharyngeal secretions, serological tests. Incubation: 3–35 days, usually 7–14. Transmission: throat secretions and faeces, asymptomatic carriers. Contagiousness: 7–10 days before and for a few days after the onset of symptoms. Occurrence: worldwide, still frequent in warm climates where it is endemic or epidemic in children. Control: no specific treatment, mechanical respiratory assistance if necessary, excretion (stool, urine) precautions for 7 days from onset. Control of epidemics by mass immunization with oral vaccine, monovalent if possible. Prophylaxis: oral live vaccine or inactivated vaccine in routine immunization programmes in infancy. Disease under surveillance by WHO. Reference: MELNICK, J. Advantages and disadvantages of killed and live poliomyelitis vaccines. *Bulletin of the World Health Organization*, **56**: 21–38 (1978).

Pontiac fever
See Non-pneumonic Legionnaires' disease.

Poxviral local cutaneous infections (ICD 051.9)
Fever and erythema may be present, the local lesion consists of vesicles or nodules, usually on a finger or hand. Caused by different poxviruses of animal origin: bovine papular stomatitis, contagious ecthyma (orf), cowpox (similar to vaccinia), goatpox, pseudocowpox, tanapox (Yaba pox). Differential diagnosis: cutaneous anthrax. Laboratory: safety precautions, electron microscopy of material from lesions, isolation of agent. Incubation: 1–2 weeks. Transmission: direct contact with animal lesions, occasionally indirect contact; tanapox may be arthropod-borne. Occurrence: worldwide, occupational, clusters of cases are possible. Control: skin precautions.

Psittacosis
See Ornithosis.

Q fever (ICD 083.0)
Sudden chills, headache, fever, weakness, severe sweating, sore throat, chest pain, cough and pneumonitis signs. Fatality rate less than 1 %. Caused by a rickettsia, *Coxiella burnetii*. Laboratory: safety precautions, isolation of agent from blood; serological diagnosis by rise in specific antibodies in paired sera. Incubation: 2–3 weeks. Transmission: contact with infected animals, dust, contaminated material (e.g., wool, fertilizer, raw milk). Occurrence: worldwide, sporadic, veterinarians, explosive outbreaks in stockyards and animal industry. Control: tetracyclines, secretion precautions, search for source of infection, pasteurization of milk.

Queensland tick typhus
See Spotted fever group.

Rabies (ICD 071)
Progressive onset, fever, headache, mental depression, restlessness, paresis, sensorial symptoms, progressing to excitement, paralysis, painful spasms of the throat (hydrophobia, salivation), convulsions, delirium, death from generalized paralysis, asphyxia in 3–10 days. Usually fatal. Caused by rabies virus. Laboratory: staining of frozen skin specimens (occipital, retroauricular) or corneal impressions with fluorescent-labelled specific antibody; virus isolation in mouse or tissue culture; high antibody level in cerebrospinal fluid, from which

the virus cannot be isolated. Incubation: 10 days to 1 year, usually 30–50 days. Transmission: bite of infected dogs or other domestic or wild animals, with or without symptoms; person-to-person transmission not confirmed. Occurrence: worldwide where infected animals are present. Control: secretion precautions (**STRICT ISOLATION** in some countries), symptomatic treatment. Prevention: postexposure active immunization, with or without immune globulin according to severity of risk, without delay after bite; pre-exposure vaccination for professionals at risk. Reference: WHO Technical Report Series, No. 709, 1984 (Seventh report of the WHO Expert Committee on Rabies).

Rat-bite fever (ICD 026.9)

May occur after the bite of an infected rat, even though wound healed normally. Sudden onset, general pains, maculopapular or petechial rash most marked on extremities. There are two separate etiological entities—streptobacillosis, caused by *Streptobacillus moniliformis* and spirillosis, caused by *Spirillum minor*. Laboratory: inoculation of blood, lymph node pus on special bacteriological medium. Incubation: 3–10 days. Transmission: rat bite or indirect contact with rats and contaminated food (milk), no person-to-person transmission. Occurrence: worldwide. Treatment: tetracyclines.

Relapsing fever (endemic, epidemic) (ICD 087.9)

Sudden onset, periods of fever during 2–9 days with general symptoms, relapses (2–10), possible delirium, transitory petechial rash during the initial period. Fatality rate: 2–10%. Caused by various species of the genus *Borrelia*. Differential diagnosis: malaria, dengue, yellow fever, leptospirosis, typhus, influenza and enteric fevers. Laboratory: spirochaetes seen in stained thick blood films or in dark-field preparations. Incubation: 5–15 days, usually 8 days. Transmission: in epidemic form, by crushing the body of an infected louse on to skin abrasion (the louse becomes infective 4–5 days after feeding on an infected person); in endemic form, by the bite of infected argasid ticks on vertebrate animals; no direct person-to-person transmission. Occurrence: epidemic louse-borne relapsing fever (due to *B. recurrentis*) in Africa, South America, Asia; endemic tick-borne relapsing fever (due to species other than *B. recurrentis*), with occasional outbreaks, in North and South America, central Asia, India, and the Mediterranean area. Control: delousing or tick control, tetracyclines. Treatment of louse-borne relapsing fever near the end of a paroxysm may cause the Herxheimer reaction, characterized by fever, headache, general malaise and rigors; it usually subsides after 1–2 hours, but can occasionally have sequelae such as hemiplegia or monoplegia. It can be prevented by administering prednisone before treatment. Louse-borne relapsing fever must be reported to WHO (disease under WHO surveillance).

Reye's syndrome (ICD 331.8)

Fatty degeneration of brain and liver occurring on about the sixth day after upper respiratory tract or exanthematous viral infection, with vomiting, hepatic dysfunction, change in mental status, progressing rapidly in severe forms to coma and respiratory arrest, which may occur in 4 days. Gastrointestinal bleeding is possible. Transmission: not from person to person. Occurrence: children under 18 years of age, clusters of cases or outbreaks linked to influenza virus B, sporadic cases after varicella, enterovirus and myxovirus infections.

Rickettsialpox (ICD 083.2)

Initial skin lesion (eschar), varicelliform rash. Fatality rate less than 1 %. Caused by *Rickettsia akari*. Incubation: 7–10 days. Transmitted by bite of an infective mouse mite, no person-to-person transmission. Occurrence: Africa, USA, USSR, probably other areas. Control: tetracyclines, elimination of house mice, miticides.

Rift Valley fever (ICD 006.3)

Dengue-like signs and symptoms with possible complications, such as haemorrhage, encephalitis and retinopathy. Caused by Rift Valley fever virus, a Bunyavirus. Differential diagnosis: dengue, yellow fever, other arthropod-borne viral fevers. Laboratory: safety precautions, isolation of virus from blood by mouse inoculation and cell culture; serological tests. Incubation: 2–7 days, usually 3. Transmission: mosquitos, mainly *Culex* genus, or direct contact with the blood of sick animals (sheep, cattle, camels); no documented person-to-person transmission. Occurrence: Africa south of the Sahara, Egypt. Control: insecticide spraying; vaccination of domestic animals (killed vaccine; live vaccine to be used only in outbreaks, after the virus has been identified); human vaccine still experimental and reserved for exposed professionals; patients to stay under bed-nets during acute phase. Reference: *Rift Valley fever: an emerging human and animal problem.* Geneva, World Health Organization, 1982 (WHO Offset Publication, No. 63).

Rocky Mountain spotted fever

See Spotted fever group.

Roseola infantum (ICD 057.8)

A disease of children. Sudden fever (40.5–41°C) of 3–5 days' duration. Transient maculopapular rash appearing first on the trunk when the fever falls in lysis. Incubation: 5–15 days, usually 10 days. Probably viral.

Rotaviral enteritis (ICD 008.8)

Gastrointestinal symptoms may be preceded by respiratory illness (cough, nasal discharge) or otitis media (red throat, inflamed tympanic membrane). Vomiting generally starts before diarrhoea, which may cause severe dehydration and rapid circulatory collapse, particularly in children aged 12–18 months (usually less severe below 12 months); occasionally fatal; subclinical infections are frequent. Caused by rotaviruses, various serotypes. Laboratory: examination of stools by electron microscopy or enzyme-linked immunosorbent assay. Incubation: 2 days. Transmission: faecal–oral, infection through respiratory routes also seems possible. Occurrence: worldwide, sporadic, winter epidemics in temperate climates, less frequent and throughout the year in tropical climates. Control: rehydration, enteric precautions; investigation of contacts and source of infection.

Rubella (ICD 056.9)

Onset with moderate fever, occipital lymphadenopathy; occasional arthralgia; maculopapular rash on 3rd–5th day in 20–50 % of cases, spreading from the face to the trunk and limbs, lasting 1–3 days. Prognosis generally benign. Complications: arthritis, encephalitis (rare), congenital malformations (infection during first trimester of pregnancy). Caused by rubella virus (family Togaviridae). Differential diagnosis: measles, scarlet fever, drug rashes, gammaherpesviral mononucleosis, erythema infectiosum, exanthema subitum, echovirus and coxsackievirus exanthems. Laboratory: isolation of virus during the first few days from blood, urine and faeces and for 2 weeks from the pharynx; serological test (fourfold rise in antibody titre in paired sera or presence of IgM in a single serum). Incubation: usually 16–18 days (range 14–21). Transmission: direct, by droplets from nose and throat and droplet nuclei (aerosols) from 1 week before onset of rash to 1 week after it has faded; infants born with congenital rubella excrete the virus for several months; indirect, through articles freshly soiled by nasopharyngeal secretions. Occurrence: major epidemics every 6–9 years in winter and spring, mainly a disease of childhood, less contagious than measles, clusters of cases in closed institutions (outbreaks have occurred in hospitals involving staff and patients). Control: no specific treatment; RESPIRATORY ISOLATION for 7 days from onset of rash; disinfection of articles freshly soiled; abortion should be considered for women who have had a possibly infective contact during early pregnancy; the value of immunoglobulin has not been established; mass immunization in schools or military groups, teachers and hospital staff. Prophylaxis by a single dose of live attenuated vaccine (contraindicated in pregnant women).

Salmonellosis (ICD 003.9)

Sudden onset, abdominal pain, fever, nausea, vomiting, diarrhoea, dehydration may be severe among infants. Complications: enteric fever, abscesses. Caused by the numerous serotypes of *Salmonella*. Laboratory: isolation of *Salmonella* from faeces. Incubation: 6–72 hours, usually 12–36 hours. Transmission: faecal–oral, person-to-person or common-source through food (meat, poultry, milk, dairy products, eggs and egg products), water, food-handlers. Occurrence: worldwide, sporadic cases, small outbreaks in the general population, large outbreaks in closed groups caused by contaminated food. Control: rehydration; use of antibiotics may lead to resistance; investigation of source and contacts; strict enteric precautions in hospitals, disinfection of faeces and soiled articles; community sanitation. Reference: WHO SCIENTIFIC WORKING GROUP. Enteric infections due to *Campylobacter, Yersinia, Salmonella* and *Shigella*. *Bulletin of the World Health Organization*, **58**: 519–537 (1980). *Salmonella* and *Shigella* surveillance: Guidelines for bacteriological clearance of *Salmonella* and *Shigella* excreters. *Weekly epidemiological record*, **57**: 156–158 (1982).

Sandfly fever
   See Arthropod-borne viral fever.

Scarlet fever (ICD 034.1)
   Sore throat, fever, vomiting, strawberry tongue, punctate rash that does not involve the face. Complications: otitis, rheumatic fever, glomerulonephritis. Fatality rate: 3% or less. Caused by *Streptococcus pyogenes,* group A. Laboratory: isolation of streptococci from throat and specific grouping of strains. Incubation: 1–3 days. Transmission: droplets, inapparent carriers are frequent. Occurs less frequently in tropical than in temperate climates. Affects the 3–12-year age group. Infective period: 10–21 days. Control: antibiotics, secretion precautions.

Schistosomiasis, intestinal (ICD 120.1)
   For early manifestations, see Acute schistosomiasis. This is followed by intermittent diarrhoea with blood and mucus. Caused by intestinal infection with *Schistosoma mansoni* in tropical Africa and America, and the Mediterranean region, *S. intercalatum* in West Africa and *S. japonicum* in Asia. Incubation: 4–6 weeks. Laboratory: repeated microscopic examination of stools. Transmission: waters with infected snails. Reference: WHO Technical Report Series, No. 728, 1985 (*The control of schistosomiasis*: report of a WHO Expert Committee).

Schistosomiasis, urinary (ICD 120.0)
   For early manifestations, see Acute schistosomiasis. This is followed by eosinophilia, lymphadenopathy, hepatosplenomegaly, cystitis and haematuria, which may be discrete. Bladder cancer may occur. Caused by *Schistosoma haematobium*, a trematode worm.

Laboratory: identification of eggs by microscopic examination of urine; enzyme-linked immunosorbent assay. Incubation period: several weeks. Transmission: contact with contaminated water in endemic zones. Occurrence: Africa, Eastern Mediterranean area. Control: specific drugs for patients and molluscicides in contaminated waters. Reference: WHO Technical Report Series, No. 728, 1985 (*The control of schistosomiasis*: report of a WHO Expert Committee).

Shigellosis (ICD 004.9)

Fever, vomiting, abdominal pains, tenesmus, diarrhoea with mucus, pus and blood. Complications: septicaemia. Fatality rate may reach 20% if untreated. Caused by several serotypes of *Shigella*. Laboratory: isolation of *Shigella* from stools, which generally contain pus cells. Incubation: 1–7 days, usually 1–3. Transmission: faecal-oral, carriers with inapparent or mild infections, water, milk, flies. Occurrence: worldwide, all ages, higher severity in children under 10 years of age, frequent in warm climates, explosive outbreaks in closed groups. Control: antibiotics (there are resistant strains), rehydration, excreta precautions, disinfection of articles soiled by faeces, investigation of source and contacts, exclusion from food handling, pasteurization of dairy products, fly control. References: WHO SCIENTIFIC WORKING GROUP. Enteric infections due to *Campylobacter, Yersinia, Salmonella* and *Shigella. Bulletin of the World Health Organization*, **58**: 519–537 (1980); *Shigella sonnei* surveillance. *Weekly epidemiological record*, **57**: 276–278 (1982).

Siberian tick typhus

See Spotted fever group.

Simian B virus disease

See Cercopithecid herpesvirus 1 disease

Sixth disease

See Roseola infantum.

Sleeping sickness

See Trypanosomiasis, African.

Smallpox (ICD 050.9)

See the description of *variola major* rash under Varicella; case-fatality rate: 20–40%. *Variola minor* has a similar rash but milder systemic symptoms and a case-fatality rate of 1%. Other forms include an attenuated disease with few lesions in partially immune persons, a fulminating haemorrhagic form, and "flat" smallpox with delayed appearance of lesions, which are superficial and do not leave scars. Caused by variola virus. Incubation: 7–17 days, usually 10–12. Transmission: airborne, respiratory droplets, contact with skin lesions, bedding and clothing. Contagiousness: until disappearance of all scabs, about 3 weeks. Control: **STRICT ISOLATION** of patients until all crusts are shed; intensive case-finding; vaccination of all categories of contacts, isolation of primary contacts (face-to-face contact with patient), medical surveillance of secondary contacts (contact with primary contact) and other possible remote contacts. **STRICT SAFETY PRECAUTIONS** for laboratory specimens (see Annex 4). **Smallpox is now considered to have been eradicated**: any suspect case should be reported as a matter of urgency to national authorities and to WHO. References: ARITA, I. & GROMYKO, A. Surveillance of orthopoxvirus infections and associated research in the period after smallpox eradication. *Bulletin of the World Health Organization*, **60**: 367–375 (1982); *Memorandum on the control of outbreaks of smallpox*, London, HMSO, 1975.[1]

Spirillosis
See Rat-bite fever.

Sporotrichosis (ICD 117.1)
Skin lesion usually on a finger, begins as a nodule then becomes an ulcer, and a series of nodules and ulcers appears on lymphatics draining the area. Complications: rarely arthritis, pneumonitis. Caused by a fungus: *Sporothrix schenkii*. Laboratory: culture of agent from lesions. Incubation: 1 week to 3 months. Transmission: pricks by thorns of infected plants, or inhalation of spores (pulmonary form); no person-to-person transmission. Occurrence: worldwide; occupational disease of farmers, gardeners, miners; may cause clusters of cases. Control: local or general fungicidal drugs (amphotericin B).

Spotted fever group (ICD 082.9)
Fever, black spot at the site of a tick bite, maculopapular rash on 3rd–5th day, sometimes petechiae. Differential diagnosis: typhus fever due to *Rickettsia tsutsugamushi*. Caused by rickettsiae. Laboratory: specific serological tests. Incubation: 3–14 days. Transmitted by ticks from animal to man; no person-to-person transmission. Occurrence: Rocky Mountain spotted fever in the Americas (due to *Rickettsia rickettsii*) (fatality rate 20% if not treated), boutonneuse fever in Africa, India, and the Mediterranean basin (due to *Rickettsia conori*), Queensland tick typhus in Australia (due to *Rickettsia australis*), and Siberian tick typhus in the USSR (due to *Rickettsia sibirica*). Control: antibiotics, repellents, protective clothing in field. Vaccine against Rocky Mountain spotted fever for persons at special risk.

---

[1] See also *Management of suspected cases of smallpox in the post-eradication period*. Unpublished WHO document, WHO/SE/80.157, Rev. 1.

Streptobacillosis
See Rat-bite fever.

Streptococcal pharyngitis (ICD 034.0)
Fever, sore throat with redness, oedema and exudate of pharynx and tonsillar pillars, petechiae, cervical adenopathy, leukocytosis, sometimes only sore throat without exudate. Complications: peritonsillar abscess, otitis media, rheumatic heart disease, glomerulonephritis. Fatality rate: zero. Caused by *Streptococcus pyogenes*, group A. Laboratory: isolation of agent on special media and determination of group and type; serological tests. Incubation: 1–3 days. Transmission: droplets, articles freshly soiled with pharyngeal discharges. Occurrence: common in 3–12-year age group in temperate climates; inapparent infections more common in warm climates; food-borne outbreaks with high attack rate have occurred on rare occasions caused by food-handlers carrying the bacteria either in the throat or on wounds on their hands. Control: secretion precautions.

Swimmers' itch (ICD 120.3)
Usually not febrile, dermatitis reaches maximum intensity in 2–3 days and heals in a week or so. Caused by intracutaneous penetration of free-swimming cercariae of bird or mammalian schistosomes which do not mature in man. May occur in many parts of the world. Reference: *Weekly epidemiological record,* **58**: 9 (1983).

Swimming-pool-associated dermatitis (ICD 686.0)
Sharp outbreaks of dermatitis associated with the use of swimming-pools and whirlpools and caused by bacteria such as *Pseudomonas aeruginosa* have been described. Patients had a maculopapular, vesicular or pustular rash.

Tetanus (ICD 037)
Painful muscular contractions beginning with masseter and neck muscles, extending to the trunk, back muscles; generalized tonic spasticity, intermittent convulsions, spasms, asphyxia, moderate fever. Fatality rate: 35–70%. Caused by the toxin of *Clostridium tetani*, a bacterium. Laboratory: isolation of the agent usually unsuccessful; no detectable antibody response. Incubation: 4–21 days, usually 10. Transmission: trivial or insignificant wounds contaminated by spores in soil or dust (horse and other animal excreta), possibly by horse and cattle bites, parenteral infections in drug addicts, umbilical contamination at birth, no person-to-person transmission. Occurrence: worldwide, sporadic or small outbreaks. Control: supportive and sedative treatment, antitoxin to neutralize unfixed toxin; immunization at time of wound, or booster dose if already immunized.

Toxic shock syndrome due to *Staphylococcus aureus* (ICD 785.5)
Sudden onset, high fever, vomiting, profuse watery diarrhoea, myalgia, a macular "sunburn-like" rash. Complication: shock within 48 hours, case-fatality rate 13%. Caused by toxin-producing *Staphylococcus aureus* associated with the use of vaginal tampons. No person-to-person transmission. Control: secretion precautions.

Toxoplasmosis (ICD 130)
Infection very common but seldom symptomatic. Mild lymphatic form resembles gammaherpesviral mononucleosis (irregular low-grade fever, malaise, cervical and axillary lymphadenopathy). A fulminating, disseminated infection may occur in immunocompromised persons. Complications: congenital toxoplasmosis transmitted transplacentally by mothers infected shortly before or during pregnancy and resulting either in abortion or congenital malformations (mainly of the central nervous system), or no symptoms. Prognosis: usually benign if not complicated. Caused by *Toxoplasma gondii*, an intracellular protozoan parasite. Differential diagnosis: other causes of lymphadenopathy. Laboratory: Sabin-Feldman test, indirect fluorescent test (confirmation requires paired sera with ascending titres, or single serum with high titre). Incubation: about 5–23 days. Transmission: direct contact with cats (cleaning litter-pans containing infective oocysts); indirect: drinking water contaminated with cat faeces, eating undercooked meat of contaminated domestic animals. Control: treatment with pyrimethamine and sulfadiazine; protection against transmission from infected cats, e.g., prevention of contamination by stray cats of sand where children play; correct cooking of meat.

Traveller's diarrhoea (ICD 009.1)
Diarrhoea, with or without fever, abdominal cramps, fatigue. Mainly caused by enterotoxigenic *Escherichia coli*, occasionally by other enteric bacteria, such as *Shigella, Salmonella,* and *Campylobacter*. Laboratory: stool culture. Incubation: 12–72 hours. Transmission: faecal–oral, person-to-person or common-source, uncooked food, fruit, vegetables, shellfish, ice-cream, water, drinks, food handlers. Occurrence: mainly in tropical areas; sporadic or clusters of cases in travellers. Control: personal hygiene; excreta precautions.

Trench fever (ICD 083.1)
Sudden or slow onset, fever, headache, muscular pains, splenomegaly, short episode (five-day fever) or relapses, sometimes with macular rash, typhoid-like. Usually non-fatal. Caused by a rickettsia, *Rochalimaea quintana*. Laboratory: culture of agent on special media, serological tests. Incubation period: 7–30 days. Infective period may be prolonged, possible recurrences. Transmission: faeces of body louse through skin breaks; man and louse are the only reservoirs; louse becomes infective after 5–12 days and remains so for life (5

weeks); no direct person-to-person transmission. Occurrence: worldwide in endemic foci, epidemic under crowded unhygienic conditions. Control: treatment with tetracyclines or chloramphenicol, delousing.

Trichinosis (ICD 124)

Mild or severe febrile disease, sometimes fatal: onset with influenza-like and gastrointestinal symptoms, continuous fever, oedema of eyelids, subconjunctival haemorrhages, muscle pain. Complications: respiratory distress, myocardial failure, hypoproteinaemia, neurological symptoms. Caused by larvae of *Trichinella spiralis* which migrate from intestine to muscles. Laboratory: a biopsy of skeletal muscle shows *T. spiralis* larvae (not earlier than 10 days after exposure); adult worms in intestinal mucosa at post mortem examination. Incubation: 1–45 days, usually 10–14 days (shorter in severe cases). Transmission: insufficiently cooked meat, chiefly pork or game: no person-to-person transmission. Occurrence: worldwide, common source, clusters or outbreaks in localized foci. Control: correct cooking of meat.

Trypanosomiasis, African (ICD 086.5)

Fever, intense headache, insomnia, usually a chancre at site of tsetse fly bite, lymph node enlargement (posterior cervical) and occasional rash. Complications: somnolence, central nervous involvement, body wasting, death. Caused by haemoflagellates *Trypanosoma brucei gambiense* and *T. b. rhodesiense*. Laboratory: detection of parasite in lymph nodes and blood during the lymphatic phase and in cerebrospinal fluid with elevated protein content during the nervous phase. Incubation: 2–3 weeks (*T. b. rhodesiense*), up to several months (*T. b. gambiense*). Occurrence: Africa between 15° N and 20° S latitude in localized foci. Transmission: tsetse fly bite. Control: Prophylaxis with pentamidine for exposed personnel; community measures: reduction of fly population. References: WHO Technical Report Series, No. 635, 1979 (*The African trypanosomiases*: report of a joint WHO Expert Committee and FAO Expert Consultation); A UNDP/WORLD BANK/WHO CONSULTATION. Control of sleeping sickness due to *Trypanosoma brucei gambiense*. *Bulletin of the World Health Organization*, **60**: 821–825 (1982); WHO Technical Report Series (*The epidemiology and control of African trypanosomiasis*: report of a WHO Expert Committee) (in press, 1986).

Trypanosomiasis, American (ICD 086.2)

Many infected persons have no clinical manifestations. Acute disease: variable fever, malaise, lymphadenopathy, hepatospleno-megaly, palpebral oedema, inflammatory lesion at the site of inoculation. Complications (later in life): myocarditis and meningo-encephalitis. Caused by *Trypanosoma cruzi*. Laboratory: demonstration of trypanosome in blood (examination, culture). Incubation: 5–14 days after bite. Transmission: by faeces of infected cone-nosed bugs; blood transfusion. Occurrence: Central and South America. Control: use of bed-nets. Reference: WHO Technical Report Series, No. 202, 1960 (*Chagas' disease*: report of a Study Group).

Tuberculosis (ICD 010.9)

Pulmonary tuberculosis (suspected on basis of X-ray examination) may be seen exceptionally as a cluster of recent cases. Caused by *Mycobacterium tuberculosis, M. africanum,* or *M. bovis.* Laboratory: tuberculin skin test, examination of smears from sputum, isolation of tubercle bacillus by cultivation. Incubation period: 4–12 weeks. Infective period: may be for years and intermittent. Transmission: by droplets from an infected person, during prolonged exposure; bovine tuberculosis may result from unpasteurized milk or exposure to infected animal. Occurrence: worldwide. Control: antibiotics, search for source and contacts by tuberculin test and X-ray screening; isolation not necessary, disposal of secretion-soiled tissues, disinfection not necessary.

Tularaemia (ICD 021)

Sudden onset, fever, chills, swollen and tender lymph nodes which often suppurate, or typhoidal and pulmonary forms. Fatality rate: untreated, 5%. Caused by a bacterium, *Francisella tularensis.* Laboratory: cultivation of material from lesions, blood, sputum; serological tests. Incubation: 2–10 days, usually 3. Transmission: contact with blood or tissue of infected wild animals, especially rabbits, hares, and some domestic animals; bites of arthropods (dog ticks, mosquitos), ingestion of insufficiently cooked rabbit or hare meat, contaminated water, inhalation of dust; no person-to-person transmission. Occurrence: North America, Europe, Japan, USSR; sporadic cases or clusters of cases in infected areas during hunting season. Control: streptomycin or tetracyclines, search for source of infection; a live vaccine is of limited use; secretion precautions.

Typhoid fever (ICD 002.0)

Gradual rise of temperature, anorexia, headache, epistaxis, abdominal pain, relative bradycardia, enlargement of spleen and rose spots on the trunk on 7th day (10% of cases). Acute phase: diarrhoea, stupor and delirium. Complications: intestinal haemorrhage or perforation (high fatality rate), pneumonia, abscesses. Fatality rate: untreated 30%, treated 1%. Caused by *Salmonella typhi* bacilli. Differential diagnosis: paratyphoid fever, salmonellosis, typhus, leptospirosis, malaria, brucellosis, tularaemia, viral hepatitis A, gammaherpesviral mononucleosis, Lassa fever. Laboratory diagnosis: repeated blood and stool cultures; Widal serological test on 7th- and 14th-day sera. Incubation: 7–21 days. Transmission: food (shellfish, vegetables, milk and milk products) or water contaminated by faeces or urine of patients or asymptomatic carriers, food-handlers and flies; exceptionally person-to-person. Occurrence: worldwide, all ages, increased in warm climates; progressive outbreaks. Control: treatment with chloramphenicol, or other antibiotics in case of resistance (laboratory test); supportive treatment may require parenteral nutrition and blood transfusion; isolation (enteric precautions); disinfection (faeces, urine and terminal cleaning); community measures (sanitary disposal of human faeces, chlorination or boiling of water, food hygiene, and fly control); prophylaxis (an oral vaccine may soon be available); notification (optional, obligatory in certain countries). Reference: *Salmonella* and *Shigella* surveillance: Guidelines for bacteriological clearance of *Salmonella* and *Shigella* excreters. *Weekly epidemiological record*, **57**: 156–158 (1982).

Typhus fever due to *Rickettsia prowazekii* (ICD 080)

Sudden onset with fever, chills, headache, general pains, prostration. On 5th or 6th day, eruption spreading gradually over the trunk and limbs, except the face, palms and soles, may become petechial and haemorrhagic; pronounced toxaemia. Complication: vascular collapse, gangrene, renal failure, coma; may recur years after as Brill-Zinsser disease. Fatality rate, untreated: 10–40%. Caused by *Rickettsia prowazeckii*. Differential diagnosis: meningococcaemia. Laboratory: differentiation from typhus fever due to *Rickettsia typhi* or to *Rickettsia tsutsugamushi*, by isolation of agent and specific serological tests. Incubation: 12 days (range 1–2 weeks). Transmission: person-to-person by the body louse, infection by rubbing faeces of crushed lice into the bite or inhalation of dust containing infected louse faeces. Occurrence: endemic foci in cold areas, including mountains in tropical areas, in louse-infested populations, outbreaks linked to crowded conditions. Control: treatment with tetracyclines or chloramphenicol and supportive care; application of effective insecticide (resistance may occur) to clothing and bedding of patients and contacts; surveillance of louse-infested contacts for 15 days after insecticide application; effective prophylactic vaccination would require an improved vaccine; notification to WHO (disease under surveillance).

Typhus fever due to *Rickettsia tsutsugamushi* (ICD 081.2)

Skin ulcers with black scab where infected mite was attached, satellite adenopathy; a few days later, sudden onset of fever, headache, conjunctival injection, generalized lymphadenopathy, followed after 5–8 days by a dull red maculopapular eruption on the trunk, spreading to the extremities, delirium, stupor. Complication: pneumonia, myocarditis. If untreated, fatality rate varies from 1% to 60%, according to rickettsial strain. Caused by *Rickettsia tsutsugamushi* (ex *orientalis*). Differential diagnosis: typhus fever due to other rickettsiae, spotted fevers. Laboratory: specific serological diagnosis. Incubation: 10–12 days (range 6–21). Transmission: bite of infected larval trombiculid mites, no person-to-person transmission. Occurrence: localized foci in Central, Eastern and South-East Asia, linked to agricultural activities, hunting, military operations, clusters of cases mainly in non-residents. Control: treatment with tetracylines, supportive care, personal protection against mites (clothes and blankets impregnated with miticidal chemicals, repellents on exposed skin surfaces).

Typhus fever due to *Rickettsia typhi* (ICD 081.0)
Similar clinically to typhus fever due to *Rickettsia prowazekii* but milder. Fatality rate 2%. Caused by *Rickettsia typhi* (ex *mooseri*). Laboratory: differentiation from typhus fever due to other rickettsiae by type-specific serological tests. Incubation: 12 days (range 1–2 weeks). Transmission: by rat fleas which defecate and contaminate the bite site, occasionally by inhalation of desiccated flea faeces. Occurrence: worldwide, clusters of cases in rat-infested dwellings of endemic areas, namely ports. Control: treatment as for typhus fever due to *Rickettsia prowazekii*, use of rodenticides after application of insecticide powders with residual action to rat runs and burrows. Reference: AL-AWADI, A. R. ET AL. Murine typhus in Kuwait in 1978. *Bulletin of the World Health Organization*, **60**: 283–289 (1982).

Varicella (ICD 052)
For some time during the smallpox post-eradication era, the clinical features of varicella should be carefully differentiated from smallpox, as shown in Table A3.2.

Varicella (chickenpox) is usually benign except in immunocompromised patients, but is more severe in adults than in children. Complications: pneumonia in infants and elderly or immunocompromised adults, encephalitis, streptococcal or staphylococcal infection of the vesicles; zoster (shingles) after a long latent period; congenital malformation in early pregnancy. Caused by varicella-zoster virus (herpesvirus group). Differential diagnosis: smallpox, generalized vaccinia (should disappear with the interruption of vaccination), impetigo, drug rashes. Laboratory: scrapings of floor of vesicles show multinucleated giant cells coloured by Giemsa stain (not in smallpox); vesicle fluid shows round particles by electron-miscroscopy in chickenpox (brick shape in smallpox) and may be used for cultivation of virus (in maximum-containment laboratory in WHO collaborating centre if smallpox is suspected);[1] serology is used mainly for epidemiological surveys. Incubation: 13–17 days (range 13–21 days). Transmission: person-to-person, directly very easily by droplets from

---

[1] See Annex 5.

Table A3.2. Clinical features of varicella and smallpox

Clinical feature	Varicella	Smallpox
Onset	Progressive, moderate fever	Sudden, high fever, intense malaise (as in meningitis)
Rash	Appears on 2nd day, with continuing fever (in children the rash is often the first sign)	Appears on 3rd–4th day with transient fall of fever for 2–3 days
	Begins on the trunk, where it will stay dense, not on palms and soles	Begins on the face and extremities of the limbs including palms and soles, where it will stay dense
	Macules become rapidly papular and produce clear vesicles which form crusts without going through the pustular stage	Macules require 4–6 days to transform into papules, vesicles and pustules before producing scabs
	Successive crops appear during 4–5 days in the same area, which shows lesions at different stages	Single crop only: all lesions are at the same stage in a given area
Vesicles	Soft, superficial, "teardrop", not umbilicated	Hard, deep-seated, umbilicated, transform into pustules with rise of fever and prostration
Crusts	Fall off rapidly leaving temporary granular scabs	Healing is slow and leaves permanent pockmarks
Lethality	Exceptional	Case-fatality rate, 20–40% (variola major)

the nose and throat starting 1–2 days before rash, less easily from vesicles of shingles, indirectly by articles freshly soiled; scabs are not infectious; mild, atypical and inapparent infections are contagious. Occurrence: in winter and early spring in 3–4-year cycles; 75 % of the population has had chickenpox by the age of 15 years; outbreaks are progressive in households, schools and other closed communities. Control: no specific treatment (antiviral drugs are under consideration), cleanliness of skin; RESPIRATORY or **STRICT ISOLATION** until 6 days after onset of rash; disinfection of articles soiled by nose and throat discharges and content of shingle vesicles; immunocompromised contacts should be given specific immune globulin. No international measures, except if smallpox is suspected, in which case telegraphic notification to local authorities and dispatch of vesicle fluid or scabs to WHO (see Annex 5).

Verruga peruana
See Bartonellosis.

Viral hepatitis A (ICD 070.1)

Sudden onset, fever, malaise, anorexia, nausea, abdominal pains followed within 3–10 days by jaundice, dark urine, discoloured stools, altered liver function, elevated serum enzyme tests, asthenia and prolonged convalescence. Complete recovery is the rule (fatality rate less than 0.1 %), except for severe forms leading to hepatic coma. Caused by hepatitis A virus (HAV), now considered to be an enterovirus. Laboratory: serological test for detection of specific IgM. Incubation: 15–50 days, usually 28–30. Transmission: faecal–oral, personal contact, contaminated water and food (dairy products, uncooked meat, vegetables, shellfish), transfusion of infected blood. Carriers with mild or asymptomatic infection are frequent, especially children. Occurrence: worldwide, sporadic or epidemic, high prevalence in warm climates in areas with low standards of sanitation, and in certain institutions; explosive outbreaks after exposure to common source of infection, such as food-handlers or water supply contamination. Control: no specific treatment, excreta and blood precautions; investigation of source and contacts; usual personal and community measures against faecal risk; prophylaxis with standard immune serum globulin for contacts and travellers at risk.

Viral hepatitis B (ICD 070.3)

Insidious onset, with anorexia, fever mild or absent, abdominal pains, nausea, vomiting, sometimes arthralgia, followed by jaundice as for hepatitis A. Complications: chronic active hepatitis, cirrhosis, hepatocellular carcinoma, liver necrosis, fulminating cases, hepatic coma. Fatality rate: 1 % (6–12 % in post-transfusion cases). Caused by hepatitis B virus (HBV). The delta agent is a defective virus which has often been found associated with hepatitis B virus in fulminant hepatitis outbreaks. Laboratory: detection of surface (HBs), core (HBc), and e (HBe) antigens, or anti-HBc and anti-HBs antibodies; these markers follow different courses during the successive phases of the disease. Diagnosis of superimposed delta agent is made by detection of the antigen in the blood or liver, or demonstration of specific IgM in serum. Incubation: 45–160 days (average 2–3 months). Transmission: parenteral, infected blood of patients and carriers, scarifications, toilet articles, injections with contaminated syringes (drug addicts are particularly at risk), blood transfusion and blood products from infected donors, sexual transmission. Occurrence: worldwide, children and adults in developing countries (carrier rate up to 20 %), mainly young adults in developed countries (carrier rate less than 1 %); sporadic cases or outbreaks in certain groups (homosexuals, prostitutes) and closed institutions; occupational risk in medical professions. Control: no specific drug, prevention with hepatitis B immune globulin for close contacts; an inactivated vaccine is now available; identification of source of infection among carriers; barrier nursing in specialized wards (renal dialysis); screening for carriers before blood donation; excreta and blood precautions.

Viral hepatitis, non-A, non-B (ICD 070.5)

Epidemiologically, there are two distinct entities: blood-transmitted hepatitis and epidemic hepatitis.

(a) Blood-transmitted hepatitis, non-A, non-B

Resembles viral hepatitis B epidemiologically but is generally less severe. Complications: chronic form in 50% of cases, only 10% of which progress to cirrhosis. Possibly caused by more than one virus, not yet identified. Laboratory: exclusion of hepatitis A and B and other causes of jaundice. Incubation: possibly as for hepatitis B. Transmission: infected blood and direct contact. Occurrence: worldwide, accounts for up to 90% of all cases of post-transfusion hepatitis; may also be transmitted by certain batches of clotting factors VIII and IX concentrates which cannot withstand inactivation of hepatitis B; "sporadic" cases may account for 20% of clinical hepatitis. Control: excreta and blood precautions.

(b) Epidemic hepatitis, non-A, non-B

Epidemiologically resembles hepatitis A but serological evidence of HAV or HBV etiology lacking. May be caused by several viruses not yet identified. Incubation: 30–40 days. Transmission: faecal–oral, and blood transfusion. Occurrence: sporadic cases or explosive outbreaks may be caused by ingestion of contaminated food or water; has occurred on several occasions after flooding of rivers. Control: usual personal and community measures against faecal risk; excreta and blood precautions.

Whooping cough

See Pertussis.

Yaws (ICD 102.9)

Initial papilloma (which may ulcerate) for several weeks or months on the face or extremities, followed by dissemination of secondary papillomas in successive crops with periostitis and hyperkeratoses on the palms and soles. Complications: destructive lesions of skin and bones. Caused by *Treponema pertenue*, a spirochaete. Laboratory: dark-field examination of exudates, syphilis serological tests. Incubation: 2 weeks–3 months. Infective period: several years, may be intermittent. Transmission: direct contact with exudates, probable role of flies. Occurrence: children in humid tropical forests. Control: treatment with penicillin, mass treatment in active foci.

Yellow fever (jungle or sylvatic: ICD 060.0; urban: 060.1; unspecified: 060.9)

First phase is dengue-like followed by a short remission on the 3rd day and a hepatonephrotoxic phase with haemorrhages, which are more obvious than jaundice. Bleeding from nose and gums, black vomit, blood (black or fresh) in stools, anuria, progressive proteinuria, uraemic coma, hypotension, shock, death within 10 days of onset. Fulminating forms: death in 3 days. Fatality rate: up to 80 % in severe cases and about 1 % if mild and asymptomatic forms are included. Caused by yellow fever virus, a flavivirus. Laboratory: safety precautions, personnel should have been vaccinated at least 10 days earlier; isolation of virus from blood in early stage of the disease or from necropsy specimens up to 12 days after onset and from

Fig. A3.2. Yellow-fever endemic zone in Africa

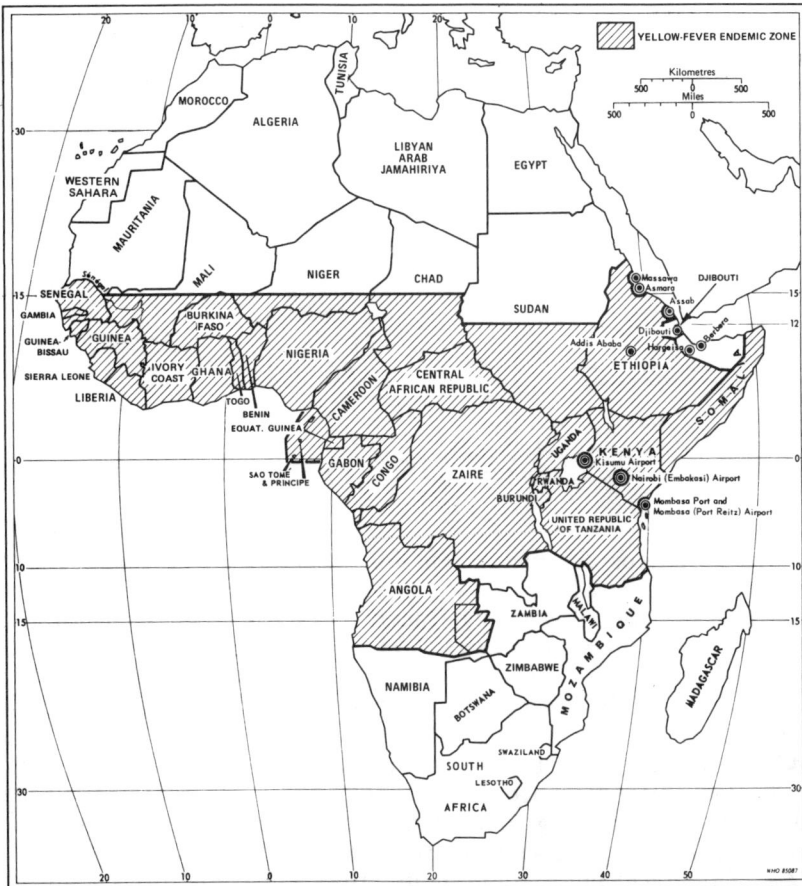

Fig. A3.3. Yellow-fever endemic zone in the Americas

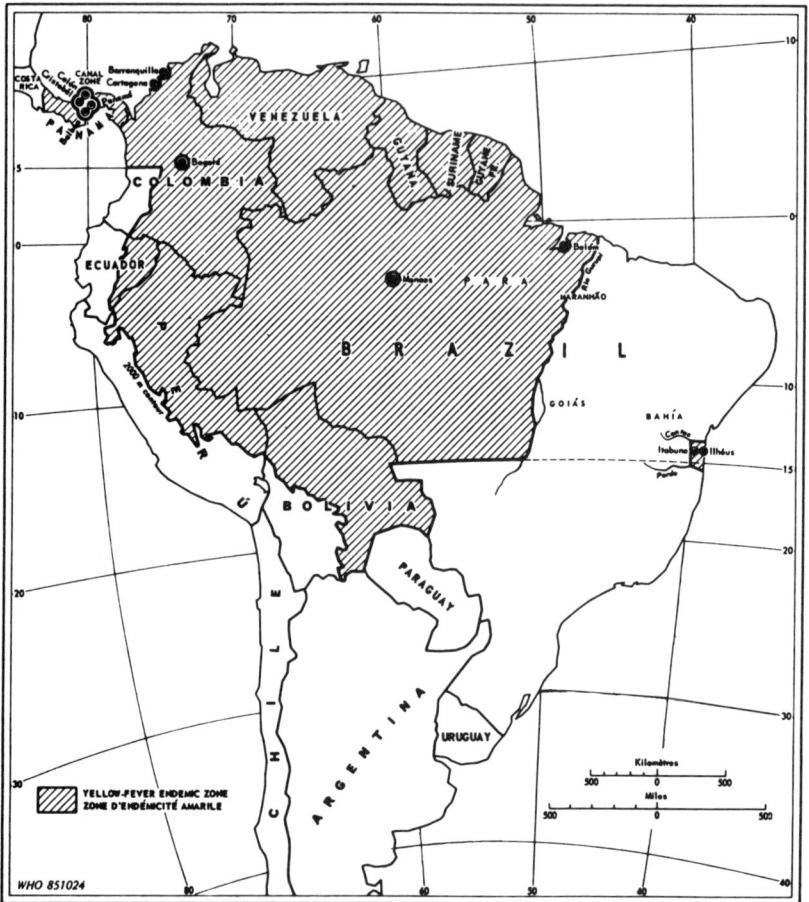

vector mosquitos; serological tests for specific IgM in single serum or rising IgG in paired sera. Liver biopsy is contraindicated because of the risk of internal bleeding. Incubation: 3–6 days. Transmission: from monkeys to man by certain forest mosquitos (jungle or sylvatic yellow fever) and from person to person by certain domestic mosquitos, mainly *Aedes aegypti* (urban yellow fever). Occurrence: all age groups in tropical zones of Africa and Americas (Fig. A3.2 and A3.3). Control: bed-nets to avoid contact of patients with mosquitos; individual protection from mosquitos; insecticide spraying during epidemics and breeding source reduction. The live attenuated vaccine requires 7 days to give protection and must be kept in the cold (4–8 °C). Urgent notification to authorities and WHO (disease subject to the International Health Regulations). References: WHO Technical Report Series, No. 479, 1971 (*Yellow fever*: third report of the WHO Expert Committee on Yellow Fever); *Prevention and control of yellow fever in Africa*. Geneva, World Health Organization, 1986.

Yersiniosis (ICD 027.8)
Watery diarrhoea in young children (blood streaks in 5 % of cases), fever, leukocytosis, enterocolitis and lymphadenitis; mimics appendicitis in older children, low-grade fever. Complication: erythema nodosum, arthritis in adults. Caused by *Yersinia enterocolitica* and *Y. pseudotuberculosis*. Laboratory: blood cultures in generalized infections, isolation from stool cultures after refrigeration of specimens. Incubation: 3–76 days. Transmission: faecal–oral; asymptomatic carriers. Occurrence: worldwide; sporadic, food- and water-borne outbreaks, person-to-person transmission, outbreaks in schools, contact with household pets. Control: antibiotic treatment; enteric precautions; investigation of common source. Reference: WHO SCIENTIFIC WORKING GROUP. Enteric infections due to *Campylobacter, Yersinia, Salmonella* and *Shigella*. *Bulletin of the World Health Organization*, **58**: 519–537 (1980).

ANNEX 4

Standard precautions, isolation and medical evacuation for diseases with person-to-person transmission

If the agent responsible for an outbreak and its mode of transmission from person to person are known, precautions can be taken against its excretion by both patients and healthy carriers. While the agent remains unidentified, the protection desirable should be based on the mode of transmission, the attack rate and the severity of the disease as judged by the case-fatality rate, sequelae ratio, or socioeconomic impact. The minimal protection procedures for diseases transmitted from person to person are known as standard precautions, but additional measures may be required, such as enteric or respiratory isolation or, exceptionally, strict isolation. The same levels of protection may also be required for medical evacuation.

A4.1 Standard precautions

A4.1.1 General principles

The purpose of standard precautions is to prevent the spread of a contagious agent to other patients, hospital personnel and visitors. Standard precautions should achieve this objective for moderately transmissible diseases without unnecessary waste of time and money.

A4.1.2 Equipment

This consists mainly of protective clothing, as follows:

—gown: should be of washable material, buttoned up at the back and protected if necessary by a plastic apron;
—gloves: cheap plastic gloves are available;
—mask: surgical masks made of cloth or paper may be used;
—caps and overshoes.

Other necessary equipment includes sinks for hand-washing (operated by foot), disinfectants (see Annex 7), plastic bags, an autoclave, and an incinerator.

A4.1.3 Procedures

Washing hands before and after each contact with potentially infected patients or materials is the most important and efficient precaution that can be taken. Rinsing hands with alcohol (700 ml/litre) or iodine solution in alcohol may cause skin damage and is not always necessary.

Warnings, in the form of coded colour cards fixed to the door or the bed, should indicate the specific type of precautions to be taken.

The double-bagging technique should be used whenever contagious material (including laboratory samples) is to be transported. Transparent plastic bags are used. The bag containing the contaminated material is placed in a second bag, which should be handled only with clean hands or a new pair of gloves; a label should be inserted between the bags to identify the material and indicate the precautions to be taken. Personnel should not smoke or eat while on duty.

Visitors are generally admitted (except for children, pregnant women and immunocompromised persons) after this has been authorized, but must be given advice on self-protection.

When indicated, gowns should be changed after each patient has been visited (individual gown technique).

Masks, whether of paper or cloth, are not effective when wet and should not be kept around the neck when not in use.

Standard precautions may be directed more specifically against excreta, secretions, skin discharges and blood, and appropriate procedures are indicated in Table A4.1.

Table A4.1. Procedures for protective precautions

Type of precautions	Procedures
Standard precautions	
Excreta, secretions and skin discharges	Wearing gloves and/or hand-washing
	Change gloves and gown after dealing with infective discharges
	Mask when dealing with oral secretions
	Excreta disposal with disinfection, or without, in communities with a modern sewage system (unsuitable for certain diseases—see Annex 3)
	Oral secretions: same precautions as for excreta in certain diseases, e.g., poliomyelitis
	Ocular secretions: when indicated, double-bagging techniques and incineration of contaminated material

Table A4.1 (*continued*)

Type of precautions	Procedures
Excreta, secretions and skin discharges (*continued*)	Discharges and dressings: double-bagging techniques
	Freshly soiled articles: double-bagging techniques and sterilization or incineration
Blood[a]	"Needle" precautions to avoid creating bubbles in emptying the syringe
	Contaminated articles: double-bagging and incineration or autoclaving
Enteric isolation	Private room (or ward for patients with same disease), isolated toilets
	Change gloves and gown after dealing with infective material
	Standard precautions for excreta and oral secretions, when indicated
	Standard precautions for freshly soiled articles
	Visiting restricted
Respiratory isolation	Private room, negative pressure (exhaust fan), anteroom desirable
	Discard gown, gloves, mask and cap after dealing with patient
	Nasopharyngeal secretions: disinfection
	Standard precautions for freshly soiled articles
	Visiting restricted
Strict isolation	Private room with anteroom and sink, airflow controlled by negative pressure and exhaust filtered (high efficiency particulate air (HEPA) filters)
	Special devices for microbiological barrier:
	—high-security, disposable, protective clothing and full-face or half-face microbiological mask, or positive-pressure hood-respirator; or plastic-film bed isolator (Trexler's tent type)
	Decontamination of sewage and disinfection of excreta, discharges and blood
	Terminal disinfection
	Medical personnel under surveillance
	Visiting prohibited

[a] A risk of transmission of hepatitis B may be present and should be borne in mind in handling blood.

A4.2 Enteric and respiratory isolation

A4.2.1 General principles

Isolation of a patient may become necessary when transmission of the agent is possible even when standard precautions are taken, as is the case with a limited number of diseases (see Annex 3 and Table 44). This procedure is time-consuming and increases the cost of hospitalization. However, under field conditions, there is room for improvisation, and simple techniques may be capable of limiting the spread of a disease by isolating the patient just as effectively. When the number of patients exceeds the number of hospital beds available, some improvisation will also be necessary to enable other rooms to be used. Field hospitals or fever clinics may also be set up temporarily with the same objective. The isolation techniques differ somewhat for patients with enteric as compared with respiratory diseases.

A4.2.2 Equipment

A private room is normally required when a patient has to be isolated. In emergency situations, at least temporarily, however, patients with enteric infections may be cared for on a ward rather than in a private room if all the patients admitted require the same care and precautions and are at the same stage of the disease. For respiratory isolation, grouping several patients together could expose them to cross-infections, thereby complicating the original disease.

In addition to gowns and gloves, masks, caps and overshoes may be necessary, a separate set being required for use in each individual patient's room.

Enteric diseases that can spread easily require disinfection of excreta, even if the sewage system is considered safe, because of the quantity of agents that may be evacuated.

A4.2.3 Procedures

General procedures as described in section A4.1.3 are applicable. Additional special procedures are indicated in Table A4.1.

A4.3 Strict isolation

A4.3.1 General principles

Strict isolation is required for a small number of exceptionally highly contagious diseases (see Annex 3 and Table 44), and is designed to avoid any direct or indirect contact with the patient and to protect medical personnel and the community from possible transmission through droplet nuclei (aerosols) which might be carried some distance. It places a barrier around the patient that no microbial agent can pass through.

Even if it is known that the epidemic is caused by a highly contagious agent, it may be appropriate, for logistic reasons, to admit suspect patients initially to standard isolation facilities, either of the enteric or respiratory type, or even a combination of both, until the presence of the agent has been confirmed or is strongly suspected.

Although strict isolation requires special rooms and specially trained personnel, it is possible to improvise effective procedures whenever appropriate facilities are not available locally. It should not be forgotten that good barrier nursing practices provide a reliable level of safety.

Under field conditions, a practical solution is to isolate patients at home, providing protective equipment and giving the bare minimum of instruction to a member of the family, with supervision by medical personnel.

A4.3.2 Equipment

Facilities. Strict isolation requires a separate building or a completely separate part of a building without any common air flow. Strict isolation facilities consist of service rooms fitted with autoclaves and direct access to an incinerator, sewage decontamination systems, patients' rooms with anterooms, and a direct entrance for ambulances, and a ventilation system providing an airflow from other areas to the anterooms, to the patients' rooms and finally to an exhaust pipe fitted with a high efficiency particulate air (HEPA) filter. A HEPA filter retains 99.97% of particulates 0.3 μm in diameter.

Two systems have been in use for isolating patients from personnel. The first is the plastic-film bed isolator (Fig. A4.1), which is operated at a pressure below atmospheric and is equipped with HEPA filters and a lock system for evacuating contaminated material in sealed plastic bags. Nursing personnel do not need special suits, since the patient is surrounded by the microbiological barrier. In the second system, the patient is in a normal bed and personnel are protected by high-security protective clothing, i.e., the microbiological barrier is around the person who is taking care of the patient. The anteroom then plays an important role, and is divided into clean and contaminated areas. Contaminated articles are first placed in bags in the patient's room and transferred to the contaminated area, where the health worker also leaves his contaminated suit in a bag. In between the two areas, the health worker decontaminates the outside of the bag containing contaminated material with hypochlorite solution, washes his hands, inserts the bag into another one taken from the clean area and moves into the clean area. The clean area contains a stock of material, and a basin for washing hands is located

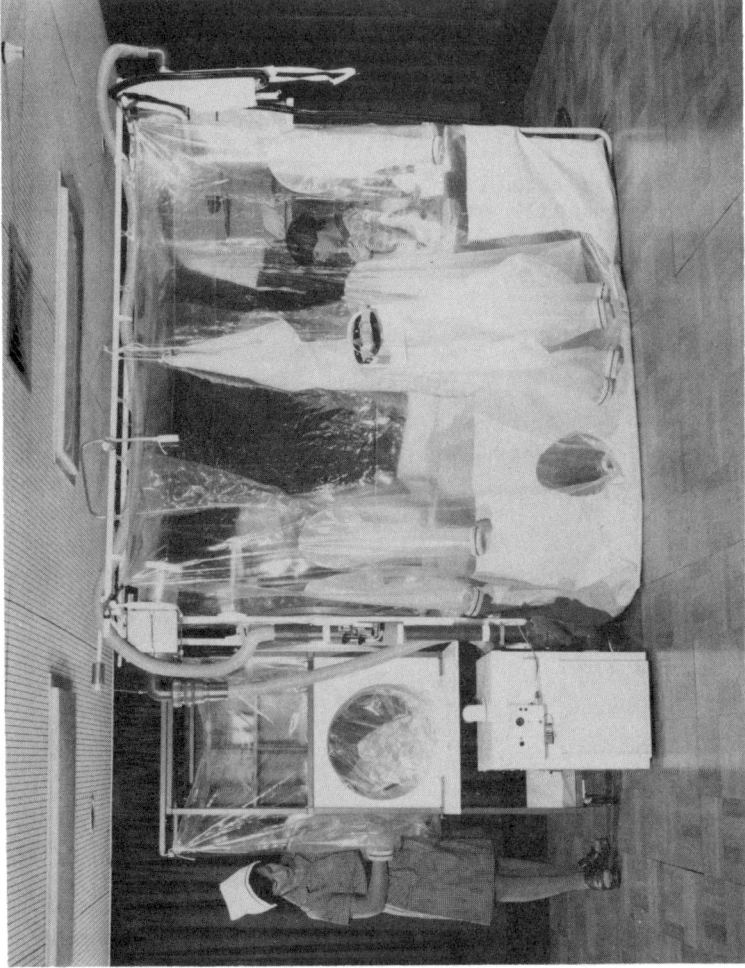

Fig. A4.1. Plastic-film bed isolator (Trexler's tent) for highly contagious patients (by courtesy of Vickers Medical, London, England)

between the two areas. Both inside and outside doors of the anteroom should be locked. Glass windows are convenient since they permit personnel to see the patient from the corridor of the clean area. The patient's room should be provided with a minimal amount of furniture, privies, bath, and alarm devices. All instruments such as thermometers, sphygmomanometers, etc., should be used only for one particular patient.

Protective clothing. Two types of protective clothing are available. The first (Fig. A4.2) is used for medical care and consists of gown, apron, hood and boots. The face is protected by a plastic visor, or

Fig. A4.2. High-security protective clothing (disposable): washable plastic apron over plastic gown, gloves, surgical cloth mask and face visor

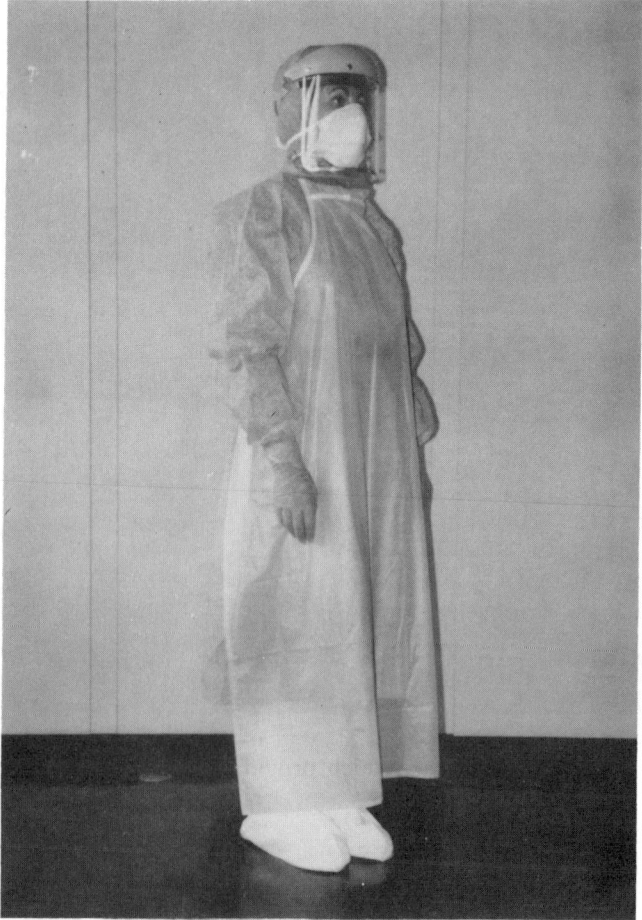

Fig. A4.3. Positive-pressure hood-respirator with back-pack HEPA filter
(by courtesy of Vickers Medical, London, England)

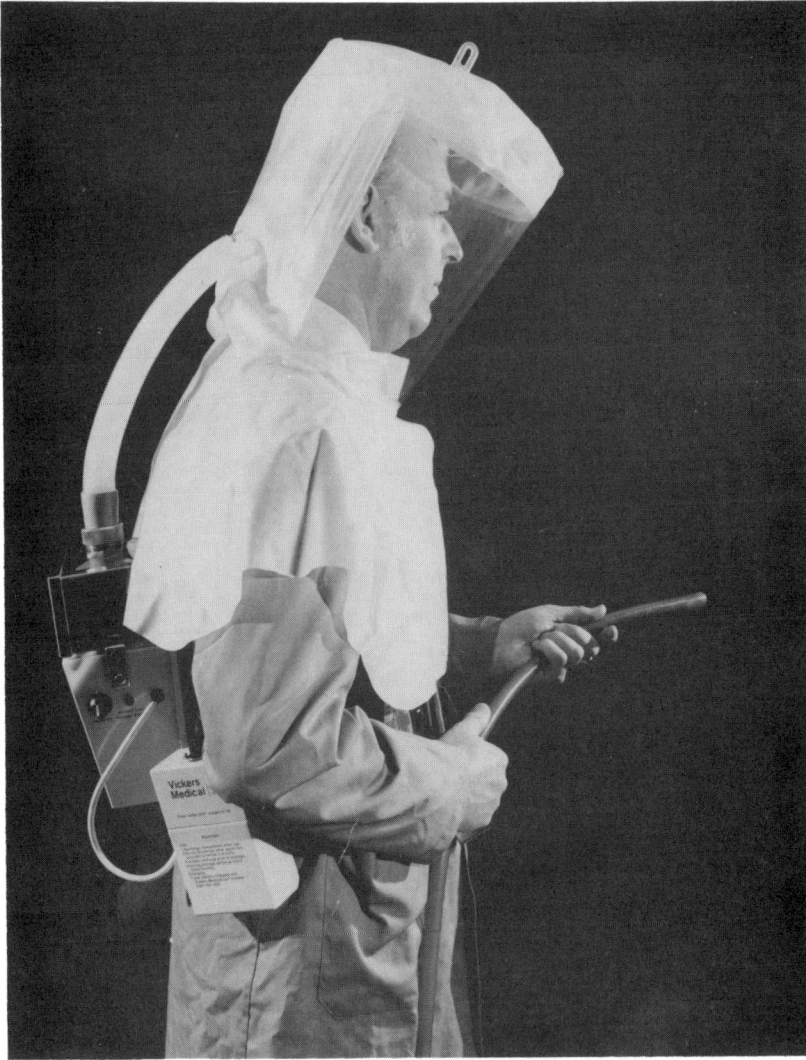

goggles. Air is filtered through a surgical mask, or a half-face or full-face mask with a cartridge, which provides a microbiological barrier. A positive-pressure hood-respirator (Fig. A4.3) with a back-pack HEPA filter may also be used.

The second type (Fig. A4.4), consisting of an overall and boots, is used for high-risk operations, such as visiting a highly contagious

Fig. A4.4. High-security protective clothing (disposable): plasticized one-
piece uniform and full-face biological respirator

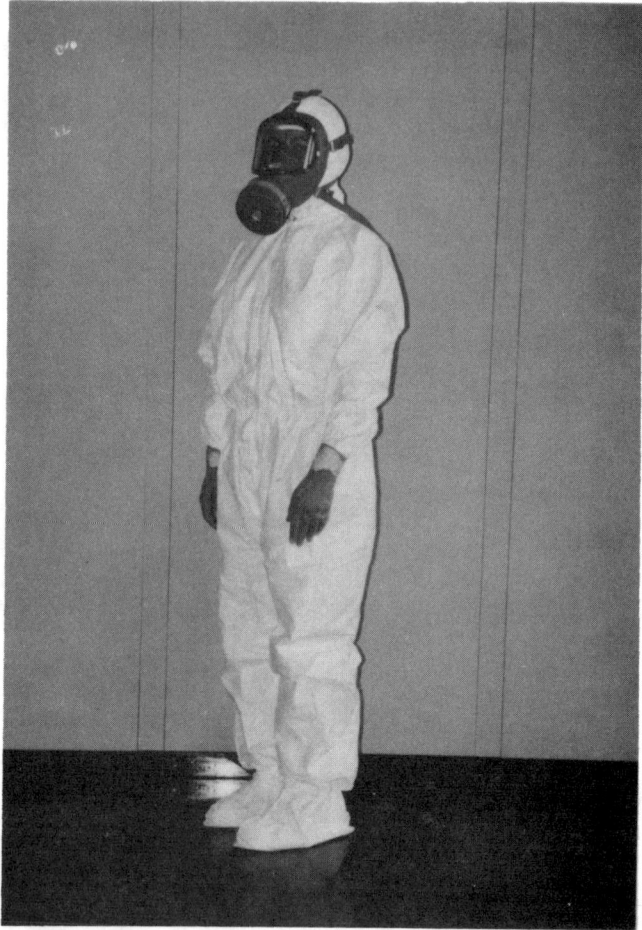

patient at home, performing necropsies, taking laboratory specimens,
or carrying out high-risk laboratory examinations. It should be made
of waterproof fabric.

Disposable protective clothing may be incinerated after use, which
avoids the problem of sterilization. It also permits new suits to be
used as often as necessary. WHO keeps an emergency stock of such

items. However, they are rather expensive and cotton equipment may also be used but must be sterilized before being washed.

Protective clothing may also be improvised with plastic materials, which will then also be disposable. Plastic bags of various sizes may be transformed into aprons, gloves, boots and hoods.

Whatever the material used for the protective clothing, the way that it is removed is of great importance in avoiding self-contamination. The procedure is described in Table A4.2. **Potentially contaminated surfaces should never touch either the operator or any uncontaminated material.**

A4.3.3 Procedures

These are indicated in Table A4.1.

A4.4 Medical evacuation

The level of precautions to be taken in the medical evacuation of acutely ill patients is shown in Table 44 (p. 109).

When strict isolation is recommended, all persons handling the patient or in close contact with him should be equipped with protective clothing and respirators or masks. The procedure for removing such clothing is shown in Table A4.2.

Pressurized stretcher transit isolators with HEPA filters are produced by commercial companies and provide the same microbiological barrier as the bed isolator (Fig. A4.5).

Medical care during evacuation will consist mainly of supportive treatment for the circulatory and respiratory functions. Ringer lactate infusions should be kept ready for use, but formation of bubbles in the ampoule resulting from the motion of the vehicles may present a difficulty.

Table A4.2 Procedure for removing protective clothing

1. In the contaminated area of the anteroom, rinse gloved hands in a sodium hypochlorite solution
2. Remove apron, head cover and overshoes and place in a plastic bag
3. Remove gown and gloves in a single operation, folding the gown and gloves inside out in doing so, or remove overall, gloves and overshoes in a single operation, turning the overall, gloves and overshoes inside out
4. Put on a fresh pair of gloves; place gown and contaminated gloves in a bag, or discard overall, gloves and overshoes into a plastic bag
5. Remove the respirator, sponge off with sodium hypochlorite solution and replace it in its container
6. Remove the second pair of gloves, place them in the bag and close it
7. Wash hands, move to the clean area of the anteroom and place the bags in an outer bag (double-bag technique) and label either for autoclaving, incineration or laboratory examination

Fig. A4.5. Pressurized stretcher transit isolator (by courtesy of Vickers Medical, London, England)

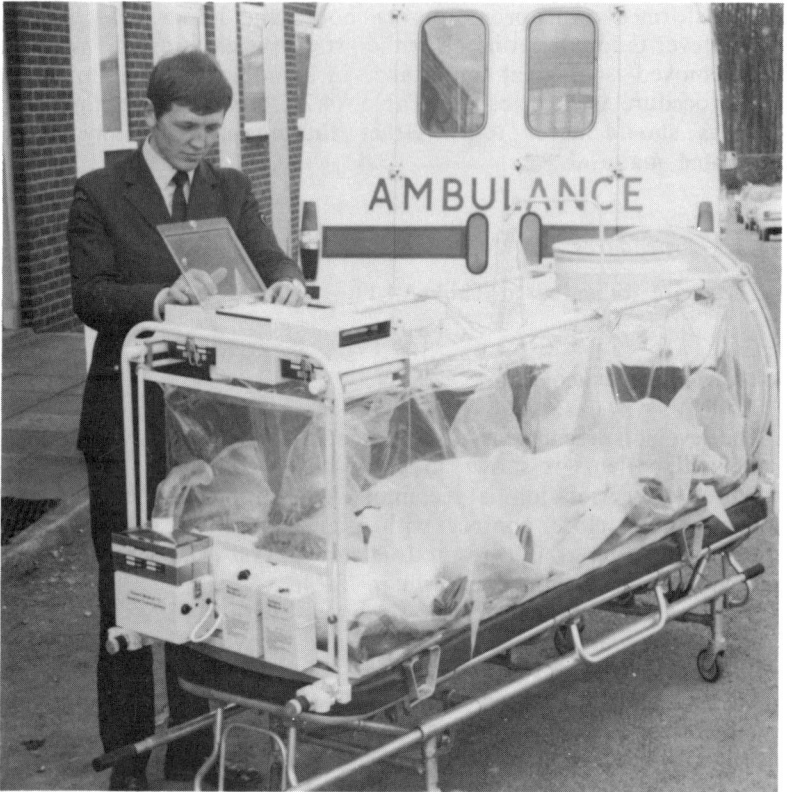

The stretcher transit isolator is suitable for transferring patients by ambulance to the main hospital. Note the cones for tubes and wires and the evaginated sleeve for supporting an infusion bag.

Methods of disinfecting the vehicle, during transport or on arrival, are described in Annex 7.

Official arrangements for medical evacuation must be made with the hospital at the destination and with the local authorities at places where it is intended to stop en route.

BIBLIOGRAPHY

CLAUSEN, L. ET AL. Isolation and handling of patients with dangerous infectious diseases. *South African medical journal*, **53**: 238–242 (1978).

CONTROL OF INFECTION GROUP, NORTHWICK PARK HOSPITAL AND CLINICAL RESEARCH CENTRE. Isolation systems for general hospitals. *British medical journal*, **2**: 41–44 (1974).

DUNSMORE, D. J. *Safety measures for use in outbreaks of communicable disease.* Geneva, World Health Organization, 1986.

EMOND, R. T. D. High security isolators. *Postgraduate doctor—Middle East*, (11): 473–478 (1981).

HUTCHINSON, J. G. ET AL. The safety of the Trexler isolator as judged by some physical and biological criteria: a report of experimental work at two centres. *Journal of hygiene*, **81**: 311–319 (1978).

Isolation techniques for use in hospitals, Washington, DC, US Department of Health, Education, and Welfare, Centers for Disease Control, 1975 (DHEW Publication No. (CDC) 76–8314).

Laboratory biosafety manual. Geneva, World Health Organization, 1983.

Practical guide to the prevention of hospital-acquired infections. Unpublished WHO document, WHO/BAC/79.1.

TREXLER, P. C. ET AL. Negative pressure plastic isolator for patients with dangerous infections. *British medical journal*, **2**: 559–561 (1977).

ANNEX 5

Collection and shipment of laboratory specimens

As mentioned in sections 4.1.5 and 4.2.6, the correct collection of specimens for laboratory examination is an important part of any investigation. Specimen collection should be carefully planned; this requires consideration of the selection of appropriate samples, the preferred method of collection, safety precautions, requirements for packaging and shipment, and the competence of the laboratory to which the specimens will be sent.

A 5.1 Collection of specimens

A5.1.1 Human population

If it is not clear what disease has caused the outbreak, specimens should be taken as outlined in Table A5.1.

The specimens required when certain specific agents are suspected are indicated in Table A5.2. It should be noted that liver biopsy is contraindicated in yellow fever and haemorrhagic fevers because of the risk of internal bleeding.

Methods for the collection of specimens are outlined in Table A5.3 and shown for blood in Fig. A5.1.

A5.1.2 Food-borne diseases

Advice on collecting clinical specimens and samples of suspected foods is given in Table A5.4. It is most important to collect remnants of suspected food but it may also be wise to take samples of all other foods, even though they do not seem to be contaminated, and even if there is only a remote possibility that they have caused the outbreak.

A5.1.3 Vertebrate animals

The collection of specimens may present hazards from contact with the sick animal or infectious aerosols produced by it; whenever this possibility exists, the safety precautions described above are recommended. Blood may be taken with vacuum blood-collecting tubes

(*Text continues on page 243.*)

Table A5.1. Specimens to be collected according to the disease or the principal body system affected

Disease or affected system	For direct examination	Specimens required[a]	
		For isolation[b]	For serology
General	Thick and thin blood films	Heparinized blood, throat swabs, faeces	Paired sera[c] (blood without additive or with heparin)
Exanthems	Skin lesions	Heparinized blood, throat swabs, skin lesions, faeces	
Lymphadenopathy	Pus from gland, or tissue taken with a biopsy needle	Heparinized blood, bubo fluid	
Haemorrhagic fever (strict safety precautions)	Heparinized blood (taken aseptically) (electron microscopy)	Heparinized blood, urine (taken aseptically)	
Nervous system	Cerebrospinal fluid, corneal impressions	Heparinized blood, cerebrospinal fluid, throat swabs, faeces	
Respiratory tract	Nasopharyngeal aspirates, throat swabs	Throat swabs	
Gastrointestinal tract	Faeces, vomit	Faeces, heparinized blood	
Jaundice	—	Heparinized blood	
Eye infections	Conjunctival scrapings or swabs	Conjunctival scrapings or swabs, heparinized blood	

[a] Adequate safety precautions are necessary in collecting all specimens. Blood for isolation should be taken aseptically.
[b] Some specimens require enrichment or transport media.
[c] For some diseases, detection of IgM antibody in a single serum specimen taken early after onset is sufficient.

Table A5.2. Laboratory specimens required for tests for particular causative agents

Suspected agent or disease	Specimen	Test
Arbovirus	Blood or brain (−70 °C)	Isolation
	Blood or serum (+4 °C)	Serology
Cholera	Rectal swabs or stool specimens in transport medium, as recommended by the laboratory	Culture
Gastroenteritis	Stool	Culture (bacterial, viral), electron-microscopy, ELISA[a]
	Blood or serum (+4 °C)	Serology
Hepatitis	Serum (+4 °C)	ELISA[a]
Legionella	Blood, sputum in enrichment broth	Culture; FA[b]
Malaria	Blood (thick and thin smears)	Staining
Meningococcal meningitis	Spinal fluid, blood, pharyngeal swabs (all on transport media)	Culture, counter-immunoelectrophoresis
Plague	Bubo fluid, blood (in broth or on blood agar slants)	Culture, FA[b]
Rabies	Brain (−70 °C)	FA[b] and isolation
Salmonella typhi	Blood (early in disease) in enrichment broth	Culture
Shigella	Faecal specimens or rectal swabs in enrichment broth	Culture
Typhus	Blood	Inoculation
	Serum (+4 °C)	Serology
Varicella and suspected smallpox	Lesion fluid, crusts	Electron-microscopy, cell culture

[a] Enzyme-linked immunosorbent assay.
[b] Fluorescent antibody test.

Table A5.3. Methods to be employed in collecting specimens

A. Safety precautions

Purpose	Precautions
Protection of operator	Depending on estimated risk: surgical mask, gloves, gown, plastic apron, and goggles or face shield
Decontamination of material	Disposable material: place in plastic bags and send for incineration
	Reusable material:
	—syringes: draw up hypochlorite or 1 % formaldehyde solution into the needle and syringe; leave for 20 minutes, wash, sterilize
	—other instruments: immerse in disinfectant solution, leave for 20 minutes
	Vials containing specimens: wash outside with cotton soaked in disinfectant or immerse in disinfectant solution

B. Collection of blood[a]

Method or type of blood	Equipment and procedure
Venepuncture	*Equipment* —10-ml vacuum blood-collecting tubes, 21/22 gauge needle, with or without heparin (see Fig. A5.1) —5–10-ml syringes (preferably disposable), 21/22 gauge needle —plastic screw-cap vials
	Procedure —As usual for venepuncture
	—For serum separation: clot formation, 1 hour at room temperature clot retraction, 4 hours at +4° C or room temperature aspirate serum with another Vacutainer, syringe, or pipette with bulb (do not use mouth pipette)
	—Storage: heparinized blood at +4°C (unless otherwise specified) serum at +4°C clot at +4°C for inoculation

Table A5.3 (*continued*)

Method or type of blood	Equipment and procedure
Capillary blood	*Equipment* —disposable sterile lancets —tubes *Procedure* —Adults: clean skin of finger or ear with alcohol, allow to evaporate, and prick skin —Babies under 6 months of age: prick on side of heel (Fig. A5.1), about 2 mm deep, cutting very slightly sideways —Older infants: prick on thumb —Collect blood either in heparinized capillary tube or on strip of absorbent paper —If absorbent paper (Whatman No. 3 for chromatography) is used, cut strips of 14 × 9 cm, allow drops of blood to fall on the paper, mark spots with reference number; collect drops from other patients sufficiently far away on the strip (samples from up to 5 suspects may be collected on one strip), allow strips to dry, standing on their sides inside a covered bowl at room temperature before transport; dry thoroughly later on for long storage and keep at + 4° C or − 20° C in polythene bags.
Blood for parasitology or haematology	Prepare thick and thin blood films as usual (heparinized blood may be used for cell counts); observe filariasis microfilariae in a drop of fresh blood diluted with normal saline solution

[a] Aseptic precautions are necessary for blood inoculation or cultivation and good preservation of serum.

C. Specimens of skin lesions[a]

Stage or purpose	Procedure
Macular-papular stage	Scrape the lesions with a lancet until the surface becomes moist but without blood. The material on the lancet should be rubbed on to slides, and further material absorbed on a swab which is then placed in a screw-cap vial
Vesiculo-pustular stage	Open the lesions with the lancet. Absorb the fluid from at least 6 lesions on the swab. Place the swab and lancet in the plastic container and screw the top on securely. If no plastic container is available: —fill at least 4 capillary tubes and seal the ends with plasticine —take the contents of 3–4 vesicles with a swab with wooden applicator, rub the swab on 2 slides with a circular motion, covering an area about 1 cm in diameter

Table A5.3 (*continued*)

Stage or purpose	Procedure
Crusting stage	With the lancet, take off a minimum of 6 crusts and place them in a plastic screw-top bottle
Parasitology	Observe trichinellosis parasites in muscle biopsy and onchocerciasis microfilariae in cutaneous snip

^a Specimens for direct examination and cultivation can be taken directly from skin lesions of vesicular rashes. In other exanthemata (macular/papular), the agent may be isolated more easily from blood, throat swabs or faeces than from skin lesions. The WHO specimen collection kit (Fig. A5.3) may be used, particularly for suspected varicella, monkeypox or smallpox lesions (with strict safety precautions).

D. Respiratory tract specimens

Purpose	Procedure
Bacteriology, mycology or parasitology	Direct examination of sputum: thin smear on a slide for Gram staining
	Cultivation: make a cough swab. Fragile bacteria require special media and particular precautions (ask laboratory for guidance)
Virology	Direct examination by immunofluorescence: cough swab transported in Hanks' medium at $+4\,^{\circ}$C, or preferably nasopharyngeal aspirate obtained with a suction apparatus
	Cultivation: same specimens. Fragile viruses require special media and particular precautions (ask laboratory for guidance)

E. Specimens of faeces

Purpose	Procedure
All examinations	3 ml (or equivalent in solid) in screw-cap "bijou" bottle (capacity 7 ml). Store at $+4\,^{\circ}$C or normal temperature
Parasitology	3 parts of 10% formaldehyde solution are added to 1 part of stool for dispatch
Bacteriology	Use special transport medium for cholera, other vibrios, *Salmonella*, *Shigella*, etc.; store at room temperature in shade, not in refrigerator. If medium not available, consult laboratory
Virology	A suitable virus transport medium may be provided by the laboratory

Table A5.3 (*continued*)

F. Specimens of cerebrospinal fluid[a]

Purpose	Procedure
All examinations	Collect in 2 tubes, one containing 6–7 ml, the other 2 ml; transfer contents of latter tube aseptically to a sterile bijou bottle
Cytology, biochemistry, or parasitology	Use specimen from first tube (examine without delay)
Bacteriology or virology	Use bijou bottle, do not put in refrigerator, keep at +37° C if possible, in shade. Transport medium is needed for meningococci (ask laboratory), but not for viruses

[a] Like the viruses of most encephalitides, the rabies virus cannot be isolated from the CSF; cutaneous biopsy in the retroauricular region and corneal impressions may give rapid results by immunofluorescence.

G. Eye specimens

Purpose	Procedure
Direct examination	Conjunctival scraping with a fine spatula, smear on clean dry microscope slide for staining to check for bacteria and chlamydiae
Cultivation	Bacteria and viruses require special media for transport (ask laboratory for guidance)

H. Specimens of urine

Purpose	Procedure
Parasitology, bacteriology, or virology	After centrifugation, parasites may be observed; the pellet can be cultivated if it has been obtained aseptically

I. Post-mortem specimens[a]

Specimen or disease	Procedure
Blood	The most important sample needed, it can be taken from the heart cavities
Liver	The second sample needed and obtainable without autopsy by use of a biopsy needle. Several fragments are needed, some in fixative for histopathology,[b] others in saline (aseptically) for bacteria and viruses

Table A5.3 (*continued*)

Specimen or disease	Procedure
Spleen, kidneys, lungs, heart	If necessary, pieces of these organs may be prepared both for histopathology[b] and for bacteria and viruses, as for liver
Encephalitides	Pieces of brain (cortex, thalamus, Ammon's horn) should be taken aseptically for isolation, and a cortical smear made for detection of *Plasmodium falciparum*

[a] Safety precautions must be taken when death is due to a communicable disease and must be strict for septicaemia, encephalitides and haemorrhagic fevers; direct contact and aerosol transmission must be avoided. Virus titres decline rapidly after death while bacteria rapidly increase in number. Post mortem material should therefore be collected as soon as possible.

[b] The fixative fluid (saline formol) for use in histopathology is made up as follows:

Formol, commercial grade	120 ml
Distilled water	880 ml
Sodium chloride	9 g

Material fixed in saline formol can be utilized in electron microscopy.

from the jugular vein in large animals, with a syringe from the humeral vein in birds, with a capillary tube from the ocular sinus in small rodents, or by cardiac puncture in post-mortem examinations. Serum from animals that have been shot is often anticomplementary in complement-fixation tests. Parasites may be found in faeces, but their immature stages in animals may be different morphologically from the mature forms in man, and vice versa.

Special techniques are required for certain diseases. For rabies in a dog, the animal should be killed and the head removed and placed in a plastic bag in a container packed with wet ice. For plague, rodents should be captured in a cage-type trap, which should then be sent to the laboratory so as not to lose the rodent's arthropod parasites. Snap traps are not recommended since infected fleas would leave the dead rodent.

A few hints on rodent identification are given in Annex 6.

A5.1.4 Arthropods

Arthropods are best captured and identified by an entomologist. Table A5.5 gives some brief advice on methods of capture; some information on identifying arthropods is given in Annex 6.

Fig. A5.1. Collection of blood (by courtesy of Becton-Dickinson, Vacutainer Systems Europe, Meylan, France)

(a) Use of vacuum blood-collecting tubes.

I. A – evacuated tube
(sterile interior)
B – protected sterile
needle
C – holder

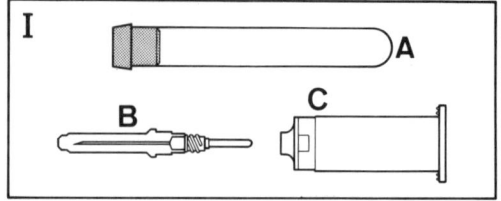

II. Screw protected needle into holder; insert tube into holder, making sure that the needle is slightly embedded in the stopper (the stopper then meets the guideline on the holder).

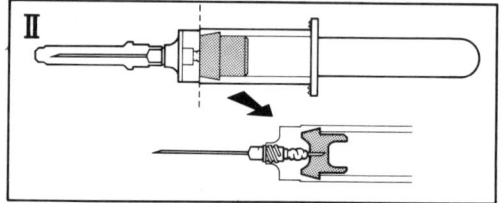

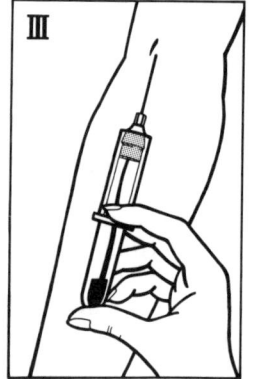

III. When the needle is in the vein, push the tube to insert the needle through the stopper; the blood flows. It is possible to fill several tubes, keeping the needle and holder in place. To obtain drops, hold the tube vertically and tap the bottom of the tube. To transfer serum, insert a second tube as if performing a venepuncture, or remove stopper and collect serum with a syringe or pipette.

(b) Collection of capillary blood from babies under 6 months of age.

IV. Prick the foot where indicated in the diagram.

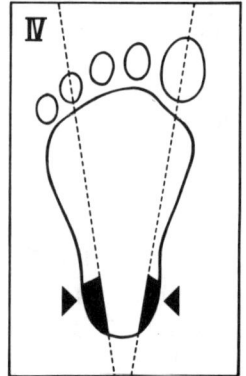

245

Table A5.4. Food-borne diseases: methods of collecting specimens

A. Body products and organs

Type of specimen	Method[a]
Blood	Collect specimens for isolation of agent and serology as for bacteriology (see Table A5.3B)
Vomit	Collect 50–200 g with a sterile spoon; put into a sterile jar
Faeces	Place 2-ml or 2-g (bean-size) portion in two sterile screw-cap bottles, one containing transport medium for bacteria and one for viruses (ask laboratory for special transport medium)
Urine	Collect 50 ml of mid-stream urine, and preserve with a few drops of diluted formalin (40 g/l formaldehyde solution)
Autopsy	Collect the stomach and its contents (tightly bound at both extremities), the liver, kidney, brain; samples of fat may be useful and can be taken with a biopsy needle

[a] The collection of specimens for use in official inquiries may be governed by legal provisions.

B. Food and other materials

Type of specimen	Method
Liquid food	Shake, pour 200 ml into a sterile container, refrigerate but do not freeze
Solid or mixed food	Separate portions with sterile knife, transfer to a sterile glass jar (e.g., jam jar); take samples from periphery to central laboratory; refrigerate
Meat and poultry	Cut portion of meat or skin aseptically from different parts of carcass; alternatively, wipe large portions of carcass with sterile gauze squares or swabs; place in transport medium
Water	See Table A5.6
Other	Collect any fabric, e.g. sheets or towels, known or suspected to contain poison, vomit, urine, faeces

Table A5.5. Capture of arthropods

A. Mosquitos

Stage	Method of capture
Adults	Collection in resting places in houses, with a collecting tube (aspirator) or after knock-down with pyrethrum insecticide spray
	Biting collections on volunteer human "bait"
	Light-trap collections, with or without carbon dioxide
	Animal bait trap collections
	Mosquito-net collections in grassland
Larvae[a]	Collection in breeding places by using dipper in water that has collected in jars, cisterns, refuse (old tyres, bottles, cans), rocks, plant and tree holes, ponds, banks of streams, etc., or in ovitraps (container in which *Aedes* females lay eggs)

[a] The following special density indexes are used for domestic *Aedes aegypti*:
— house index = percentage of houses positive for larvae;
— container index = percentage of water-holding containers positive for larvae;
— Breteau index = number of positive containers per 100 houses.

B. Other arthropods

Arthropod	Method of capture and characteristics
Bedbugs	Inspection of mattresses and corners of bed-frames, cracks in walls
Biting midges (*Culicoides*)	Pests of man and livestock. Great diversity of larval breeding habitats (soil, sandy beaches, low-humus-content or high-organic muck, saltwater beaches, swamps, tidal pools, freshwater bogland, rice fields, pools, small streams, whether polluted or not, edges of larger streams and lakes, crab holes, tree holes, plant axils, decomposing plants). Collection of adults with hand-operated sweep nets, light traps with carbon dioxide
Blackflies (*Simulium*)	Feed on man, domestic and wild animals, birds. Adults 1.5 mm long. Immature stages in slow- to fast-flowing streams, attached to plant axils. Adults fly in swarms. Capture with standard insect net
Fleas	Collect by brushing the animal over a white enamelled basin, probing rodent burrows with a rubber rod covered with white flannel or introducing a "sentinel" mouse attached to a long string. A "sentinel" guinea pig can be released in human dwellings, or a white enamelled tray containing water may be placed on the floor, with a piece of brick in the middle and a lighted candle placed on it
Horse flies	Collect with hand-net

Table A5.5 (*continued*)

Arthropod	Method of capture and characteristics
Houseflies	Collect with sticky fly paper
Sandflies (phlebotomines)	Adults are active from dusk to dawn. During daylight they rest in a variety of well protected sites: tree trunks, animal burrows, tree holes, crevices in walls and in the ground, piles of rocks, animal shelters, forest litter. Light traps and sticky paper are most useful for their capture
Ticks	Worldwide, two families: Argasidae (soft ticks) which feed on multiple hosts (up to 3 at each developmental stage) and Ixodidae (hard ticks) which feed on a single host. Collect parasitic stage on animal skin and free-living stages by dragging a square piece of flannel across the ground
Tsetse flies	In Africa only. Attracted by movement, e.g., by people on foot or on bicycles, or by slowly moving vehicles. Capture with hand-net when they alight

A5.1.5 Environment

Investigations of diseases thought to have originated in the environment should cover:

—sources of water used for drinking and other domestic purposes at the point where contamination may have originated;
—water for recreational or agricultural use;
—facilities for faeces disposal;
—unusual situations, such as large amounts of bird droppings, caves inhabited by bats, contamination of ventilation/air-conditioning systems, etc.

Methods of collecting water samples are shown in Table A5.6. However, the detection of pathogens in water, air, dust and ground samples calls for complicated procedures and sometimes for special devices and is better achieved with the cooperation of a laboratory. Water and other specimens to be sent to the laboratory should preferably be kept at the temperature of wet ice.

A5.2 Shipment of infectious substances

A5.2.1 Packaging

Packaging must comply with national and international safety regulations for the transport of infectious material by air freight, airmail or surface mail; a suitable package fulfilling these requirements is shown in Fig. A5.2. The principle is to provide material that

Fig. A5.2. Packaging for transport of infectious material and diagnostic specimens

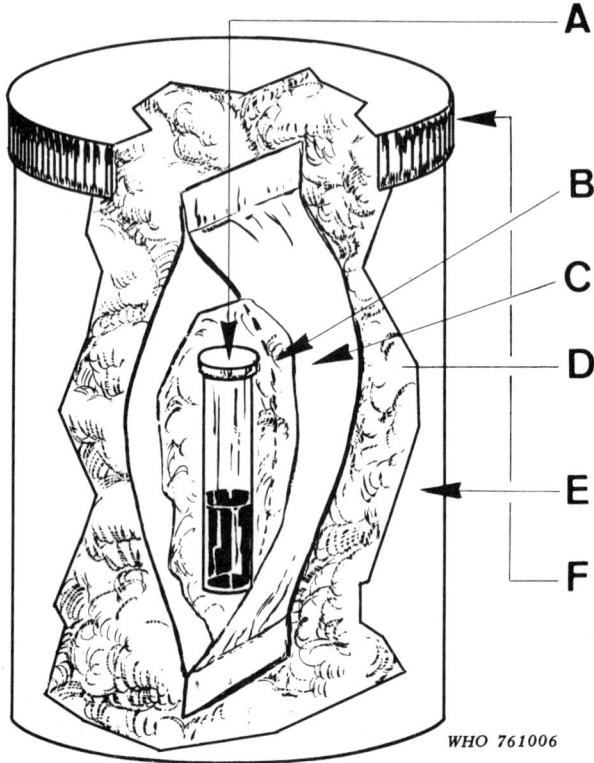

WHO 761006

A: Ampoule containing the specimen: screw-capped vial (illustrated) with a nontoxic rubber liner and *taped shut,* or flame-sealed glass ampoule. } Primary receptacle

B: Absorbent material – e.g., tissue paper or absorbent cotton wool—sufficient to absorb all the specimen should leakage occur.

C: Plastic bag, *heat-sealed or taped over* (not stapled). } Secondary packaging

D: Shock-absorbing padding – e.g., loosely packed paper or absorbent cotton wool.

E: Rigid waterproof outer container.

F: Tight-fitting lid – e.g., screw-on or push-on (paint-can typé) – *taped shut or clipped.* } Outer packaging

Table A5.6. Collection of water samples[a]

Type of water	Method of collection
Tap-water	(1) Disinfect the mouth of the tap with a burning cotton wool swab soaked in 700 ml/litre alcohol (2) Let the water flow for 2 minutes (3) Fill the bottle
Well-water	Weight a sterile bottle with a sterile stone attached with sterile string and dip into well
Open water[b]	Plunge the bottle neck down into the water and then turn it upwards with the mouth facing the current

[a] Water should be collected in sterile bottles (1–5 litres).
[b] Water from springs, streams, rivers and lakes.

will absorb liquids in case of leakage and protect against shocks, as described in Table A5.7.

A special kit is available from WHO for the collection and transport of material suspected of containing varicella, monkeypox or smallpox viruses (see Fig. A5.3).

Table A5.7. Instructions for packaging infectious material

Item	Instructions
Primary container	Use watertight test tube or vial (screw cap fixed with adhesive tape), or flame-sealed ampoule, together with absorptive material
Secondary container	Use watertight container (metal or sealed plastic bag) which may contain several primary containers if there is no risk of shock and breakage
Outer shipping container	Must be waterproof, rigid to resist crushing; use expanded polystyrene to provide adequate thermal insulation (picnic box)
Refrigerant	Place outside secondary container; use dry ice (will leave space after melting) or wet ice in sealed plastic bag (vacuum jars are not recommended as they often break)
Labels	Should include both sender's and receiver's name and carry the special tag for infectious material (see Fig. A5.4)
Letter	Include list of specimens in a sealed plastic bag and mail a duplicate list separately

Fig. A5.3. WHO specimen collection kit used for material suspected of containing varicella, monkeypox or smallpox viruses

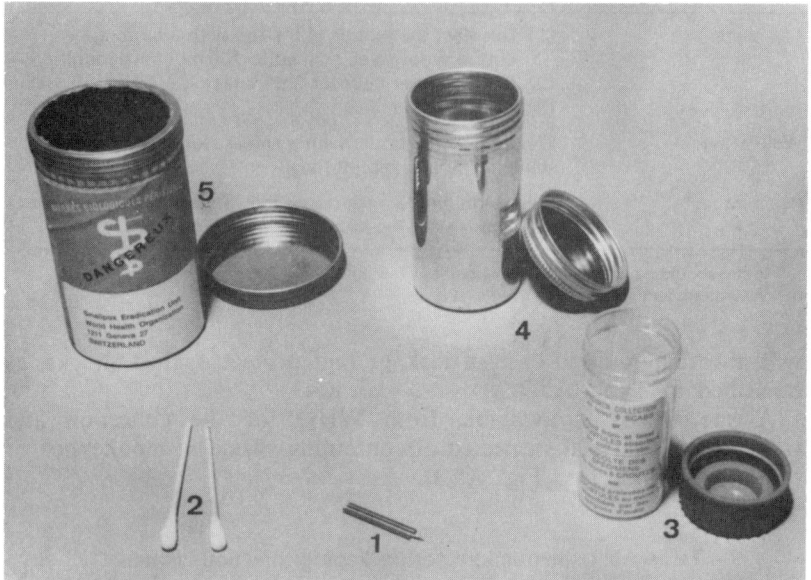

1. Lancet (sterile); 2. Sterile swabs; 3. Plastic specimen collection container; 4. Metal tin; 5. Outer cardboard mailing container.

A5.2.2 Refrigeration

In general, infectious agents should be kept at a low temperature during storage and transport. The types of refrigeration required to achieve various temperatures are as follows:

Temperature (°C)	Type of refrigeration
+ 10	Domestic refrigerator
+ 4	Wet ice or frozen pads (cold dogs)
− 8	Freezer of domestic refrigerator
− 20	Freezer cabinet
− 70	Deep freezer or dry ice
− 163	Liquid nitrogen

Repeated freezing and thawing should be avoided as this rapidly kills all living agents. Some respiratory viruses cannot be kept under cold conditions and special instructions should be sought from the receiving laboratory. Whole blood should not be frozen as this will haemolyse the red blood-cells.

The different methods of refrigeration during shipping have various advantages and disadvantages, as shown in Table A5.8.

Table A5.8. Advantages and disadvantages of refrigeration methods

Refrigeration method	Advantages	Disadvantages
Wet ice	Universally available, re-plenishment easy	Melts rapidly, messy unless in sealed plastic bag
Frozen pads (cold dogs)	Pads are dry	Refrigerate for a short time; freezing the pads takes a long time
Dry ice (solid carbon dioxide)	Material may be kept for several days at $-70\,^{\circ}C$	Gives off carbon dioxide gas which is noxious to some agents (the receptacle used for the specimen must be airtight and space must be left in the package for the carbon dioxide gas produced to evaporate)
Liquid nitrogen	Material may be kept for a long period at $-160\,^{\circ}C$	Special container (open) for transport, not accepted by all airlines

A5.2.3 Air-freight and airmail requirements

A package containing infectious substances must be identified by means of a special label, as shown in Fig. A5.4.

The sender should fill in the form for air-freight or airmail required by the International Air Transport Association (see Fig. A5.5).

Both the sender and the receiver of packages containing infectious material have certain responsibilities. The sender must:

—obtain the agreement of the transport company;
—contact the laboratory by telephone or cable to confirm acceptance and obtain advice on arrangements for shipment and refrigeration;
—obtain an import permit, if required;
—notify the receiver of the transportation data (company, flight, transit point(s), airway bill number, estimated time of arrival);
—avoid sending packages during holiday periods;
—send separately a description of the material concerned;
—ensure that the refrigerant is replenished in transit, if necessary.

Similarly, the receiver must:

—obtain the agreement of the national authorities, if necessary;
—send the import permit;
—arrange for prompt delivery by the transportation company and customs;
—check the acceptability of transit points;
—inform the receptionist, give instructions for cold storage;
—send an acknowledgement of receipt to the sender.

Fig. A5.4. Label for packages containing infectious substances

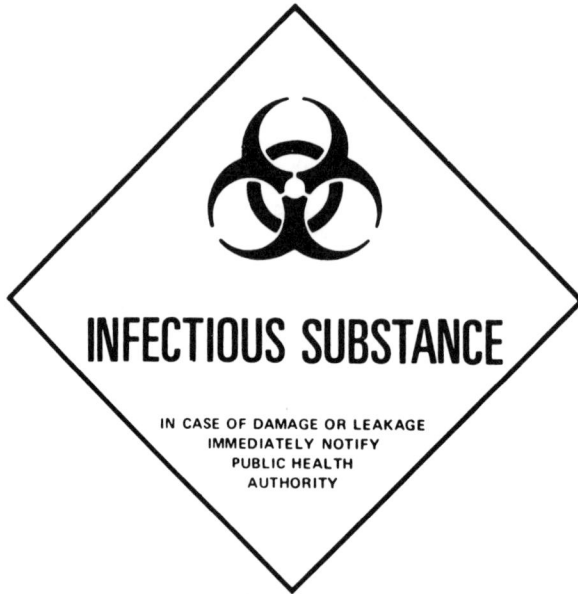

Regulations governing shipments by airmail and air-freight are very strict. Even when these have been complied with, difficulties may be encountered with airlines if the pilot refuses to carry infectious material on a passenger aircraft. WHO can assist with transportation, particularly of highly dangerous materials to be sent to the WHO collaborating centres for special pathogens.

A5.3 Shipment of other materials

A5.3.1 Shipment of specimens collected in connection with food-borne diseases

Refrigeration is necessary to preserve samples from putrefaction; unpreserved samples may undergo chemical changes that may interfere with the identification of the poison. It should be noted that a number of plastics and rubbers contain impurities that may be difficult to distinguish chemically from certain toxic substances; glass receptacles are therefore preferred. However, imperfect specimens are better than none at all.

Specimens should be carefully labelled and should indicate the nature of the material, the weight of the sample, the time and date of collection, the nature of the transport medium, etc. Those suspected to be heavily contaminated should be kept apart from others.

Samples that may be of medicolegal importance must be sealed in the presence of a representative of the law and transported with great care.

Fig. A5.5. Form to be completed for shipment of infectious substances by air

SHIPPER'S DECLARATION FOR DANGEROUS GOODS

Shipper	Air Waybill No
	Page of Pages
	Shipper's Reference Number
	(optional)

| Consignee | |
| | **IATA** |

| Two completed and signed copies of this Declaration must be handed to the operator | WARNING |

| **TRANSPORT DETAILS** | Failure to comply in all respects with the applicable Dangerous Goods Regulations may be in breach of the applicable law, subject to legal penalties. This Declaration must not, in any circumstances, be completed and/or signed by a consolidator, a forwarder or an IATA cargo agent. |

This shipment is within the limitations prescribed for *(delete non-applicable)* | Airport of Departure

| PASSENGER AND CARGO AIRCRAFT | CARGO AIRCRAFT ONLY |

| Airport of Destination | Shipment type *(delete non-applicable)* NON-RADIOACTIVE RADIOACTIVE |

NATURE AND QUANTITY OF DANGEROUS GOODS

Proper Shipping Name, Class, UN Number or Identification Number, number of packages, packing instructions and all other required information as detailed in sub-Section 8 1 of IATA Dangerous Goods Regulations

Additional Handling Information

I hereby declare that the contents of this consignment are fully and accurately described above by proper shipping name and are classified, packed, marked and labelled, and are in all respects in the proper condition for transport by air according to the applicable International and National Government Regulations.	Name/Title of Signatory
	Place and Date
	Signature *(see warning above)*

8

477

A5.3.2 Shipment of arthropods

Arthropods may be shipped in Barraud cages made of muslin and nylon organdie suspended on a wire frame. Cages, which should contain some food (slices of fruit with sugar), should be placed inside insulators containing wet towels. Tin cans provided with a screened hole for ventilation and plaster of Paris as a humidifier may also be used.

BIBLIOGRAPHY

DEPARTMENT OF HEALTH AND SOCIAL SECURITY. *Code of practice for the prevention of infection in clinical laboratories and post-mortem rooms.* London, HMSO, 1978.

GOMPERTS, E. D. ET AL. Handling of highly infectious material in a clinical pathology laboratory and in a viral diagnostic unit. *South African medical journal,* **53**: 243–248 (1978).

Guidelines for biological safety cabinets. Unpublished WHO document, CDS/ SMM/81.21.

Laboratory classification. Unpublished WHO document, CDS/SMM/79.11.

Laboratory safety for arboviruses and certain other viruses of vertebrates. *American journal of tropical medicine and hygiene,* **29**: 1359–1381 (1980).

MADELEY, C. R. *Guide to the collection and transport of virological specimens.* Geneva, World Health Organization, 1977.

Manual for rapid laboratory viral diagnosis. Geneva, World Health Organization, 1979 (WHO Offset Publication, No. 47).

Rapid diagnosis in acute bacterial respiratory infections. Unpublished WHO document, WHO/BAC/ARI/81.5.

VAN DER GROEN, G. ET AL. Negative-pressure flexible film isolator for work with class IV viruses in a maximum security laboratory. *Journal of infection,* **2**: 165–170 (1980).

WHO/CAMR meeting on guidelines for laboratory facilities and containment equipment and isolation facilities for persons infected with dangerous pathogens. Unpublished WHO document, WHO/SMM/80.17.

Identification of arthropod and rodent vectors of communicable diseases and use of insecticides and rodenticides

A6.1 Identification of arthropods and rodents

Determination of the species of arthropod or rodent incriminated in an outbreak is important because the potential for transmission of a disease to man, and hence the control measures required, may vary from species to species, and even locally from biotype to biotype (a biotype is a population within a species, with its own particular behaviour and environment). This determination can be made only by a specialist in entomology or mammalogy. However, a few simple indications may be useful for the epidemiologist so as to enable him to recognize arthropods or rodents that could transmit the agent suspected of causing the outbreak.

A6.1.1 Arthropods

The main arthropod vectors and some of their taxonomic characteristics are indicated in Table A6.1 and Fig. A6.1.

Mosquitos that can transmit diseases to man belong to about a dozen genera, but only certain species of a given genus can transmit specific diseases. Furthermore, the same disease may be transmitted by different mosquito species in different geographical areas. The epidemiologist should at least be able to identify the *Anopheles* and *Culex* genera and, more particularly, to recognize some of the *Aedes* species. The distinctive characteristics that may be used for this purpose are indicated in Fig. A6.2.

Among fleas, the human flea and the oriental rat flea may be distinguished from other species as indicated in Fig. A6.3.

The bionomics and methods of controlling arthropods of medical importance, other than mosquitos, are described in Table A6.2.

Table A6.1. Arthropods of public health importance

A. Class Insecta

Characteristics: 3 pairs of legs; 3 body regions: head, thorax, abdomen; 1 pair of antennae; 1 or 2 pairs of wings (may be rudimentary)

Species	Characteristics
(i) One pair of wings	
Mosquitos[a] Order: Diptera Family: Culicidae	Body length 3–6 mm Scales on wing veins and the posterior margin Elongated proboscis (see Fig. A6.1A)
Sandflies (phlebotomine flies) Order: Diptera Family: Phlebotomidae	Body length 1.5–4 mm Wings are held upward and outward at an angle of about 60° Wings without cross veins beyond the basal third (Fig. A6.1B)
Culicoides (biting midges, punkies) Order: Diptera Family: Ceratopogonidae	Body length 0.6–5 mm Narrow wings Costal vein ending before wing tip Few wing veins Vestiture of wing very sparse (Fig. A6.1C)
Blackflies Order: Diptera Family: Simuliidae	Body length 1–5 mm Variable in colour Antennae short Posterior veins fine (Fig. A6.1D)
Domestic flies Order: Diptera Family: Muscidae	Body length 6–9 mm Wings not covered with scales (Fig. A6.1E)
Tsetse flies Order: Diptera Family: Glossiinidae	Body length 6–11 mm, (Fig. A6.1E)
(ii) Two pairs of wings	
Triatoma (kissing bugs, cone-nosed bugs) Order: Hemiptera Family: Reduviidae	Up to 2 cm in length Elongated body, dorsally flattened Wings not covered with scales Mouthparts consisting of an elongated proboscis directed backward between front legs, adapted for sucking (Fig. A6.1F)
Cockroaches Order: Dictyoptera	12–30 mm in length Possess the power of flight but are typically runners Front wings leathery or paper-like with a network of veins, usually overlapping in the middle, serving as covers for membranous hindwings Mouthparts adapted for biting and chewing (Fig. A6.1G)

Table A6.1 (*continued*)

Species	Characteristics
(iii) Wings absent or rudimentary	
Fleas[b]	1.5–6 mm in length
Order: Siphonaptera	Body strongly flattened from side to side
	Wings absent
	Antennae small, fitting into grooves in head (Fig. A6.1H)
Sucking lice	3–5 mm in length
Order: Phtiraptera	Body strongly flattened from top to bottom
	Wings absent
	Mouthparts retracted into head
	Tarsi having 1 or 2 segments (Fig. A6.1I)
Bedbugs	4–5 mm in length, 3 mm in breadth
Order: Hemiptera	Body flattened horizontally
Suborder: Heteroptera	Wings rudimentary
	Mouthparts consisting of tubular jointed beak (Fig. A6.1J)

[a] For identification of individual species, see Fig. A6.2.
[b] For identification of individual species, see Fig. A6.3.

B. Class Arachnida

Characteristics: 4 pairs of legs in the adult stage; 1 or 2 body regions (sack-like leathery appearance); antennae absent; wings absent

Species	Characteristics
Hard-bodied ticks (Ixodidae)	Up to 20 mm in length
	Terminal capitulum (mouthparts)
	Scutum, plate covering the anterior part of the dorsum (smaller in females)
	Festoons on the posterior part of the dorsum
	Engorged females are bean-like (Fig. A6.1K)
Soft-bodied ticks (Argasidae)	About 8 mm long and 6 mm wide
	Capitulum subterminal, palpi leglike
	Scutum absent
	Festoons absent (Fig. A6.1L)
Mites (Chigger mites)	Adults about 1 mm long, oval or figure-eight shaped
(Trombiculidae)	*Only larvae parasitic* — 0.5 mm in length, difficult to see with the naked eye, feed on vertebrates

Fig. A6.1. Taxonomic characteristics of main arthropod vectors (see also Table A6.1)

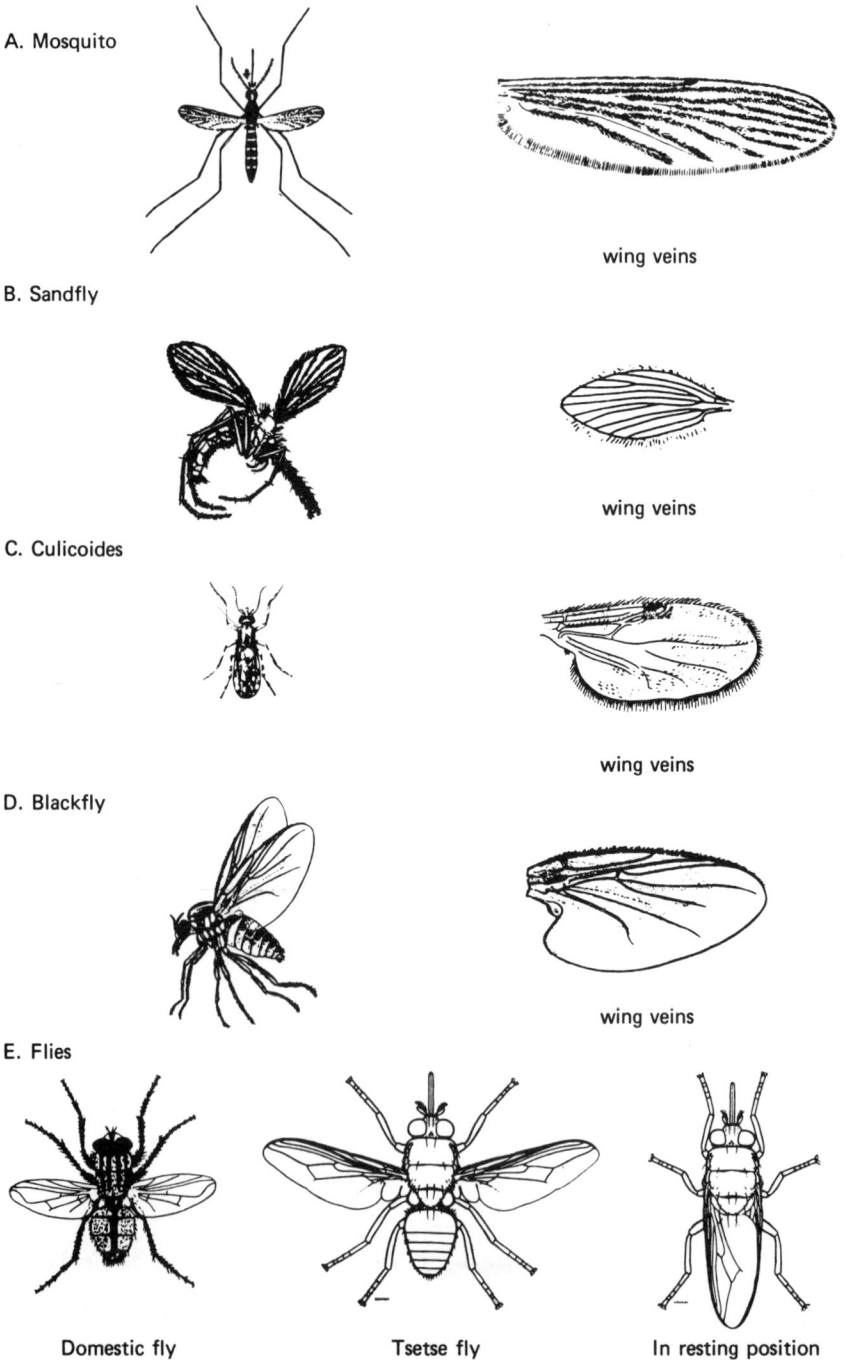

A. Mosquito

wing veins

B. Sandfly

wing veins

C. Culicoides

wing veins

D. Blackfly

wing veins

E. Flies

Domestic fly · Tsetse fly · In resting position

Fig. A6.1 (*continued*)

F. Triatoma

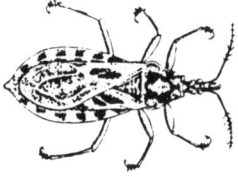

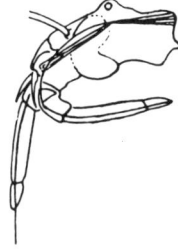

mouthparts

G. Cockroach

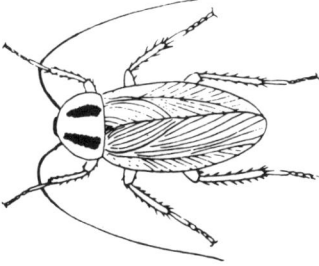

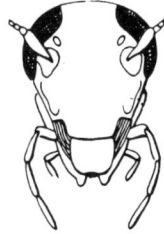

mouthparts

H. Flea   I. Sucking lice

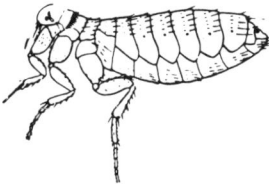   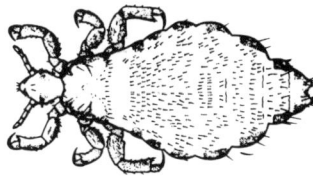

J. Bedbug

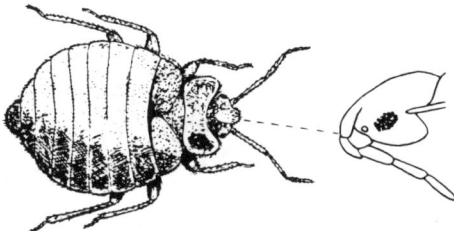

WHO 851252

Fig. A6.1 (*continued*)

K. Hard tick

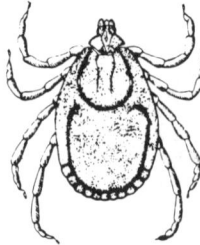

L. Soft tick

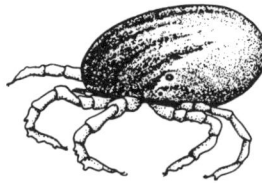

M. Mite

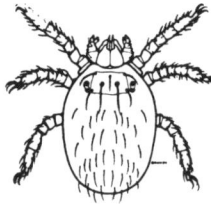

WHO 851253

A6.1.2 Rodents

Several diseases are transmitted by direct contact with certain domestic or wild rodents or by contact with their excreta. Fig. A6.4 shows the characteristics used to identify the most frequently incriminated rodents, namely the roof rat (*Rattus rattus*), the Norway rat (*Rattus norvegicus*), and the house mouse (*Mus musculus*); the field rat *Mastomys natalensis* (the multimammate rat) is a vector of Lassa fever.

In moving from their nest or burrow, rodents tend to use the same routes or "runs" when visiting feeding and drinking sites. Indoors, these runs are often revealed by the presence of black, greasy "smears" along overhead pipes and beams. Outdoor runs may

Fig. A6.2. Distinctive characteristics of *Anopheles, Culex and Aedes aegypti*

Anopheles

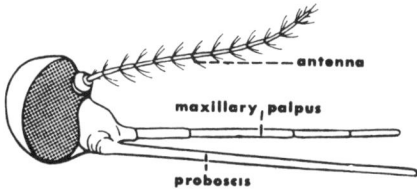

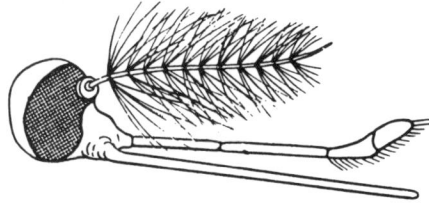

Head of *Anopheles* female

Head of *Anopheles* male

Culex

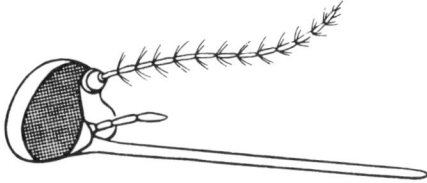

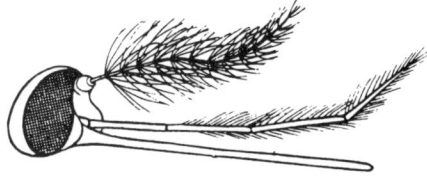

Head of *Culex* female

Head of *Culex* male

Aedes aegypti

Head

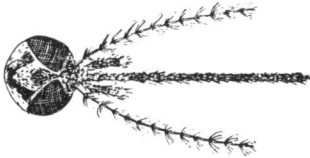

Leg

Thorax

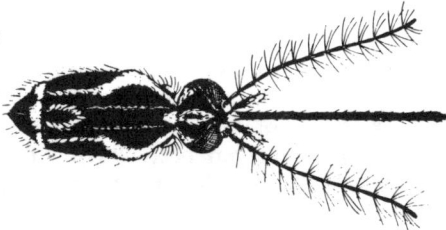

WHO 851254

Fig. A6.3. Distinctive characteristics of human flea and oriental rat flea

A. Heads of human flea and oriental rat flea

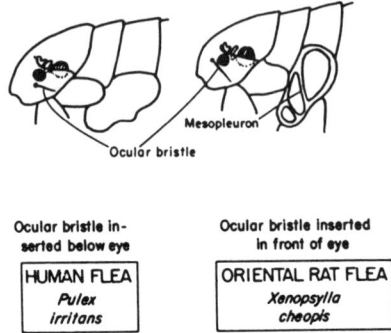

Ocular bristle inserted below eye	Ocular bristle inserted in front of eye
HUMAN FLEA	ORIENTAL RAT FLEA
Pulex irritans	*Xenopsylla cheopis*

B. Heads of other fleas

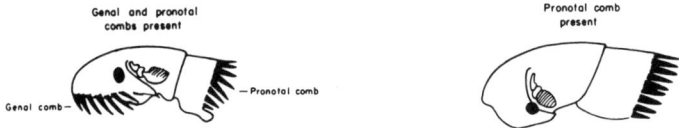

WHO 851255

sometimes be found on open ground, but they are generally seen more clearly on low-growing vegetation, where continual running has worn a path. The presence of rodents may also be detected by their smell and the noises they make. Whereas the roof rat is strictly domestic, the Norway rat may be found both in towns and in burrows in agricultural areas, marshlands and forests, although in warmer climates it tends to be confined to cities.

A6.2 Use of pesticides

As far as possible, in referring to pesticides, names approved by the International Organization for Standardization have been used and listed alphabetically in the various tables; the order does not imply any preference for one compound over another. Similarly, the presence or absence of any given pesticide in no way constitutes a recommendation by the World Health Organization, for or against its use.

Fig. A6.4. Identification of the roof rat, Norway rat and house mouse

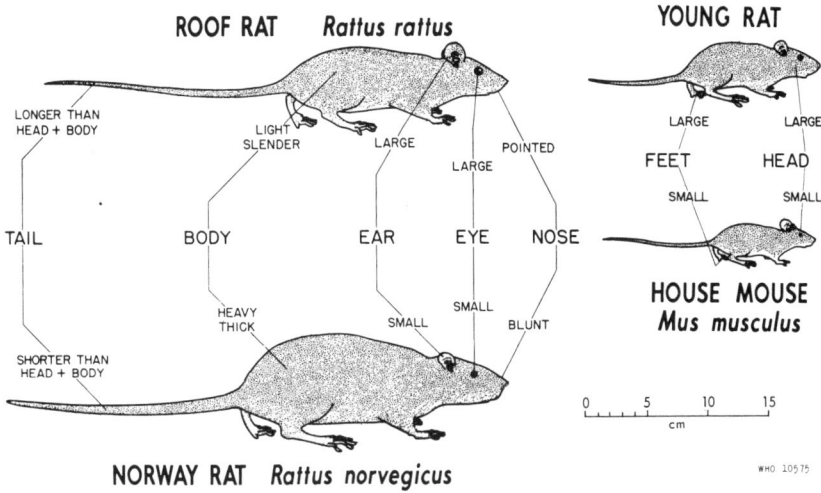

ROOF RAT   *Rattus rattus*

YOUNG RAT

LONGER THAN
HEAD + BODY

LIGHT
SLENDER   LARGE   POINTED

LARGE

LARGE   LARGE

FEET   HEAD

SMALL   SMALL

TAIL   BODY   EAR   EYE   NOSE

HEAVY
THICK   SMALL   SMALL   BLUNT

HOUSE MOUSE
Mus musculus

SHORTER THAN
HEAD + BODY

0   5   10   15
cm

NORWAY RAT   *Rattus norvegicus*

WHO 10575

A6.2.1 Common formulations

Most chemical insecticides have a low solubility in water and require specific formulations for their use.

Technical grade insecticide is the purest form of the product, although it may contain up to 10 % of other products. It may be used either by direct application at ultra-low volume (ULV) dispersion with special equipment, or diluted in different ways.

Solutions can be made with a suitable solvent. Oil solutions remain on the surface of water where mosquito larvae come to breathe, but may damage plants.

Emulsifiable concentrates are prepared by diluting the technical grade insecticide with a suitable organic solvent plus an emulsifier, which makes it possible to mix the concentrate with water to form a stable emulsion suitable for spraying.

Wettable powders consist of an inert substance impregnated with the insecticide and a wetting agent which keeps it in suspension when the mixture is agitated in water. Unlike solutions and emulsions, this suspension is not harmful to plants.

Dusts are fine, inert, solid carrier substances impregnated with insecticide, and applied in a dry form which floats on the surface of water.

Granules are slightly larger (sand-like) particles which sink down into water and release the insecticide progressively.

Baits can be prepared by incorporating the insecticide into a material on which insects like to feed, e.g., peanut granules for ants and cockroaches.

Table A6.2.　Bionomics and control methods for the main arthropods of medical importance other than mosquitos

Arthropod	Bionomics and control methods
Bedbugs	Adults hide in crevices of walls or in beds during the day, and bite man during the night. They are able to endure long fasts. Although they have sometimes been suspected of transmitting disease, they have not yet been demonstrated to be natural vectors of human disease. Eliminated by spraying or dusting insecticides into cracks and crevices where they hide during the day.
Blackflies	Adults of the genus *Simulium* occur in swarms near water and the bite of the females is painful. Immature stages are aquatic and live in fast-running water. Adults are active during the day, and transmit onchocerciasis (river blindness) to man in warm climates in Africa and the Americas. Treatment is directed against aquatic larvae in streams, either by the drip method or by using plaster blocks impregnated with DDT, but can damage aquatic fauna. Temephos has also been shown to be effective.
Cockroaches	Closely associated with man and play the same vectorial role as flies. They occur mainly in food-handling areas but also feed on any organic matter, such as fabrics, starchy book binding, excrement and sputum. Food-storage areas should be treated with insecticides. The organophosphorus compounds and carbamates are generally effective for shorter periods than are chlordane and dieldrin. Resistance to insecticides has been encountered. Care must be taken to avoid the contamination of food with insecticides offered as bait or applied as residual sprays or dusts inside and behind furniture, and where pipes pass through walls or floors. Food should be stored in tight or screened containers and all kitchen scraps eliminated.
Culicoides	"Biting midges" (females) suck the blood of man and vertebrate animals during the evenings in warm climates. They are able to pass through the fine mesh of ordinary window screens or bed-nets and transmit arboviruses and filarial worms. They may be controlled by fogging as for mosquitos but this has only a transient effect. Window screens and bed-netting can be treated with DDT.
Fleas	Bubonic plague and murine typhus are transmitted by fleas which are parasites of rats. Control is effected by application of DDT powder (50–100 g/kg, 5–10%) to rodent burrows, runs, living areas of commensal rats and burrows of field rats. Where DDT resistance has developed, organophosphorus compounds should be used. Control measures against fleas must precede rodent control, otherwise the fleas will leave dead rats and bite man more actively.
Flies	Domestic flies breed in any accumulation of moist organic matter, e.g., human and animal excreta, animal carcasses, etc. They are vectors of a number of pathogenic bacterial, viral, and parasitic agents excreted in animal and human faeces. Chemical control procedures include the appli-

Table A6.2 (*continued*)

Arthropod	Bionomics and control methods
	cation of residual insecticides to surfaces in and around houses and animal shelters, and the placing of poisoned bait around farms and food-handling establishments; space sprays should be directed towards exterior sites, such as alleys, refuse dumps, cargo-storage areas and food-handling establishments. Resistance to DDT has been found.
Lice	Body lice are vectors of rickettsiae causing typhus fever and of spirochaetes causing epidemic relapsing fever. The eggs of the body louse are attached to fibres of the under-clothing, and hatch in about a week, the nymphs developing to the adult stage in about 18 days. Clothing and bedding require treatment. Insecticide powder should be applied evenly over the inner surface of the underwear. Resistance to DDT may occur. Pyrethrins may be applied as a 10 g/kg dusting powder but a second application is necessary after 8 days when eggs have hatched.
Mites	Vectors of typhus fever due to *Rickettsia tsutsugamushi.* Control measures consist of the application of residual acaricides, such as dieldrin or lindane, in woodland or bush-land where infestations occur. Individual protection can be achieved by using clothing impregnated with acaricides (benzyl benzoate) in conjunction with application of repellents. Burning of undergrowth surrounding villages and camps, or the use of defoliants and herbicides may be indicated.
Reduviids (triatomid bugs)	Found in warm areas of North and South America. They are active at night and spend the daylight hours in shelters such as crevices of walls and wood piles. They transmit American trypanosomiasis. Screening houses is the best method of protection. Treatment of dwellings with residual insecticides, such as HCH, which is inexpensive, has produced a marked reduction of infestation by these bugs.
Sandflies (phlebotomine flies)	Transmit visceral and cutaneous leishmaniasis and sandfly fever to man. Insecticides are difficult to apply in jungle or forest environments, but should be used in temporary camps. Clearing away bush around villages and camps is indicated. Individual protection can be achieved by applying repellents on exposed parts of the body, especially after sunset. Application of residual insecticides, such as DDT, in and around dwellings, during malaria control campaigns, has given excellent results against sandflies. Spraying should be carried out in places where the vector breeds, such as animal shelters, rock faces, refuse dumps, cracks in walls, and on vegetation and other surfaces where they make frequent stops.
Ticks	Reservoirs and vectors of several bacterial, rickettsial and viral diseases, mainly endemic relapsing fever, Q fever, tularaemia, spotted fevers (boutonneuse fever and Rocky Mountain spotted fever) and several arboviral infections. The numerous tick species have a complicated development cycle in the ground or on vertebrate hosts and can

Table A6.2 (*continued*)

Arthropod	Bionomics and control methods
	bite man and reservoir animals in either the larval or adult stages, or both. Accordingly, protection is mainly individual, by the use of special protective clothing and repellents in tick-infested areas.
Tsetse flies	Vectors of African trypanosomiasis. Control is difficult as it requires clearance of undergrowth along the banks of rivers and lakes (the flies' habitat) and reducing the fly population by application of insecticides.

The appropriate dilution to be used must be adjusted for each individual case and a specialist will have to be called upon to determine the optimum concentration of insecticide to be used. Information for use in preparing dilutions is given in Table A6.3.

A6.2.2 Spraying equipment

A number of different types of spraying equipment are available. *Space-spraying equipment* includes:

—thermal foggers (portable or vehicle-mounted), which deliver a powerful blast of visible fog and are useful in areas of dense vegetation;

—mist blowers (portable, vehicle- or aircraft-mounted), which deliver relatively large droplets in the form of a cold mist and are suitable for use around houses and for treating large areas; they can be used both for adult vector control and for larvicidal applications;

—aerosol applicators (portable, vehicle- or aircraft-mounted), which deliver very fine droplets of ULV insecticide concentrate; these remain suspended in the air and kill flying insects. They are suitable for use around and inside houses. As low volumes of insecticides are used, they are relatively cost-effective for treating large areas from the air.

Hand-operated compression sprayers include the ubiquitous "spray pump" used for residual treatment of houses, mainly against malaria vectors, and for larviciding. In general, fan-shaped nozzles are used for residual spraying and cone-nozzles for larviciding.

Dusting equipment exists in various forms, either manual or power-operated, for application of pesticide dust formulations, and is widely used for mosquito control.

Details of specifications for different types of spraying equipment, their modes of action and use in the field, are given in the WHO publication *Equipment for vector control*, copies of which should be

Table A6.3. Preparation of dilutions of insecticides

A. Preparation of emulsifiable concentrates from technical material

Concentration desired (%)	Weight of technical material required to make the given volumes of concentrate: [a]		
	100 litres	100 gal (US)	100 gal (UK)
35	35 kg	292 lb	350 lb
25	25 kg	208 lb	250 lb
15	15 kg	125 lb	150 lb
12.5	12.5 kg	104 lb	125 lb
6.25	6.25 kg	52 lb	62.5 lb

[a] Two parts of emulsifier should be added to every 100 parts of concentrate.

B. Preparation of emulsions from emulsifiable concentrates of different strengths

Percentage of a.i.[a] in emulsifiable concentrate	Parts of water to be added to 1 part of EC[b] for given final concentration				
	5%	2.5%	1%	0.5%	0.25%
80	15	31	79	159	319
60	11	23	50	119	239
50	9	19	49	99	199
25	4	9	24	49	99
10	1	3	9	19	39

[a] a.i. = active ingredient.
[b] EC = emulsifiable concentrate.

C. Amount of spray formulation required to give specific weights of active ingredient per unit area

Dosage		Litres[a] of spray required per 100 m² (1000 ft²) using given concentrations of technical insecticide				
g/m²	mg/ft²	0.25%	0.5%	1.0%	2.5%	5.0%
2	200	—	—	20	8	4
1	100	—	20	10	4	2
0.5	50	20	10	5	2	1
0.2	20	8	4	2	0.8	0.4

[a] 1 litre is approximately equal to 0.25 gal(US) or 0.2 gal(UK).

Table A6.3 (*continued*)

D. Amount of emulsifiable concentrate or dust required per unit area to give specific weights of active ingredient

Dosage		Amount of 25% concentrate[a] required		Amount of 5% dust[b] required	
kg/ha	lb/acre			kg	lb
4.54	10	18.2 litres	4.8 gal (US) 4.0 gal (UK)	90.8	200
2.27	5	9.1 litres	2.4 gal (US) 2.0 gal (UK)	45.4	100
1.36	3	5.5 litres	1.4 gal (US) 1.2 gal (UK)	27.2	60
1.0	2.2	4.2 litres	1.1 gal (US) 0.9 gal (UK)	20.0	44
0.45	1	1.8 litres	1.9 qt (US) 1.6 qt (UK)	9.1	20
0.23	0.5	900 ml	1.9 pint (US) 1.6 pint (UK)	4.5	10
0.045	0.1	200 ml	6.1 fl oz (US) 6.4 fl oz (UK)	–	–

[a] Containing 0.25 kg/litre (2.1 lb/ gal (US); 2.5 lb/ gal (UK)).
[b] Containing 50 g of active ingredient per kg.

E. Dilution factors for 25% concentrate

Required concentration (mg/l) (ppm)	Volume of 25% concentrate[a] needed for the given volumes of water		
	1 million litres of water	1 million gal(US) of water	1 million gal(UK) of water
1	4 litres	4 gal(US)	4 gal(UK)
0.1	400 ml	3.2 pint(US)	3.2 pint(UK)
0.01	40 ml	5.1 fl oz(US)	6.5 fl oz(UK)
0.001	4 ml	0.5 fl oz(US)	0.6 fl oz(UK)

[a] Containing 0.25 kg/litre (2.1 lb/gal(US); 2.5 lb/gal(UK)).

F. Concentrations of active ingredient equivalent to one part per million

1 part per million (ppm)	= 1 mg (0.015 grain) per kg
	= 1 g (15.4 grain) per tonne
	= 0.007 grain (0.45 mg) per lb
	= 1 ml (0.035 fl oz (UK)) per 100 litres
	= 0.16 fl oz(UK) (4.5 ml) per 1000 gal (UK)
	= 0.13 fl oz(US) (3.8 ml) per 1000 gal (US)

available at the government or regional office responsible for coordination of vector control measures in emergency situations. Information on supplies of spraying equipment can also be obtained from WHO and should be kept at hand. In addition, it is recommended that at least one manual of spare parts should be available for each type of spraying equipment in store to facilitate rapid identification and supply of spare parts.

A6.2.3 Mosquito control operations

Chemical insecticides are used in emergencies to control mosquito vectors of epidemic diseases, and can rapidly reduce the density of the adult vector population and thus quickly stop, or drastically reduce, transmission. A quick-acting formulation, applied for a short period to cover the epidemic or epizootic area, is required. Space sprays are ideal for this purpose because the flying vectors collide with the insecticide droplets suspended in the air. Two or three such applications, separated by intervals of a few days, quickly interrupt transmission and can therefore halt an epidemic. Indoor application of residual contact insecticides against endophilic vectors and larvicidal applications may take several days or weeks if a large area has to be treated.

(a) Space-spraying operations. These are appropriate for the following situations:

—in emergencies, as already mentioned, to produce rapid reduction in vector densities;
—when the vector is exophilic and/or exophagic, so that indoor residual spraying is not cost-effective;
—when there is an immature mosquito population in inaccessible or widely dispersed habitats;
—when highly built-up urban areas are involved, so that residual or larval applications are operationally complicated and therefore costly;
—when they are economical compared with other methods of vector control that require larger labour forces.

The forms of space-spray generally used are:

(i) *Thermal fogs*, produced by special equipment in which the insecticide, usually dissolved in an oil with a suitably high flash-point, is vaporized by being injected into a high-velocity stream of hot gas. When discharged into the atmosphere, the oil carrying the pesticide condenses in the form of a fog. In thermal-fogging operations, 4–5% malathion in diesel oil is generally the insecticide and concentration of choice, applied at a target dosage rate of 430 ml/ha;

(ii) *ULV aerosols (cold fogs) and mists*, i.e., the application of the minimum quantity of concentrated liquid insecticide that will provide efficient control of the target arthropod vector. Although not precisely defined, the use of less than 4.6 litres/ha (0.5 gal(US) per acre) of an insecticide concentrate is considered as a ULV application.

During an emergency, the rapid application of adulticides would appear to be the ideal measure. Although ground application of insecticide aerosols or thermal fogs at the recommended dosage rates should be considered, aerial spraying might be appropriate if the area to be treated is large. Two applications at an interval of 3–5 days (in view of the incubation period of the virus in the mosquito) would be more effective. Several types of portable and vehicle-mounted thermal-fogging equipment are available. Details of suitable equipment and insecticides are available from the Division of Vector Biology and Control, World Health Organization, 1211 Geneva 27, Switzerland.

The following estimates have been made of the average coverage per day with certain aerosol and thermal-fog producers, from both the ground and the air:

Twin-engined aircraft or large helicopter	6000 ha
Light fixed-wing aircraft or small helicopter	2000 ha
Vehicle-mounted cold-fog generator	225 ha
Vehicle-mounted thermal fogger	150 ha
Back-pack mist blower	30 ha
Hand-carried thermal fogger	5 ha

Applications from the ground using portable equipment. When the area to be treated is not very large, or in areas where vehicle-mounted equipment cannot be used, portable back-pack equipment can be used to apply insecticidal mists. One operator may be able to treat up to 100–150 premises per day, but the weight of the machines and the vibrations caused by the engine make it necessary to allow the operators to rest, so that 2–3 operators are needed per machine. For speedy and extensive coverage, area treatment (rather than house or room treatment) is essential. Several types of portable ULV equipment are available, and a list can be obtained on request from the Division of Vector Biology and Control, World Health Organization, 1211 Geneva 27, Switzerland.

Applications from the ground using vehicle-mounted equipment. Vehicle-mounted aerosol generators are very useful in urban or suburban areas with a good road system because of their sturdiness, reliability and ability to cover large areas; one machine can cover up to 1500–2000 houses per day. It is necessary to calibrate the equipment, vehicle speed and swath width to determine the coverage obtained by a single pass. A good map of the area showing all the roads, houses, etc., is of great help in carrying out operations. A great deal of health education may be required to persuade the inhabitants to cooperate by having their windows and doors open and by not obstructing the vehicles carrying out these treatments.

A wide range of vehicle-mounted ULV equipment is available, details of which may be obtained on request from the Division of Vector Biology and Control, World Health Organization, 1211 Geneva 27, Switzerland.

Aerial application. This is often the method of choice in emergency situations when an extensive area must be treated in a short time. Although the equipment used (aircraft equipped with a spray system) may have a high initial cost, this form of application may be cost-effective since very large areas can be treated.

Insecticides for use against mosquitos. Insecticides that may be used in ULV applications against mosquitos are shown in Table A6.4 together with the approximate dosages recommended.

Table A6.4. Insecticide formulations and dosages for use in control of adult mosquitos

Insecticide	Formulation	Approximate dosage
Bioresmethrin	20% ULV concentrate	10 g of active ingredient per ha
Chlorpyrifos	24% active ingredient ULV concentrate	430 ml/ha
Fenitrothion	95% active ingredient	500 ml/ha
Fenthion	100 g/litre	70 ml/ha
Jodfenphos	20% ULV concentrate	1.5–3.0 litres/ha
Malathion	96% active ingredient	220–430 ml/ha
Naled	Technical ULV concentrate	70 ml/ha
Propoxur	ULV concentrate	53 g of active ingredient per ha

(b) Residual contact insecticides. In areas where epidemiological surveillance indicates that an outbreak is likely to occur via house-resting species, the vector population should be reduced by applying a residual insecticide in the form of a water-dispersible powder formulation or as an emulsion, at 1–2 g of active ingredient per m^2, to the interior of buildings used as resting places. This should be done before the period at which it is predicted that outbreaks are likely to occur. The susceptibility of the adult vector to the candidate insecticide should be assessed beforehand. Malathion, as a water-dispersible powder or emulsion, may be suitable in certain areas but alternative insecticides, such as fenitrothion, will be required where resistance to malathion occurs. The choice of an alternative compound should be based on a number of factors including cost, availability, and possible adverse effects, e.g., toxicity to birds and animals. Insecticides that should be considered for use as residual sprays are indicated in Table A6.5. The most frequently used type of spraying equipment is the hand-operated compression sprayer, which should conform to the WHO specification (see unpublished document WHO/EQP/1.R3).

Table A6.5. Insecticides suitable for use in residual spray applications for control of mosquitos

Insecticide	Chemical type[a]	Dosage of a.i.[b] (g/m²)	Duration of effective action (months)	Insecticidal action	Toxicity:[c] oral LD$_{50}$ of a.i.[b] to rats (mg/kg of body weight)
Bendiocarb	C	0.4	2–3	Contact and airborne	55
Chlorphoxim	OP	2	1–3	Contact	500[d]
Cypermethrin	PY	0.5	4 or more	Contact	>4 000[e]
DDT	OC	1–2	6 or more	Contact	113
Deltamethrin	PY	0.05	2–3	Contact	>2 940[e]
Fenitrothion	OP	1–2	3 or more	Contact and airborne	503
Lindane (gamma-HCH)	OC	0.2–0.5	3 or more	Contact and airborne	100
Malathion	OP	1–2	2–3	Contact	2 100
Permethrin	PY	0.5	2–3	Contact	>4 000[e]
Pirimiphos-methyl	OP	1–2	2–3 or more	Contact and airborne	2 018
Propoxur	C	1–2	2–3	Contact and airborne	95

[a] OC = organochlorine compound; OP = organophosphorus compound; C = carbamate; PY = synthetic pyrethroid.
[b] a.i. = active ingredient.
[c] Toxicity and hazard are not necessarily equivalent.
[d] Dermal toxicity.
[e] Dermal toxicity. Because this is low, and on the basis of experience with its use, the product has been included in the WHO Hazard Classification in Class III, Table 5 (products unlikely to present acute hazards in normal use).

(c) Larviciding operations. Larviciding operations must be directed against *all* breeding sites, so that thorough preparations and studies are necessary before such operations. Subject to the results of insecticide-susceptibility tests, larvicides suitable for use in polluted water include chlorpyrifos at 11–16 g of active ingredient per ha, the high dosage being applied to the most heavily polluted waters. Temephos, at 56–112 g of active ingredient per ha, should be reserved for use in water that may be consumed by animals and/or man, as it is less effective than chlorpyrifos in polluted water. Where *Aedes aegypti* is found to be breeding extensively in domestic stored water, temephos 1 % sand granules, applied at 1 mg/litre, have been found to be effective for 8–12 weeks.

Insecticides that should be considered for use as larvicides are indicated in Table A6.6. Various types of spraying equipment are used for larviciding operations, e.g., compression sprayers, dusters, and granule-applicators. Aircraft application of larvicides is also possible, using boom and nozzle, or ULV equipment. Details of insecticides and equipment for larval control operations have been published by WHO (see Bibliography, page 280).

Table A6.6 Insecticides suitable for use as larvicides in mosquito control

Insecticide	Chemical type[a]	Dosage of a.i.[b] (g/ha)	Formulation[c]	Duration of effective action (weeks)	Toxicity:[d] oral LD$_{50}$ of a.i.[b] to rats (mg/kg of body weight)
Chlorphoxim	OP	100	EC	2–7	500[e]
Chlorpyrifos	OP	11–25	EC, GR, WP	3–17	135
Deltamethrin	PY	2.5–10[f]	EC	1–3	>2 940[g]
Diflubenzuron[h]	—	25–100	GR, WP	1–4	4 640
Fenitrothion	OP	100–1000	EC, GR	1–3	503
Fenthion	OP	22–112	EC, GR	2–11	330[e]
Fuel oil	—	[i]	Solution	1–2	Negligible
Jodfenphos	OP	50–100	EC, GR	7–16	2 100
Larvicidal oil	—	[j]	Solution	1–2	Negligible
Malathion	OP	224–1000	EC, GR	1–2	2 100
Methoprene[h]	—	100–1000	SRS	4–8	34 600
Paris green[k]	—	840–1000	Dust, solution in oil	2	22
Permethrin	PY	5–10[f]	EC	5–10	>4 000[g]
Phoxim	OP	100	EC	1–6	1 000
Pirimiphos-methyl	OP	50–500	EC	1–11	2 018
Temephos	OP	56–112	EC, GR	2–4	8 600

[a] OP = organophosphorus compound; PY = synthetic pyrethroid.
[b] a.i. = active ingredient.
[c] EC = emulsifiable concentrate; GR = granular formulation; WP = water-dispersible powder; SRS = slow-release suspension.
[d] Toxicity and hazard are not necessarily equivalent.
[e] Dermal toxicity.
[f] The lower levels are recommended for use in fish-bearing waters.
[g] Dermal toxicity. Because this is low, and on the basis of experience with its use, the product has been included in the WHO Hazard Classification in Class III, Table 5 (products unlikely to present acute hazards in normal use).
[h] Insect growth regulator.
[i] Apply at 142–190 1/ha, or 19–47 1/ha if spreading agent added.
[j] Apply at 19–47 1/ha.
[k] Copper–arsenic complex.

A6.2.4 Control of other arthropods of medical importance

To be effective, control measures must be adapted to the bionomics of the vector species incriminated. A few hints with regard to certain species are given in Table A6.2; textbooks of medical entomology should be consulted if further information is required. Insecticide formulations for use against flies are shown in Table A6.7, for fleas in Table A6.8, for cockroaches in Table A6.9 and for human lice in Table A6.10.

A6.2.5 Poisoning by insecticides

Organophosphorus, carbamate and organochlorine insecticides may be toxic to man, so that inhalation, ingestion and contamination of

Table A6.7. Insecticides for use against flies

Insecticide	Chemical type[a]	Concentration of formulation (%) as applied	Dosage of a.i.[b] (g/m²)	Toxicity[c] oral LD_{50} of a.i.[b] to rats (mg/kg of body weight)	Remarks
Azamethiphos	OP	1.0–5.0	1.0–2.0	750	Can also be used in dairies, restaurants and food stores
Bromophos	OP	1.0–5.0	1.0–2.0	1 600	
Cypermethrin	PY	0.25–1.0	0.025–0.1	>4 000[d]	
Deltamethrin	PY	0.015–0.030	0.0075–0.15	>2 940[d]	
Diazinon	OP	1.0–2.0	0.4–0.8	300	
Fenchlorphos	OP	1.0–5.0	1.0–2.0	1 740	
Fenitrothion	OP	1.0–5.0	1.0–2.0	503	
Jodfenphos	OP	1.0–5.0	1.0–2.0	2 100	
Permethrin	PY	0.0625–0.125	0.025–0.05	>4 000[d]	
Pirimiphos-methyl	OP	1.25–2.5	1.0–2.0	2 018	
Dimethoate	OP	1.0–2.5	0.046–0.5	150	Animals must be removed during treatment. Not to be used in dairies
Fenvalerate	PY	1.0–5.0	1.0	300	
Malathion	OP	5.0	1.0–2.0	2 100	Only premium-grade malathion can be used in dairies and food-processing plants
Naled	OP	1.0	0.4–0.8	430	Not to be used in dairies. At 0.25% strength can be applied to chicken roosts, nests, etc., without removing the birds
Bendiocarb	C	0.24–0.48	0.1–0.2	55	Animals must be removed during treatment
Propetamphos[e]	OP	1.0–2.0	0.25–1.0	75	—

[a] OP = organophosphorus compound; PY = synthetic pyrethroid; C = carbamate.
[b] a.i. = active ingredient.
[c] Toxicity and hazard are not necessarily equivalent.
[d] Dermal toxicity. Because this is low, and on the basis of experience with its use, the product has been included in the WHO Hazard Classification in Class III, Table 5 (products unlikely to present acute hazards in normal use).
[e] If applied by non-commercial operators, it should be supplied, for safety reasons, in a diluted form containing not more than 5% of the active ingredient.

Table A6.8. Insecticides for use on pets for flea control

Insecticide	Chemical type[a]	Formulation	Concentration (%)	Toxicity:[b] oral LD$_{50}$ of a.i.[c] to rats: (mg/kg of body weight)
Carbaryl	C	Dip or wash	0.5	
		Dust[d]	2.0–5.0	300
Coumaphos[e]	OP	Dip	0.2–0.5	16
		Dust[f]	0.5	16
Deltamethrin	PY	Spray or shampoo	0.0025	>2 940[g]
Jodfenphos	OP	Dip	0.5	2 100
Lindane[e]	OC	Dust	1.0	100
Malathion	OP	Dip	0.25	
		Dust	5.0	
		Spray	0.5	2 000
Natural pyrethrins + synergist		Dust, spray or shampoo	0.2 + 2.0	200–2 600
Permethrin	PY	Dust	1.0	>4 000[g]
		Spray or shampoo	1.0	
		Wash	0.1	
Propetamphos	OP	Collar	10.0	75
Propoxur	C	Spray	1.0	95
		Dust	1.0	
Rotenone[h]		Dust	1.0	132–1 500

[a] OC = organochlorine compound; OP = organophosphorus compound; C = carbamate; PY = synthetic pyrethroid.
[b] Toxicity and hazard are not necessarily equivalent.
[c] a.i. = active ingredient.
[d] Do not use on cats under 4 weeks old.
[e] Do not use on dogs under 2 months old or on cats.
[f] Also contains 1% trichlorfon.
[g] Dermal toxicity. Because this is low, and on the basis of experience with its use, the product has been included in the WHO Hazard Classification in Class III, Table 5 (products unlikely to present acute hazards in normal use).
[h] Extract of derris root.

the skin should be avoided. For some pesticides, skin absorption is a more important route of entry than inhalation. Protective clothing can be worn but is passive protection and should be regarded as secondary to the use of safe working methods. Substantial protection against pesticide sprays is afforded by ordinary clothing and headgear. A set of working clothes that is changed at the end of the working day and is washed sufficiently frequently to prevent it from becoming grossly soiled with spray deposit will effectively limit exposure during almost all pesticide applications.

In an emergency resulting from exposure to a toxic insecticide, successful treatment depends on the rapid and simultaneous application of measures for:

(1) alleviation of life-threatening effects;
(2) removal of non-absorbed material; and

Table A6.9. Insecticides commonly employed in control of cockroaches

Insecticide	Chemical type[a]	Formulation	Concentration (%)	Toxicity[b] oral LD$_{50}$ of a.i.[c] to rats (mg/kg of body weight)
Bendiocarb	C	Spray	0.24–0.48	55
		Dust	1.0	
		Aerosol	0.75	
Chlorpyrifos	OP	Spray	0.5	135
Deltamethrin	PY	Spray	0.0075	>2 940[d]
		Dust	0.0005	
		Aerosol	0.02	
Diazinon	OP	Spray	0.5	300–850
		Dust	2.0	
Dichlorvos	OP	Spray	0.5	56
		Bait	1.9	
Dioxacarb	C	Spray	0.5–1.0	90
Jodfenphos	OP	Spray	1.0	2 100
Malathion	OP	Spray	3.0	2 100
		Dust	5.0	
Permethrin	PY	Spray	0.125–0.25	>4 000[d]
		Dust	0.5	
Pirimiphos-methyl	OP	Spray	2.5	2 018
		Dust	2.0	
Propetamphos[e]	OP	Spray	0.5–1.0	75
		Dust	2.0	
		Aerosol	2.0	
Propoxur	C	Spray	1.0	95
		Bait	2.0	

[a] OP = organophosphorus compound; C = carbamate; PY = synthetic pyrethroid.
[b] Toxicity and hazard are not necessarily equivalent.
[c] a.i. = active ingredient.
[d] Dermal toxicity. Because this is low, and on the basis of experience with its use, the product has been included in the WHO Hazard Classification in Class III, Table 5 (products unlikely to present acute hazards in normal use).
[e] If applied by non-commercial operators it should be supplied, for safety reasons, in a diluted form containing not more than 5% active ingredient.

(3) symptomatic treatment and the administration of antidotes if these exist.

It may also be necessary to take samples of the insecticide, if its nature is not known.

Alleviation of life-threatening effects. For the removal of secretions and maintenance of a patent airway, the patient should be placed in a prone position with head down and to one side, the mandible extended, and the tongue pulled forward. The mouth and pharynx should be cleared with a cloth or by suction, and an oropharyngeal or nasopharyngeal airway or endotracheal intubation used if airway obstruction persists. Artificial ventilation should be applied if required. Mouth-to-mouth respiration is to be avoided when it is suspected

Table A6.10. Insecticides commonly employed in control of human lice

Insecticide	Chemical type[a]	Formulation	Concentration (%)	Toxicity[b] oral LD_{50} of a.i.[c] to rats (mg/kg of body weight)
Bioallethrin	PY	Lotion	0.3–0.4	500
		Shampoo	0.3–0.4	
		Aerosol	0.6	
Carbaryl	C	Dust	5.0	300
DDT	OC	Dust	10.0	113
		Lotion	2.0	
Deltamethrin	PY	Lotion	0.03	>2 940[d]
		Shampoo	0.03	
Jodfenphos	OP	Dust	5.0	2 100
Lindane	OC	Dust	1.0	100
		Lotion	1.0	
Malathion	OP	Dust	1.0	2 100
		Lotion	0.5	
Permethrin	PY	Dust	0.5	>4 000[d]
		Lotion	1.0	
		Shampoo	1.0	
Propoxur	C	Dust	1.0	95
Temephos	OP	Dust	2.0	8 600

[a] OC = organochlorine compound; OP = organophosphorus compound; C = carbamate; PY = synthetic pyrethroid.
[b] Toxicity and hazard are not necessarily equivalent.
[c] a.i. = active ingredient.
[d] Dermal toxicity. Because this is low, and on the basis of experience with its use, the product has been included in the WHO Hazard Classification in Class III, Table 5 (products unlikely to present acute hazards in normal use).

that the patient has been intoxicated by mouth, because vomited material may contain dangerous amounts of toxic substances.

Removal of non-absorbed material. Toxic material may be present in the gut or on the skin, from which absorption may continue for days. The condition of intoxicated patients who have become free of symptoms may deteriorate when newly absorbed toxic material reaches the circulation. Where intoxication has occurred by mouth, gastric lavage is essential. If the clothing or exposed skin is contaminated by insecticide or by vomit, the clothing must be removed and the skin washed with soap and water for at least 10 minutes. Contamination of the eyes should be treated by irrigation of the conjunctiva with water for 10 minutes.

Antidotes. These are available for organophosphorus compounds and carbamates but not for organochlorine compounds. The use of antidotes is a delicate matter and requires the advice of a specialist. Normally, those using insecticides should be instructed on the action to be taken in case of poisoning, antidotes should be provided, and personnel trained in their use.

Sampling. If the nature of the insecticide is not known, samples should be collected and sent to a laboratory so that it can be identified. These samples should include:

—the incriminated product, taking care to avoid any possible contact (direct or indirect) with other specimens;
—blood, urine, stool specimens, skin washings, expired air, bile, vomit, and subcutaneous fat, which can be taken from a living patient by needle biopsy without danger;
—clothing or sheets contaminated by the product, vomit or urine.

In fatal cases, the toxicologist may need various tissue samples (e.g., the stomach and its contents) for precise identification of the product.

Solid and liquid specimens should be collected in glass bottles or jars with ground-glass stoppers or screw caps lined with aluminium foil. Rubber or plastic stoppers contain extractable impurities which may complicate the analytical procedure. The specimens should be refrigerated but freezing must be avoided.

If a number of patients are found to be exhibiting symptoms of poisoning by an insecticide (or other chemical) without a history of exposure, the possibility that the cause is gross contamination of a food item or drinking-water should be borne in mind.

A6.3 Use of rodenticides

Several products are available. The first-choice rodenticides against commensal rodents, in most control operations, are the anticoagulant poisons since these are slow-acting compounds. Some anticoagulants in current use are shown in Table A6.11.

Table A6.11. Recommended dosage levels[a] for anticoagulant rodenticides

Rodenticide	R. norvegicus	R. rattus	M. musculus
Brodifacoum	0.001	0.005	0.01
Bromadiolone	0.005	0.005	0.01
Chlorophacinone	0.005–0.01	0.005–0.01	0.01
Coumatetralyl	0.03–0.05	0.03–0.05	0.05
Difenacoum	0.005	0.005	0.01
Diphacinone	0.005–0.01	0.005–0.01	0.0125–0.025
Fumarin	0.025	0.025	0.025–0.05
Isovaleryl-indandione	0.055	0.055	—
Pival	0.025	0.025	0.025–0.05
Warfarin	0.025	0.025	0.025–0.05

[a] Percentage concentration in finished bait.

Table A6.12. Acute and subacute rodenticides for rapid reduction of rodent populations

Rodenticide	Lethal dose (mg/kg of body weight)[a]	Concentration used in baits (%)	Effective against:[b] Rn	Rr	Mm	Acceptance in baits	Solvent	Hazard to man	Antidote	Restrictions on use
Calciferol	40	0.1	+	+	+	Good	Oil	Moderate	Calcium disodium edetate (orally)	—
Castrix (Crimidine)	1–5	0.5	+		+	Poor	Oil	Extreme	Sodium pento-barbital	—
Fluoroacetamide	13–16	2.0	+	+	+	Good	Water	Extreme	—	Only by licensed personnel
Red squill	500	10.0	+			Fair	Water/oil	Low	—	—
Scilliroside	0.42	0.015	+			Fair	Water/oil	Moderate	—	—
Sodium fluoroacetate	5–10	0.25	+	+	+	Good	Water	Extreme	—	Only by licensed personnel
Zinc phosphide	40	1.0	+	+	+	Fair	Oil	Moderate	—	—

[a] LD_{50} for R. norvegicus.
[b] Rn= R. norvegicus; Rr = R. rattus; Mm= M. musculus.

In contrast to the slow-acting multiple-dose anticoagulants, the acute (single-dose, quick-acting) rodenticides are principally employed in situations demanding a rapid reduction of high-density rodent populations. When an acute poison is used, it is essential to survey the infested area thoroughly and number the baiting points to be used. Poison bait is generally accepted and an improved kill obtained by laying pre-bait (unpoisoned food) a few days beforehand. Acute and subacute rodenticides available are shown in Table A6.12. Acute rodenticides are hazardous to man and their application should only be carried out by qualified and experienced operators. Brodifacoum, although an anticoagulant, can provide effective control as a single-dose rodenticide and can be used together with zinc phosphide. During an outbreak of bubonic plague, control of vector fleas should precede any measures taken against rodents, otherwise a further increase in plague cases may occur as a result of large numbers of fleas leaving dead rodent hosts to seek new sources of blood.

BIBLIOGRAPHY

BURGESS, N. *John Hull Grundy's arthropods of medical importance*. London, Noble Books Ltd, Curwen Press, 1981.

Chemical methods for the control of arthropod vectors and pests of public health importance. Geneva, World Health Organization, 1984.

Emergency vector control after natural disaster. Washington, DC, Pan American Health Organization, 1982 (Scientific Publication No. 419).

Equipment for vector control, 2nd ed. Geneva, World Health Organization, 1974.

JAMES, T & HARWOOD, F. *Herm's medical entomology*, 6th ed. London, Macmillan, 1969.

Manual on environmental management for mosquito control. Geneva, World Health Organization, 1982 (WHO Offset Publication No. 66).

Manual on practical entomology in malaria. Geneva, World Health Organization, 1975 (WHO Offset Publication No. 1).

Revision of *Guide to chemical methods for the control of vectors and pests. Weekly epidemiological record*, **58**: 103–107 (1983).

The control of Aedes aegypti-*borne epidemics*. Unpublished WHO document, WHO/VBC/77–660.

The WHO recommended classification of pesticides by hazard. Unpublished WHO document, VBC/84.2.

Ultra-low-volume application of insecticides: a guide for vector control programmes. Unpublished WHO document, WHO/VBC/79.734.

WHO Technical Report Series, No. 603, 1977 (*Engineering aspects of vector control operations*: first report of the WHO Expert Committee on Vector Biology and Control).

WHO Technical Report Series, No. 634, 1979 (*Safety of pesticides*: third report of the WHO Expert Committee on Vector Biology and Control).

WHO Technical Report Series, No. 649, 1980 (*Environmental management for vector control*: fourth report of the WHO Expert Committee on Vector Biology and Control).

WHO Technical Report Series, No. 655, 1980 (*Resistance of vectors of disease to pesticides*: fifth report of the WHO Expert Committee on Vector Biology and Control).

ANNEX 7

Decontamination procedures

A7.1 General procedures

The following general procedures may be used for decontamination purposes.

Boiling
Immersion in water at "rolling boil" (100 °C) for 20 minutes.

Autoclaving
The temperature reached under pressure (120 °C) must be maintained for 20 minutes. The material for sterilization should be packed loosely enough to permit good circulation of steam, which forces out the air as the temperature rises. Bacterial spores are unlikely to resist this treatment. A household pressure cooker containing a little water achieves the same effect but the pressure relief indicator is not accurate, and there is no thermometer, so that it is impossible to check that the temperature has reached 120 °C.

Dry heat
The temperature must reach 160 °C in a special oven and be maintained for at least 45 minutes; this can be used only for glass and not for rubber, paper or fabric.

Incineration
A field incinerator improvised from a 200-litre drum can be used to protect the operator and the environment.

As an alternative to the foregoing, the following liquid disinfectants may be used.

Alcohol (70%, 700 ml/litre)
Alcohol may be employed as a routine antiseptic but has no effect on bacterial spores or on certain viruses.

Chlorine (sodium hypochlorite)
Chlorine is a universal disinfectant active against all microorganisms, including hepatitis B virus. It is a strong oxidizing agent, corrosive to metals, but may be inactivated to some extent by organic matter. Chlorine solutions gradually lose strength so that fresh solutions must be made frequently. Liquid sodium hypochlorite is commonly available as household bleach but the amount of available

chlorine can vary between 5 % and 15 %, depending on the brand, and is not always known or stated on the container. In general, the use of a 1:100 aqueous solution of household bleach is recommended for most decontamination purposes. As a means of checking that the solution is of the correct concentration, there should be a strong chlorine odour and a "slippery feel", but it should not be strong enough to "burn" the fingers. If necessary, the stock solution can be titrated and the dilution adjusted to give the concentration required for medical use, depending on the purpose.

Phenol (phenolic compounds)

Phenolic compounds may be used if chlorine is not available. Clear phenolics are inactivated only to a small extent by organic matter and do not attack metals. They have a wide range of applications but are not effective against hepatitis B virus.

Iodine

Iodine kills vegetative organisms, spores, viruses and fungi. The combination of iodine and alcohol (1.6 g of available iodine in each litre of 44–50 % ethanol) is a most effective antiseptic for use in washing hands, leaving them 80–90 % free from bacteria after soaking for 2 minutes in the solution. However, skin irritation may result from frequent use.

Iodophors

Iodophors are water-soluble complexes of iodine with organic compounds. They cause less skin reaction but are less effective than iodine–alcohol.

Formaldehyde (formalin)

Formaldehyde is marketed as formalin, a solution of the gas in water (370 g/litre). Diluted to 50 g/litre, it makes an effective liquid disinfectant.

Alternatively, material for decontamination may be placed in a plastic bag to which is added, before sealing, a pledget of cotton soaked in formalin and a small open container of water. An exposure time of at least 8 hours is necessary (see also room disinfection in section A7.2).

A7.2 Procedures for specific items, rooms and vehicles

The following procedures may be used for items of clothing, bedding, rooms, aircraft, etc.

Gloves

Dip gloved hands in 0.5 % hypochlorite (household bleach) solution and rub together; repeat this operation in clean water.

Hands
Wash with soap, rinse in a 1.6 g/litre solution of iodine in 50 % alcohol and then in water.

Protective clothing
With the appropriate precautions, disposable equipment is placed in sealed plastic bags and incinerated. Reusable equipment is placed in sealed plastic bags and boiled or autoclaved prior to washing.

Masks, respirators
The face piece is wiped down with a damp cloth that has been soaked in hypochlorite solution (1:100 dilution of household bleach with a wetting agent or 85 % alcohol) and the excess squeezed out. The mask is then thoroughly rinsed with warm water and left to dry for 30 minutes. Before reuse, the functioning of valves and the tightness of fit should be checked. The high-efficiency particulate air (HEPA) cartridge should be changed, when necessary, in accordance with the instructions.

Excreta
Use a 2 % sodium hypochlorite solution (household bleach) and allow 15 minutes for contact. Do not discharge to septic tank.

Thermometers
Clean after use with 70 % alcohol. Store dry.

Mattresses and pillows
Incinerate if autoclaving is not feasible.

Surfaces (floors, walls)
Rub with a cloth soaked in 0.1 % hypochlorite solution; rinse with clean water after contact time of 5–10 minutes.

Rooms and laboratory isolators
All openings from the room should be sealed with masking or similar tape. Fumigate with formaldehyde gas, which may be generated by heating formalin (0.5 ml per cubic foot of space). The gas has a poor penetrating power and should be allowed to remain in the room for 8 hours. Even then disinfection may not be complete. The room surfaces should be dry, as formaldehyde gas is soluble in water and will be rapidly absorbed if any is present. The use of air-circulating fans is recommended. Where electricity is not available, formaldehyde may be generated by reacting formalin (60 %) with potassium permanganate (40 %), as follows. Formalin is placed in a small open container, placed inside a larger container that will hold any mixture that boils over; the operator should add potassium permanganate to the formalin and immediately leave the room.

Aircraft
Formaldehyde gas must not be used in aircraft because of the risk of chemical reactions with aircraft equipment. The use of special

gases for disinfection (e.g., carboxide, ethylene oxide and Freon II, betapropiolactone vapour) does not give an absolute guarantee of security, and disinfection must be carried out by the airline. Contaminated parts may be rubbed with 0.1 % hypochlorite solution or preferably with a clear soluble phenolic fluid, and rinsed after 30 minutes contact. Exposed parts should be protected with plastic sheets before suspected infected persons are transported. Alternatively, transit isolators with HEPA filters are recommended, if available.

Other vehicles

As for aircraft, but gas disinfection may be used.

A7.3 Precautions

Concentrated liquid disinfectants should be handled with caution, and gloves and aprons should be used so as to avoid contact with the skin (burns or allergic sensitization) and mucous membranes (goggles should be worn to protect the eyes). Clean water for washing or showering should be readily available when concentrated disinfectants are being used. Proper labelling of containers is recommended and labels should stress the need to avoid absorption of disinfectants.

Appropriate respirators must be worn by personnel required to enter rooms disinfected with gas before they have been properly ventilated.

ANNEX 8

Informal Consultation on Strategies for the Control of Emergencies Caused by Epidemics of Communicable Disease, 9–13 November 1981

Participants

Dr J. Aashi, Assistant Director-General, Preventive Medicine, Ministry of Health, Riyadh, Saudi Arabia

Dr E. G. Beausoleil, Director of Medical Services, Ministry of Health, Accra, Ghana

Dr J. G. Breman, Special Programs Officer, Office of the Director, Centers for Disease Control, Atlanta, GA, USA

Dr P. Brès, 41 chemin M. Duboule, Geneva, Switzerland (*Rapporteur*)

Dr P. N. Burgasov, Deputy Minister of Health, Ministry of Health, Moscow, USSR

Dr L. J. Charles, Sr, St. John's, Antigua, West Indies

Dr B. El Tahir, Head, Department of Virology, National Health Laboratory, Khartoum, Sudan

Dr J. Etienne, Chief, Laboratory of Microbiological Research, Institute of Tropical Medicine of the Health Service of the Armed Forces, Marseilles, France

Dr S. Fernando, Director-General of Health Services, Directorate of Health Services, Colombo, Sri Lanka

Dr H. Gelfand, Associate Dean, School of Public Health, University of Illinois at the Medical Center, Chicago, IL, USA

Dr H. Groot, National Institute of Health, Ministry of Public Health, Bogotá, D. E., Colombia

Dr F. Jurji, Director of Epidemiology and Quarantine, Ministry of Health, Baghdad, Iraq

Dr W. Koinange Karuga, Director of Medical Services, Ministry of Health, Nairobi, Kenya (*Chairman*)

Dr N. Kumara Rai, Chief, Malaria Control Programme, Ministry of Health, Jakarta, Indonesia

Dr J. B. McCormick, Chief, Special Pathogens Branch, Virology Division, Center for Infectious Diseases, Centers for Disease Control, Atlanta, GA, USA

Dr Mai Wen-kui, Deputy Director, Health Bureau, Guangxi Zhuang, China

Dr M. V. Mataitoga, Director of Preventive Medicine, Ministry of Health, Suva, Fiji

Dr K. Pavri, Director, National Institute of Virology, Pune, India

Dr P. Rezai, Director, Malaria Eradication and Epidemic Control, Ministry of Health, Teheran, Islamic Republic of Iran

Dr Kalisa Ruti, Director, Expanded Programme on Immunization, Kinshasa, Zaire

Dr D. I. H. Simpson, Special Pathogens Reference Laboratory, Public Health Laboratory Service, Centre for Applied Microbiology and Research, Porton Down, Salisbury, Wiltshire, England

Dr J. E. M. Whitehead, Director, Public Health Laboratory Service, London, England

Observer

Dr. D. Carter, United Nations Office of the Disaster Relief Coordinator (UNDRO), Geneva, Switzerland

WHO Secretariat

Regional Offices

Dr A. E. J. Delas, Medical Officer, Inter-country project AFR/ICP/ ESD/005, Regional Office for Africa, Brazzaville, Congo

Dr C. Tigre, Epidemiological Surveillance, Regional Office for the Americas, Washington, DC, USA

Dr M. Wahdan, Regional Adviser, Epidemiology, Regional Office for the Eastern Mediterranean, Alexandria, Egypt

Dr B. Velimirovic, Regional Adviser, Communicable Diseases, Regional Office for Europe, Copenhagen, Denmark

Dr Chaiyan K. Sanyakorn, Director, Disease Control and Prevention, Regional Office for South-East Asia, New Delhi, India

Dr C. Ross-Smith, Director, Disease Prevention and Research, Regional Office for the Western Pacific, Manila, Philippines

WHO Headquarters, Geneva, Switzerland

Dr F. Assaad, Chief, Virus Diseases

Dr I. Arita, Chief, Smallpox Eradication

Dr D. Barua, Consultant, Control of Diarrhoeal Diseases

Dr K. Bogel, Veterinary Public Health

Dr I. Carter, Chief, Epidemiological Surveillance of Communicable Diseases

Dr G. Causse, Chief, Bacterial and Venereal Infections

Mr R. F. Davies, Environmental Hazards and Food Protection, Division of Environmental Health

Dr A. Davis, Director, Parasitic Diseases Programme

Dr N. Gratz, Director, Vector Biology and Control
Dr S. Gunn, Emergency Relief Operations
Dr T. Kereselidze, Bacterial and Venereal Infections
Dr A. Koulikovskii, Veterinary Public Health
Dr T. Lepes, Director, Malaria Action Programme
Mr G. Levi, Public Information
Dr Z. Matyas, Chief, Veterinary Public Health
Dr M. Merson, Programme Manager, Control of Diarrhoeal Diseases
Dr L. Molineaux, Epidemiological Methodology and Evaluation, Malaria Action Programme
Mr G. Nickitas, Chief, Supply Services
Mr V. Oviatt, Coordinator, Safety Measures in Microbiology
Dr C. P. Pant, Ecology and Control of Vectors, Division of Vector Biology and Control
Dr P. de Raadt, Trypanosomiases and Leishmaniases, Parasitic Diseases Programme
Mr A. Schmier, Hospital and Teaching Equipment Procurement, Supply Services
Dr A. Smith, Ecology and Control of Vectors, Division of Vector Biology and Control
Dr A. Zahra, Director, Division of Communicable Diseases

WHO publications may be obtained, direct or through booksellers, from:

ALGERIA: Entreprise nationale du Livre (ENAL), 3 bd Zirout Youcef, ALGIERS

ARGENTINA: Carlos Hirsch, SRL, Florida 165, Galerías Güemes, Escritorio 453/465, BUENOS AIRES

AUSTRALIA: Hunter Publications, 58A Gipps Street, COLLINGWOOD, VIC 3066 — Australian Government Publishing Service *(Mail order sales)*, P.O. Box 84, CANBERRA A.C.T. 2601; *or over the counter from:* Australian Government Publishing Service Booshops *at*: 70 Alinga Street, CANBERRA CITY A.C.T. 2600; 294 Adelaide Street, BRISBANE, Queensland 4000; 347 Swanston Street, MELBOURNE, VIC 3000; 309 Pitt Street, SYDNEY, N.S.W. 2000; Mt Newman House, 200 St. George's Terrace, PERTH, WA 6000; Industry House, 12 Pirie Street, ADELAIDE, SA 5000; 156–162 Macquarie Street, HOBART, TAS 7000 — R. Hill & Son Ltd., 608 St. Kilda Road, MELBOURNE, VIC 3004; Lawson House, 10–12 Clark Street, CROW'S NEST, NSW 2065

AUSTRIA: Gerold & Co., Graben 31, 1011 VIENNA I

BANGLADESH: The WHO Programme Coordinator, G.P.O Box 250, DHAKA 5

BELGIUM: *For books:* Office International de Librairie s.a., avenue Marnix 30, 1050 BRUSSELS. *For periodicals and subscriptions:* Office International des Périodiques, avenue Louise 485, 1050 BRUSSELS — *Subscriptions to World Health only:* Jean de Lannoy, 202 avenue du Roi, 1060 BRUSSELS

BHUTAN: *see* India, WHO Regional Office

BOTSWANA: Botsalo Books (Pty) Ltd., P.O. Box 1532, GABORONE

BRAZIL: Biblioteca Regional de Medicina OMS/OPS, Sector de Publicações, Caixa Postal 20.381, Vila Clementino, 04023 SÃO PAULO, S.P.

BURMA: *see* India, WHO Regional Office

CANADA: Canadian Public Health Association, 1335 Carling Avenue, Suite 210, OTTAWA, Ont. K1Z 8N8. (Tel: (613) 725–3769. Telex: 21–053–3841)

CHINA: China National Publications Import & Export Corporation, P.O. Box 88, BEIJING (PEKING)

DEMOCRATIC PEOPLE'S REPUBLIC OF KOREA: *see* India, WHO Regional Office

DENMARK: Munksgaard Export and Subscription Service, Nørre Søgade 35, 1370 COPENHAGEN K (Tel: + 45 1 12 85 70)

FIJI: The WHO Programme Coordinator, P.O. Box 113, SUVA

FINLAND: Akateeminen Kirjakauppa, Keskuskatu 2, 00101 HELSINKI 10

FRANCE: Librairie Arnette, 2 rue Casimir-Delavigne, 75006 PARIS

GERMAN DEMOCRATIC REPUBLIC: Buchhaus Leipzig, Postfach 140, 701 LEIPZIG

GERMANY FEDERAL REPUBLIC OF: Govi-Verlag GmbH, Ginnheimerstrasse 20, Postfach 5360, 6236 ESCHBORN — Buchhandlung Alexander Horn, Friedrichstrasse 39, Postfach 3340, 6200 WIESBADEN

GHANA: Fides Enterprises, P.O. Box 1628, ACCRA

GREECE: G.C. Eleftheroudakis S.A., Librairie internationale, rue Nikis 4, ATHENS (T. 126)

HONG KONG: Hong Kong Government Information Services, Beaconsfield House, 6th Floor, Queen's Road, Central, VICTORIA

HUNGARY: Kultura, P.O.B. 149, BUDAPEST 62

INDIA: WHO Regional Office for South-East Asia, World Health House, Indraprastha Estate, Mahatma Gandhi Road, NEW DELHI 110002

INDONESIA: P.T. Kalman Media Pusaka, Pusat Perdagangan Senen, Block 1, 4th Floor, P.O. Box 3433/Jkt, JAKARTA

IRAN (ISLAMIC REPUBLIC OF): Iran University Press, 85 Park Avenue, P.O. Box 54/551, TEHERAN

IRELAND: TDC Publishers, 12 North Frederick Street, DUBLIN 1 (Tel: 744835–749677)

ISRAEL: Heiliger & Co., 3 Nathan Strauss Street, JERUSALEM 94227

ITALY: Edizioni Minerva Medica, Corso Bramante 83–85, 10126 TURIN; Via Lamarmora 3, 20100 MILAN; Via Spallanzani 9, 00161 ROME

JAPAN: Maruzen Co. Ltd., P.O. Box 5050, TOKYO International, 100–31

JORDAN: Jordan Book Centre Co. Ltd., University Street, P.O. Box 301 (Al-Jubeiha), AMMAN

KUWAIT: The Kuwait Bookshops Co. Ltd., Thunayan Al-Ghanem Bldg, P.O. Box 2942, KUWAIT

LAOS PEOPLE'S DEMOCRATIC REPUBLIC: The WHO Programme Coordinator, P.O. Box 343, VIENTIANE

LUXEMBOURG: Librairie du Centre, 49 bd Royal, LUXEMBOURG

MALAWI: Malawi Book Service, P.O. Box 30044, Chichiti, BLANTYRE 3

A/1/86